Bottom Line's
HEALTH
BREAKTHROUGHS

2007

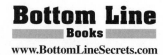

Bottom Line
Books
www.BottomLineSecrets.com

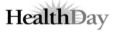

Articles in this book were written by reporters for HealthDay, an award-winning international daily
consumer health news service, headquartered in Norwalk, Connecticut.

Bottom Line Books® publishes the opinions of expert authorities in many fields.
The use of this book is not a substitute for health or other professional service. Consult a physician
or other health-care practitioner for answers to your specific questions and before you make
any decision regarding your health.

Addresses, telephone numbers and Web sites listed in this book are accurate
at the time of publication, but they are subject to frequent change.

Bottom Line Books® is a registered trademark of Boardroom® Inc.
281 Tresser Boulevard, Stamford, CT 06901

Printed in the United States of America

Contents

1

Aging & Senior Health

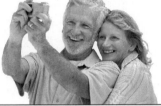

Simple Nasal Vaccine May Slow Alzheimer's

Researchers think they are close to devising a deceptively simple way to prevent the progression of Alzheimer's disease— a nasal spray vaccine.

The vaccine, which so far has only been tested on mice, is a combination of two medications— Protollin and *glatiramer acetate* (Copaxone), which has already been approved to treat other conditions, including multiple sclerosis (MS).

The spray targets the abnormal buildup of *beta-amyloid plaque* in the brain. Although scientific evidence is not sufficient to prove that this amyloid accumulation is the main cause of Alzheimer's disease, many researchers believe that it is.

THE RESEARCH

The researchers sought to design a vaccine —administered via drops in the nose—that would initiate an amyloid-cleansing process by triggering the immune system without provoking antibody development, a problem that occurred in previous trials.

Study coauthor Dr. Howard L. Weiner, codirector of the Center for Neurologic Diseases at Brigham and Women's Hospital, and his colleagues targeted *microglial* cells, which essentially eat away the amyloid build-up. The researchers tried to produce a vaccine that would stimulate these microglial cells into action.

Mice that had a similar amount of beta-amyloid plaque in their brains as what would be present in a human Alzheimer's patient, were given an initial four doses of the vaccine in the first week, followed by weekly doses for the next six weeks. The research team began monitoring the mice one week after vaccination began. They were looking for signs of disease, paralysis, limb weakness and fatigue.

Ultimately, brain tissue was dissected and examined for evidence of both amyloid quantity

Howard L. Weiner, MD, codirector, Center for Neurologic Diseases, Brigham and Women's Hospital, Boston. *Journal of Clinical Investigation* online.

and any toxic side effects that might have developed in reaction to the vaccine.

The authors found that, overall, amyloid plaque levels in the vaccinated mice were reduced by 73%. None of the vaccinated mice showed any evidence of toxic side effects.

> *I think the nasal vaccine has a good chance of working and helping Alzheimer's patients.*
>
> *Howard L. Weiner, MD*

"I'm very hopeful [that this vaccine] could stimulate the immune system to reduce this buildup among people with early signs of Alzheimer's as well as for those in later stages of the disease," says Weiner.

THE NEXT STEP

Weiner and his team say they hope to begin small-scale testing of the Alzheimer's nasal spray vaccine in people following talks with the US Food and Drug Administration (FDA). They note that the human trial process will take time, so a nasal Alzheimer's vaccine is, at best, several years away from clinical use.

Weiner notes that although there are a number of different research projects currently exploring the possibility of reducing beta-amyloid buildup in the brain, none has yet been shown to work in people. And he emphasizes that transitioning from animals to people is a tricky process that doesn't always work.

"But I'm very enthusiastic," he says. "I think it has a good chance of working and helping Alzheimer's patients—and even opening up a new avenue for developing a vaccine for MS."

info For more information on Alzheimer's disease, visit the Alzheimer's Association at *www.alz.org.*

■ ■ ■ ■

Alzheimer's Slowed by Statins

In a three-year study of 300 Alzheimer's patients, the disease progressed more slowly in those who took a cholesterol-lowering drug than it did in those who did not take the medication.

Theory: High levels of cholesterol may increase the depositing of proteins that can impair brain function.

Florence Pasquier, MD, PhD, professor of neurology, University Hospital, Lille, France.

Drug Effective for Severe Alzheimer's

Bengt Winblad, MD, director of neurology, Karolinska Institute, Huddinge, Sweden.
David B. Hogan, MD, Brenda Strafford chair, geriatric medicine, University of Calgary Health Sciences Centre, Calgary, Alberta, Canada.
The Lancet.

The medication *donepezil* (Aricept), which is typically used to treat mild to moderate Alzheimer's disease, seems to reverse some cognitive and functional deterioration in patients who have severe forms of the disease, Swedish researchers report.

Approximately 20% of Alzheimer's patients have severe dementia, but the potential benefit of using Aricept to treat them had not been studied until now.

THE STUDY

In the trial, a research team led by Dr. Bengt Winblad, director of the Karolinska Institute's neurology department, assigned 248 Alzheimer's patients who were living in nursing homes to receive either donepezil or a placebo for a period of six months.

Winblad's team found that the patients taking donepezil experienced improvements in cognitive function and in their ability to perform daily activities, compared with patients receiving a placebo.

The patients receiving donepezil were more likely to have side effects than those on a placebo, but these side effects were usually short-lived and mild to moderate in severity, according to the researchers.

HELPFUL FOR CAREGIVERS

"This drug is effective in the severe stage of Alzheimer's," Winblad says. "It greatly reduces caregiver burden."

The results are significant, Winblad continues, because the high cost of caring for Alzheimer's patients is largely due to the need for intensive caregiver attention. "You have to support the patient in every activity of life," Winblad says. "If they understand better, if they communicate better, it makes it easier for caregivers to do their job."

Dr. David B. Hogan, holder of the Brenda Strafford chair in geriatric medicine at the University of Calgary Health Sciences Centre in Alberta, Canada, agrees that the people who care for Alzheimer's patients need help. "If you can decrease the strain on families, that would be very beneficial," he says. "It would also be beneficial to the staff caring for these people in nursing homes."

However, Hogan is not impressed with donepezil's benefit to patients. "There was some effect of treatment, but it was not substantial or significant," he notes.

"Even if there was some benefit to the patients, it may not be worth the effort and cost of prescribing the medication. The money might be better spent elsewhere," such as on better nursing care to improve the patients' quality of life or on resources to help relatives cope with the loss of a loved one, Hogan suggests.

info To find out more about donepezil, visit the US National Library of Medicine's MedlinePlus Web site at *www.medlineplus.gov.* Click on "Drugs & Supplements."

Alzheimer's—Is It Really A Form of Diabetes?

Suzanne M. de la Monte, senior researcher and neuropathologist, Rhode Island Hospital, and professor of pathology, Brown University Medical School, Providence, RI.

Hugh C. Hendrie, MB, ChB, DSc, professor of psychiatry and codirector, Center for Alzheimer's Disease and Related Neuropsychiatric Disorders, Indiana University Center for Aging Research, Indianapolis.

Douglas N. Ishii, PhD, professor, department of biomedical sciences, Colorado State University, Fort Collins.

Journal of Alzheimer's Disease.

Could Alzheimer's be a form of diabetes? That is the tantalizing suggestion raised by a new study that found that insulin production in the brain declines as Alzheimer's disease advances.

THE STUDY

Senior researcher Suzanne M. de la Monte, a neuropathologist at Rhode Island Hospital and a professor of pathology at Brown University Medical School, and her team autopsied the brain tissue of 45 patients who had been diagnosed with different degrees of Alzheimer's diseases. They compared those tissues to samples taken from individuals who had no history of the disease.

There is now increasing evidence that diabetes, metabolic syndrome and insulin resistance increase the risk for Alzheimer's disease.

Hugh C. Hendrie, MB, ChB, DSc

The team analyzed insulin and insulin-receptor function in the frontal cortex of the brain, a major area affected by Alzheimer's. The discovery that the brain produces insulin at all is a recent one. The researchers found that as the severity of Alzheimer's increased, the levels of insulin as well as the brain's ability to respond to insulin decreased.

"Insulin disappears early and dramatically in Alzheimer's disease," says de la Monte. "We're able to show that insulin impairment is linked to abnormalities that contribute to the tangles [that are] characteristic of advanced Alzheimer's disease. This work ties several concepts together and demonstrates that Alzheimer's disease is quite possibly a type 3 diabetes," she says. (To understand the differences between type 1 and type 2 diabetes, see page 76.)

This study may have treatment implications, such as using certain types of antidiabetes drugs to treat and/or prevent Alzheimer's.

OTHER FACTORS

Dr. Hugh C. Hendrie, professor of psychiatry and codirector of the Center for Alzheimer's Disease and Related Neuropsychiatric Disorders at Indiana University Center for Aging Research, believes that declining insulin levels may be an important feature of Alzheimer's, but not the whole story.

"There is now increasing evidence, primarily from observational studies, that diabetes, its predecessor metabolic syndrome and insulin resistance are implicated in increasing the risk for Alzheimer's disease," he says.

"However, there are many other factors also implicated in Alzheimer's disease, such as hypertension and inflammation, so I think it's a bit of a stretch, at the moment, to describe Alzheimer's disease as an endocrinological disorder like diabetes," Hendrie says.

Another expert thinks that insulin and insulin-like growth factors may be the key to slowing the progression of Alzheimer's.

"We have shown that insulin-like growth factors regulate learning and memory," says Douglas N. Ishii, professor in the department of biomedical sciences at Colorado State University in Fort Collins. "The clinical potential is that by injecting insulin-like growth factors into patients, one might be able to prevent the loss of learning and memory."

The Nun Study— How the Sisters Ward Off Alzheimer's

Guy McKhann, MD, professor of neurology and neuroscience and founding director of the Mind-Brain Institute at Johns Hopkins University School of Medicine, Baltimore. He is author of *Keep Your Brain Young*. Wiley.

Doctors still don't know what causes Alzheimer's disease. And today's treatments are far from ideal. But thanks to the ongoing Nun Study—a one-of-a-kind examination of brain diseases in seniors—scientists are beginning to identify some of the main risk factors, which could open the door to preventive strategies and more effective treatments.

Key finding: Scientists now believe that behaviors and personality traits established early in life are strongly linked to the development of Alzheimer's in later years. Some people have a genetic predisposition to getting the disease, but other factors—such as education, staying mentally active and a history of head trauma or stroke—are thought to play a bigger role.

MANY VARIABLES

Epidemiology is the field of medicine that examines the differences between people who get sick and those who don't. The goal is to identify factors that cause or contribute to disease, such as genetics, diet, exercise and vitamin intake.

Over the years, researchers have used epidemiology to try to identify risk factors for Alzheimer's disease.

The difficulty in this approach is that populations are rarely static. Individuals within a group move away or come from different places…change their habits over time…or fail to accurately recollect their previous behavior. The greater the number of variables, the harder it is to determine which particular factors have positive or negative effects.

Example: It was once widely believed that people who had a high intake of vitamin E were less likely to get Alzheimer's. Yet these are also the people who tend to have healthier habits overall. This makes it difficult to determine if vitamin E itself is beneficial or if the lower disease rates are linked to different factors altogether.

What we have learned: A recent study of blood samples from the nuns showed that vitamin E did *not* protect against Alzheimer's.

A STABLE POPULATION

Starting in 1986, David A. Snowdon, PhD, now a professor of neurology at the University of Kentucky, Lexington, began studying nuns of the School Sisters of Notre Dame living in Mankato, Minnesota. The study was later expanded to include nuns living in the midwestern, eastern and southern US.

The researchers hoped to identify factors in early, mid- and late life that increase the risk of Alzheimer's and other brain diseases.

Now in its 19th year, the Nun Study, which initially included 678 participants ranging in age from 75 to 103, is providing answers.

Unlike most populations studied by epidemiologists, the School Sisters of Notre Dame live in small, relatively uniform communities. They get similar medical care and have similar lifestyles. And because convent archives contain detailed personal histories, researchers were able to collect accurate information spanning previous decades of the nuns' lives.

The Nun Study has revealed that even though symptoms of Alzheimer's typically appear in older adults, the underlying causes may be rooted much earlier in life. *Important findings...*

STROKE–HEAD TRAUMA RISK

When scientists examined the brains of nuns who had died, they found that nearly all of those who exhibited signs of Alzheimer's, such as brain deposits of a protein called *beta-amyloid,* showed evidence of a previous stroke or other forms of brain injury, such as head trauma from a car accident.

It's not yet certain that a history of stroke increases the risk of Alzheimer's, but it does seem likely that a stroke can accelerate the onset of symptoms and cause more rapid disease progression.

Reason: We all have brain reserves—"extra" neurons that give us the ability to maintain cognitive function after neurological damage. Those who lose some of their brain reserves early in life and then go on to develop Alzheimer's will experience mental impairment more rapidly than those who have not had previous injuries, and therefore, have greater brain reserves.

What to do: Prevent strokes by keeping the cardiovascular system strong—do not smoke, manage blood pressure and cholesterol, and get regular exercise. Protect against head injury—wear a helmet while biking, motorcycling and horseback riding, always wear seatbelts, etc.

FOLATE HELPS

A number of studies indicate that low levels of the B vitamin folate are linked to dementia and brain atrophy (shrinkage). The Nun Study indicates that a deficiency may be linked to Alzheimer's as well.

When researchers compared autopsy results with earlier blood samples, they found that nuns who had higher blood levels of folate were less likely to show signs of the brain atrophy associated with Alzheimer's.

Folate (the supplemental form is called folic acid) suppresses the amino acid *homocysteine.* Excessive homocysteine levels promote the development of atherosclerotic plaques in brain and heart arteries. These plaques increase the risk of stroke and heart attack. Homocysteine is also thought to damage neurons and increase brain atrophy in Alzheimer's patients.

What to do: Eat plenty of folate-rich foods—leafy green vegetables, legumes, fortified cereals and enriched grain products. For extra protection, take a daily multi-supplement that contains 400 micrograms (mcg) of folic acid.

STAY MENTALLY ACTIVE

Scientists have learned from autopsies that people who have brain changes that are characteristic of Alzheimer's don't necessarily exhibit impairments of cognitive function. Why do some Alzheimer's patients experience severe declines in mental abilities while others continue to function more or less normally?

When researchers analyzed the biographies that the nuns wrote decades before taking holy orders, they found that those who had a high "idea density"—a marker of education level and vocabulary—were less likely to develop Alzheimer's symptoms later in life, even when their brains showed signs of disease.

The brain continues to form neurons and connections between neurons throughout life. People who are mentally active form the most connections and develop brain reserves that can slow the onset of Alzheimer's symptoms.

What to do: Take classes at a local college. Read challenging books. Do crossword puzzles. Learn a new language. Mental activity increases the number of *synaptic pathways*—connections between neurons that enhance memory and cognitive function.

EXERCISE

Obesity and hypertension are among the leading causes of stroke. One of the best ways to reduce stroke risk—and protect brain reserves—is with daily physical activity. It's never too late to start. One of the sisters in the Nun Study, who was 91 years old when she was interviewed, attributed her longevity to an exercise program that she started when she was 70.

Exercise improves blood circulation in the brain and lowers blood pressure. It also lowers stress hormones and stimulates the release of *trophic factors*—brain proteins that repair neurons and keep them functioning at peak capacity.

What to do: Exercise daily. Even light physical activity, such as walking or yardwork, increases the release of trophic factors and promotes better cognitive function.

STRESS AND DEPRESSION

Depression, anger and stress increase the risk of cardiovascular disease as well as declines in cognitive function.

A study of the nuns' biographies showed that those who expressed negative emotions died sooner and were more likely to have declines in mental function. Stress and anxiety increase levels of *glucocorticoids*, hormones that damage the *hippocampus*, the part of the brain that controls memory.

Depression saps motivation and self-esteem and it can cause significant declines in memory. In patients who already have Alzheimer's symptoms, depression and stress can actually accelerate mental declines.

Know the signs: Insomnia, changes in appetite, increasing irritability or a loss of interest in daily activities can indicate clinically significant stress and/or depression. See a doctor or therapist right away.

What to do: Reduce stress with activities you find relaxing, such as exercise, or even simply by taking deep breaths.

Talk about your problems with friends and family. Sharing concerns with others can lower levels of stress hormones even when the source of the stress is ongoing.

■■■■

Curry May Fight Alzheimer's

The ingredient that gives curry its distinctive color, *curcumin*, is filled with potent antioxidants called *phenols* that may also have anti-inflammatory effects.

Curcumin triggers the production of an enzyme that protects against oxidative diseases—possibly including Alzheimer's. Further research is necessary to determine whether curcumin boosts health in humans.

For now, consider eating Indian food once a week or adding a teaspoon or two of curry to vegetables and meat dishes you make at home.

Nader G. Abraham, PhD, professor of pharmacology, New York Medical College, Valhalla, NY.

■■■■

What Is Dementia?

According to the National Institutes of Health (NIH), dementia refers to a broad range of intellectual impairments involving memory, problem-solving, emotional control and the overall ability to think and reason.

Dementia is not considered to be a disease in itself, but rather a collection of symptoms brought on by diseases such as Alzheimer's and, in some cases, Parkinson's.

Intellectual impairment of this sort is not considered to be a normal part of aging, despite its common occurrence among seniors.

Poor Blood Flow May Raise the Risk Of Dementia

Aart Spilt, MD, department of radiology, Leiden University Medical Center, Leiden, the Netherlands.
David Yousem, MD, director, department of neuroradiology, Johns Hopkins University, Baltimore.
Radiology.

Reduced blood flow to the brain may play a role in dementia in seniors, Dutch researchers report.

They believe that a chronic drop in cerebral blood pressure—resulting in declines in the delivery of oxygen and glucose, which are vital to brain functioning—causes brain damage that can trigger the onset of dementia.

THE STUDY

In the study, Dr. Aart Spilt, director of the department of radiology at Leiden University Medical Center in the Netherlands, and his colleagues focused on a group of 17 Dutch patients, all older than 75 years of age and all diagnosed with *late-onset dementia*.

The participants underwent blood testing and neuropsychological exams, as well as magnetic resonance imaging (MRI) to detect signs of structural brain damage and impairments in brain blood flow.

Results were compared with similar tests that were conducted on a group of 16 men and women of similar age who did not have dementia. A third group of 15 healthy young men and women (averaging 29 years of age) was also tested.

As expected, the researchers found that the younger group had greater brain blood flow and less evidence of brain damage or scarring than either of the older groups.

> *We have to be very cognizant of our cardiovascular systems as we get older, not only for the health of our hearts, but for the health of our brains.*
>
> *David Yousem, MD*

When looking solely at the elderly patients, however, those who had dementia had significantly more structural brain damage and significantly less brain blood flow than the patients who did not have dementia.

As measured in milliliters (mL), the dementia patients had an average cerebral blood flow of 443 mL per minute—108 mL per minute less than the healthy elderly group.

IMPLICATIONS

"I think it's surprising, but we see more and more evidence that blood flow is more important in the developing of dementia in older men and women than what was previously thought," says Spilt.

Dr. David Yousem, director of the department of neuroradiology at Johns Hopkins University in Baltimore, expresses confidence in the study conclusions.

"Basically, there has been a debate about the degree to which blood flow to the brain contributes to the onset and severity of dementia," Yousem notes. "And this study strongly suggests that blood flow is one of the components that has to be factored in when a patient develops dementia—be it Alzheimer's or other dementias."

Impaired brain blood flow can result from heart failure or other cardiovascular problems, such as a narrowing of either brain or neck arteries due to atherosclerosis.

"So this finding points out that we have to be very cognizant of the state of our cardiovascular systems as we get older," Yousem adds. "Not only for the health of our hearts, but for the health of our brains."

THE LOW BLOOD PRESSURE CONNECTION

According to the Dutch team, late-onset dementia shows clear associations with both structural brain damage and decreased cerebral blood flow.

"So we think the most important point is that besides hypertension—which is very important to regulate—it's also important to look at hypotension [low blood pressure], to see if elderly people with low blood pressure are at risk for dementia," Spilt says.

Although elderly patients often have reduced blood flow as a result of diminishing brain activity, Split says the normal aging process does not account for the striking differences observed in blood flow between the healthy elderly patients and the dementia patients.

FUTURE STUDIES

Ideally, future studies could follow up on this finding by tracking healthy patients over a one- to five-year period, watching to see how blood flow changes correlated to the development of dementia over time, Spilt says.

info For more information on dementia, check out the National Institute of Neurological Disorders and Stroke Web site at *www.ninds.nih. gov.* Click on "Disorders."

■ ■ ■ ■

Hidden Cause of Mental Decline

A new report from a 20-year study indicates that untreated high blood pressure is linked to mental decline even in otherwise healthy and relatively young people, ages 18 to 46. Other studies show that when high blood pressure is successfully treated by medication, the risk of mental decline is reduced by as much as half. Yet 70% of Americans who have high blood pressure don't receive treatment for it and 30% don't even know they have it.

Penelope K. Elias, PhD, associate professor, department of psychology, University of Maine, Orono.

9 Ways to Keep Your Brain and Body Young

Gary Small, MD, director, Center on Aging, University of California at Los Angeles, and author of *The Memory Prescription: Dr. Gary Small's 14-Day Plan to Keep Your Brain and Body Young.* Hyperion. *www.drgarysmall.com.*

Many people assume that memory lapses are part of the aging process. However, in recent years, we have identified important ways to stop—and sometimes reverse—the brain changes that are associated with aging.

Anyone who does not have neurological impairment can sharpen mental skills by following a four-pronged strategy of memory training, stress reduction, physical conditioning and a brain-friendly diet.

WORK YOUR BRAIN

Scientists who tracked two groups of people discovered that those in the mentally active group—who played board games, read, did puzzles, etc.—had a 63% lower risk of developing dementia compared with the group that rarely exercised their brains.

Other studies have shown that any mental activity—work or play—is associated with better brain health. *How to put mental activities to work for you…*

●**Cross-train your brain.** Mental activities should involve workouts for both the left and right side of your brain.

In right-handed people, left-brain functions include logical analysis, language and speech, reading, writing and math, as well as symbol recognition.

Right-brain functions cover spatial tasks such as reading maps, artistic and musical activities, emotional perception and a sense of humor. Functions reverse in the majority of people who are left-handed.

Choose activities that you enjoy because these are the ones that you'll stick with. Then exercise each side of your brain in a more or less alternating fashion. *Examples…*

Left-brain activities: Word games, crossword puzzles and reading.

Right-brain activities: Playing a musical instrument, jigsaw puzzles, three-dimensional spatial puzzles and games.

Many activities that combine logical, verbal and spatial tasks exercise both sides of the brain.

Examples: Canasta, bridge, chess and many board games.

●**Build up from simple activities to more demanding ones.** While an activity should be stimulating, pace yourself and keep your expectations reasonable.

Examples: Those who have mentally demanding jobs may not need more mental stimulation at home and should opt for relaxing choices instead. People who work extensively with words should consider activities that will challenge their spatial abilities rather than verbal skills, and vice-versa.

REDUCE STRESS

Severe stress causes the release of the hormone *cortisol*, which has been identified with decreased memory performance. Studies have shown that stress can shrink a key memory center of the brain. Being actively engaged mentally is a good way to relieve stress, but there is much more to the stress-relief "package." *Other important ways to lower stress…*

●**Give up multitasking.** Multitasking is often admired, but ultimately, it is counterproductive. Attempting to do several things at once is distracting and stressful. When tempted to multitask—for example, talking on a cell phone while watering the lawn or cooking while housecleaning—stop and focus on just one thing at a time until you have completed that objective.

●**Get enough sleep.** In a 14-day study, volunteers sleeping four to six hours a night—a range common to many adults—showed significant deficits in memory performance. Interestingly, the sleep-curtailed volunteers had no sense of the extent of their cognitive impairment.

To get proper sleep, avoid late-evening liquids, which cause you to get up to use the bathroom, and avoid exercise that hypes you up so much that you can't settle down. Establish a regular bedtime and wake time. Avoid daytime naps that last for more than 20 minutes.

Get enough sleep to feel rested—for most people age 50 or older, six to seven hours is enough.

•**Learn a "relaxation response."** There are many reliable ways to relax, including meditation and self-hypnosis as well as yoga, tai chi and other gentle exercises. For a real treat, have a massage. And don't forget to regularly kick back and just take it easy.

GET AND STAY FIT

Exercise is vital to well-being, including brain health. Everyone should have a regular fitness program. *Key elements...*

•**Start an aerobic activity.** Anything that gets your heart rate up for a sustained period, such as brisk walking, jogging and swimming, markedly improves the brain's frontal lobe function. This is the brain's "executive control," which handles complex reasoning, planning and memory. Such exercise also lowers the risk for Alzheimer's disease. Exercise at least 30 minutes, three times a week.

•**Build a complete program.** In addition to aerobic exercise, a good program should include strength training, stretching and balance work, because together, these will help prevent injury. Check with your doctor before starting a new exercise plan.

EAT SMART

Diet has a tremendous impact on how a brain ages. Keeping to a normal weight is also vital for your mental functioning. A high body mass index (BMI) is associated with an increased risk for Alzheimer's along with other health risks that can ultimately cause memory loss and dementia. *Key in establishing a brain-friendly diet...*

•**Get your omegas straight.** Americans eat an abundance of omega-6 fatty acids, which are found in corn oil and many other vegetable oils as well as in fried and processed foods. Atkins and other low-carb diets include a hefty portion of omega-6s, which can create health risks and may contribute to chronic brain inflammation, setting the stage for brain impairment.

What to do: Eat one serving per day of omega-3s—found in high-fat fish, such as salmon and tuna, and in avocados, olive oil, nuts and other foods. Also consider a daily supplement of 1,000 milligrams (mg) of fish oil.

•**Fight free radicals.** Free radicals, the cell-damaging byproducts of metabolism, are always present in the body, including the brain, causing cells to lose structure and function. Antioxidants are the front line for fighting off free radicals. Most fruits and vegetables—in particular prunes, raisins, blueberries and spinach—are high in antioxidants.

Vitamin E (400 international units [IU]) and vitamin C (500 mg) supplements—taken together—seem to lower dementia risk.

Note: Consult your doctor about whether vitamin E is safe for you—and how much you should take.

■ ■ ■ ■

Alzheimer's and Exercise

A recent study of subjects older than age 64 concluded that those who were doing the widest variety of exercise were the least likely to develop dementia, most commonly caused by Alzheimer's disease. The activities that were surveyed were the 15 most frequently performed by older adults, including gardening, raking, hiking and bowling.

Possible explanation: A variety of activities may keep more parts of the brain active.

Constantine G. Lyketsos, MD, MHS, codirector, division of geriatric psychiatry and neuropsychiatry, Johns Hopkins University Hospital, Baltimore.

12 Powerful Ways to Boost Your Energy

Kenneth H. Cooper, MD, MPH, a pioneer in the fields of preventive medicine and physical fitness. He is president of Cooper Aerobics Center, Dallas, and author of numerous books, including *Regaining the Power of Youth at Any Age.* Nelson. *www.cooperaerobics.com.*

As we get older, we often complain that we're "running on empty." I call this age-related loss of energy *youth drain*—but we don't have to be victims of it. At 74 years of age, I work 60 hours a week, travel widely and still feel energetic.

Youth drain can be caused by a variety of factors, including obesity...chronic medical problems, such as anemia, diabetes, emphysema or an underactive thyroid gland…depression…cancer…use of sedatives and sleeping pills… menopause…poor diet…inadequate sleep…and stress. These factors batter us over the years and drain our vitality—unless we learn how to respond to them and counter their effects.

Here are 12 revitalizing strategies for us all…

●**Eat less but more frequently.** Consuming large meals (more than 1,000 calories per sitting) makes you feel sluggish, as your body's resources are directed toward digesting all that food.

Instead, graze on small meals and snacks that contain a mix of carbohydrates and protein (but little fat) to provide a steady stream of fuel.

Examples: Yogurt smoothie (one cup light nonfat yogurt, one-half cup fat-free milk, one-half peach, blended)…peanut butter and banana sandwich (one slice whole wheat bread, one-half tablespoon peanut butter, one-half banana, sliced)…fruity cottage cheese (one-half cup 1% low-fat cottage cheese, one-half cup pineapple chunks in juice, drained).

●**Exercise.** The health benefits of exercise are well-known, but many people tell me they continue to exercise year after year because it makes them feel good and gives them more energy. I recommend at least 30 minutes of sustained activity five times a week. The best activities for most people tend to be brisk walking, jogging, swimming, cycling and aerobic dance.

●**Take a multivitamin.** In a clinical trial, people who took multivitamins daily not only had improved immunity against infectious diseases but also had more energy. In general, it is best to get vitamins from food, but many people don't get the necessary amounts, so I suggest taking a multivitamin/mineral supplement daily.

●**Prevent dehydration.** Consuming an inadequate amount of fluids, particularly if it's hot outside or you're exercising, can deplete energy and lead to weakness, dizziness and headaches. Drink at least six to eight 8-ounce glasses of water daily. On days that you exert yourself to the point of perspiring, drink up to 13 glasses.

●**Watch what you drink.** Drink no more than one caffeinated beverage a day. Coffee, tea, cola and other caffeinated beverages provide a temporary energy boost, but energy levels plunge when the stimulant's effects wear off.

Caffeinated drinks also have a diuretic effect, which may cause you to lose fluids because you urinate more frequently.

Also, limit your alcohol consumption to no more than one drink per day—any more can lead to fatigue.

●**Practice the "relaxation response."** This technique, developed by Herbert Benson, MD, of Harvard University, has been shown to reduce blood pressure and heart rate. For me, doing this for just five minutes in the middle of the day is rejuvenating.

How to do it: Sit in a chair in a quiet room. Close your eyes. Starting with your feet, begin to relax your muscles, progressively moving up the body to the top of the head. While you do this, breathe in slowly and naturally through your nose and out through your mouth. As you exhale, silently repeat a focus word or phrase that has meaning for you, such as "peace." Push away distracting thoughts by focusing on your breathing and the word you have chosen to repeat.

●**Take naps.** Surveys show that most Americans don't get as much sleep as they need (most of us require seven to eight hours a night). Daily naps of 15 to 20 minutes are energizing—and longer naps can help you catch up if you are sleep-deprived. I sleep only five to six hours a night, so I often take a two-hour nap on Saturdays.

●**Don't immerse yourself in bad news.** The glut of negative information coming our way from TV, radio, newspapers, the Internet, etc., can hurt the psyche, causing stress and fatigue. Reduce the amount of time you spend watching, listening to or reading the news, and focus on things that bring you joy.

●**Be social.** Studies show that isolation can lead to depression and early death. We gain energy by being with others (both humans and animals). Make time for family, friends and pets.

●**Explore your creativity.** Boredom leads to a lack of motivation and energy. Finding a creative outlet that absorbs you is invigorating. Developing your creativity also teaches you new skills…challenges your brain…and leads to the release of *endorphins*, feel-good brain chemicals. Take up a new hobby…learn a musical instrument…take on an unusual project at work.

Added benefit: Activities that are mentally stimulating can lower your risk of developing Alzheimer's disease.

•**Laugh.** Laughter appears to release endorphins just as creative pursuits do. By improving your outlook, you'll feel more energetic and ready to tackle life.

Helpful: Watch funny movies…read cartoons …share humorous stories and jokes with your family and friends.

•**Think young.** To a large extent, your own mindset dictates how much energy you have as you age. If you expect the worst, you're likely to feel tired and unwell. On the other hand, if you expect to stay vital, you'll fight off disease that can sap energy and well-being—and you'll add years to your life.

■ ■ ■ ■

A Simple Exercise Routine

Follow the program outlined here six days a week. Progress to the next level only after you're very comfortable with the current one.

Level one: Work your way (at your own pace) up to 45 minutes of aerobic (heart-pumping) exercise without discomfort. Get your heart rate up to 60% to 65% of your maximum heart rate (approximately 220 minus your age) and try to keep it there for, say, a 45-minute bike ride or hike at a pace where you're still able to have a conversation.

If you stay at level one forever, that's OK—you'll still be fitter than most people and fit enough to feel younger than you are.

Level two: Do aerobic exercise for 45 minutes four days a week…45 minutes of weight training two days a week.

Caution: Get help from a trainer (available at most gyms) until you know what you're doing in the weight room.

Level three: Do aerobic exercise for 45 minutes one or two days a week. Do more intense aerobic exercise—reaching 70% to 85% of your maximum heart rate—on your remaining days of aerobic activity (a total of four days a week). Do weight training two days a week. One day a

month, take a two-hour hike, a three-hour bike ride or an equivalent exercise that's fun.

Caution: Check with your health-care provider before attempting any new exercise program. If you keep working to stay fit, your body will go along.

Henry S. Lodge, MD, Columbia University College of Physicians and Surgeons, New York City.

Proven Ways to Keep Your Memory Very Sharp

Lynn Stern, MSW, senior clinical social worker who helps people overcome memory problems, University of Michigan Health System, Ann Arbor. She is coauthor of Improving Your Memory: How to Remember What You're Starting to Forget. Johns Hopkins University.

Unlike the memory experts who perform tricks on stage and television, Lynn Stern spends many hours each week actually helping people who have memory problems. In her 20 years at the University of Michigan's Turner Clinic, Stern has learned what works—and what doesn't—to improve memory.

She says that scientists do not understand exactly how it happens, but as we get older, nearly everyone's memory slowly undergoes certain changes…

•**It becomes harder to remember words that were once familiar to you**—a friend's maiden name, for example, or the type of dog your uncle had as a pet.

•**Learning something new takes more effort** than it used to.

•**You increasingly forget items on your schedule,** such as the need to pay a bill by a certain date.

•**You have more difficulty paying attention to more than one thing at a time**—carrying on a conversation while you are watching TV, for example.

While these memory changes are common, it still may be wise to consult your physician. In most cases, the doctor will reassure you that some memory difficulties are normal as you age. In some cases, he/she may recommend medical tests if they suspect the onset of Alzheimer's disease or another serious condition.

PROTECTING MEMORY

You can't reverse memory changes, but following are five sure ways to dramatically slow them down...

●**Learn something new.** Scientists aren't certain of the reason, but research indicates that learning a new language, craft, game or other skill slows memory loss.

It's generally more effective to learn a new skill than to enhance one you already have. An accountant, for instance, probably wouldn't benefit as much from learning calculus as from studying a foreign language, while a person who already knows two languages would not benefit as much from studying a third one as he/she would from, say, learning to play bridge.

Challenge: Motivating yourself to learn something new. Choose a skill that you'll enjoy using once you learn it. If you learn a language, plan a trip to a country where it's spoken. If you learn bridge, join a bridge club where you can meet new people.

●**Play challenging games.** Games such as bridge, Go (an ancient Chinese board game), crossword puzzles and Scrabble can strengthen memory, especially the type of memory required for the game itself.

Working crossword puzzles, for example, has been proven to help with verbal recognition. But such proficiency at crosswords is unlikely to help you remember the phone numbers of close friends and relatives. If that's a problem for you, devise a challenge by writing down the phone numbers and then trying once or twice a week to repeat them from memory.

Or if you have trouble recalling names of new people you meet, jot them down and test yourself periodically in the same way.

●**Socialize with friends, new and old.** Socializing—no matter how you do it or how often—helps slow down memory changes because it always requires the use of memory. It's all but impossible to carry on a conversation without referring to people and events that you have stored in memory.

Moreover, talking to friends about what you've read in the newspaper or seen on TV reinforces those facts in your mind.

●**Stay physically active.** According to researchers at the University of Michigan and elsewhere, people who engage in physical activity—regardless of the type or amount—are more likely to maintain their memory and other mental abilities.

●**Organize important activities around your most alert time periods.** Almost everyone has a time of day when he/she is most alert. It's usually impossible to cram all important activities into that time slot, but try to reserve that period for important tasks, such as caring for a grandchild or driving.

Also try to learn new skills during your most alert times. For example, if you want to study acting and have a choice between a morning or an afternoon class, choose the time when you usually feel more alert.

Smart move: Ask your doctor whether any medication you're taking can impair memory. This effect occurs most often with prescription medications for sleeping problems, anxiety, muscle tension, allergies, colds and pain.

If the answer is "yes," ask if another drug without this side effect is available. Should you opt to continue the medication, at least you'll know that related memory problems are likely to stop when you stop taking it.

MEMORY TRIGGERS

Fortunately, most memory changes occur over a period of many years, and this usually gives you time to adapt before they become serious. *Successful strategies...*

●**Do something unusual to trigger your memory.** For example, to remember to stop at the grocery store on the way home from work, switch your watch from one wrist to the other earlier in the day. The mild but nagging discomfort acts as a reminder.

Yes, you may occasionally forget what it was you were supposed to remember, but with a little thought it usually will come back.

Other memory triggers: Be organized—always put your glasses, keys, etc., in the same place. Say what you want to remember aloud or write it down—both actions will reinforce it in your memory.

●**Write down information you may need in the future** in one compact notebook. If you order a product over the phone, jot down the phone number and the name of the person you spoke with. And if you meet interesting people at a party, put their names and phone numbers in the notebook.

Information like this too often winds up on scraps of paper stored in dozens of places around the house. By using a single notebook, however, you can easily refer to it as the information becomes necessary.

Also helpful: A date for each entry to make it easier to look up information. And when one book fills up, store it in a designated place and start another.

●**Jot down information next to names in your personal phone book,** such as birthdays, anniversaries and the names of children that are too easy to forget as families grow larger and grow apart, too.

●**Avoid procrastination.** If you put off doing something, chances increase that you will forget it altogether.

There's no simple way to change the habits of a lifetime, but if you're prone to procrastination, post reminders of appointments and upcoming events on the bathroom mirror and in other places where you regularly look.

■ ■ ■ ■

Remember Your Medicine

Do you keep forgetting to take your medication? *If so, here are some suggestions to help you remember from the National Heart, Lung, and Blood Institute…*

●**Put a picture of yourself on the refrigerator** with a post-it-note saying, *Remember to take your medication.*

●**Keep your medication on the nightstand** next to your bed.

●**Take your pills right after brushing your teeth** and keep them with your toothbrush.

●**Ask a friend to leave a reminder** on your answering machine and don't erase it.

●**Put your medicine in a weekly pillbox.**

●**Establish a buddy system** with a friend and arrange to call each other every day.

Get Hooked! Fish Lowers Dementia Risk

Martha Clare Morris, ScD, epidemiologist, Rush University Medical Center, Chicago.
Greg M. Cole, PhD, neuroscientist, Greater Los Angeles VA Healthcare System, and associate director, Alzheimer's Disease Research Center, David Geffen School of Medicine, University of California, Los Angeles.
Archives of Neurology online.

Your mother probably told you that fish is brain food. Apparently, she was right. A new study has found that older people who regularly eat fish reduce the amount of cognitive decline they experience.

THE STUDY

In the study, Martha Clare Morris, an epidemiologist at Rush University Medical Center in Chicago, and her team collected data on 6,158 people age 65 and older who lived on the south side of Chicago and were part of the Chicago Health and Aging Project.

The participants filled out a questionnaire about what they ate, and had their cognitive ability tested every three years during the six-year study.

People who ate fish once a week had a 10% slower decline in thinking ability over time than people who consumed fish less than weekly. Those who ate two or more fish meals per week had a 13% slower decline in thinking ability. "The rate reduction is the equivalent of being three to four years younger in age," Morris says.

THE DHA CONNECTION

Fish is a source of omega-3 fatty acids, which have been shown to be essential for neurocognitive development and normal brain functioning. In addition, fish consumption has been associated with a lower risk of dementia and stroke. Some recent studies have discovered that one omega-3 fatty acid in particular, *docosahexaenoic acid* (DHA), is important for memory in older animals.

Morris believes that increased levels of DHA may be responsible for the slower decline in thinking ability. In a previous study, Morris found that DHA reduced the risk of developing Alzheimer's disease. "DHA is very important for the communication between neurons and the overall functioning of neurons," she explains.

THE JURY IS STILL OUT

At least one expert thinks this study does not make a conclusive case that DHA—or any other omega-3 fatty acid, for that matter—is the reason that fish consumption appears to slow a decline in thinking ability.

Greg M. Cole, associate director of the Alzheimer's Disease Research Center at the David Geffen School of Medicine at the University of California, Los Angeles, says that although Morris's study "also finds reduced cognitive decline associated with increased fish intake, it doesn't find much evidence to relate this to greater omega-3 fatty acid intake.

"One problem is that the questionnaires on fish intake were not that highly correlated with actual blood levels of omega-3," Cole says. "These new results suggest that the jury is still out on whether it is the oil in the fish, specifically the omega-3 fatty acids, that we should try to increase."

info The University of California, San Francisco, has more information on aging and cognitive decline at *http://memory.ucsf.edu*. Click on "Normal Aging" under "Topics" in the pull-down menu under "Education."

■ ■ ■ ■

Memory-Boosting Supplement

The US Food and Drug Administration (FDA) allows *phosphatidylserine* (PS) makers to claim that their products can reduce the risk of both dementia and cognitive dysfunction in the elderly.

If you want to try PS supplements, start with a dose of 300 milligrams (mg) per day—the amount used in many studies. After a few months, you may be able to reduce this to a dose of 100 mg per day.

Caution: Pregnant or nursing women should not take PS before discussing it with an obstetrician or pediatrician.

Thomas H. Crook III, PhD, clinical psychologist and president, Psychologix, Inc., Fort Lauderdale, FL.

Master of Memory: How to Fight Forgetfulness ...and Win!

Scott Hagwood, founder and president of The Center for Creative Memory Leadership, a corporate training center in Fayetteville, NC. He is author of *Memory Power: You Can Develop a Great Memory—America's Grand Master Shows You How*. Free Press.

Scott Hagwood had an average memory growing up. Then, at age 36, the chemical engineer learned that he had cancer and that the radiation treatments he needed often cause forgetfulness.

Determined to ward off memory loss, Hagwood performed mental exercises for several hours a day. He would do such things as remember the exact order of cards in a shuffled deck and all the names of the doctors and nurses on his hospital floor.

Hagwood became so proficient that he entered the US National Memory Championships in 2001 and won. He is now one of 50 Grand Masters of Memory in the world. *Here are his solutions to common memory problems...*

Problem: **You call directory assistance for a phone number, but you don't have a pen to write it down.**

Solution: After you hang up, repeat the number out loud. There's something about hearing yourself say what you want to remember that resonates in the brain and enhances recall.

Speak slowly. The faster you go, the less you remember. It's much more effective to say the phone number once or twice in a deliberate rhythm than to repeat it over and over in a hurried manner.

Problem: **You can't remember the name of a coworker's spouse even though it is on the tip of your tongue.**

Solution: Your forgetfulness is caused by stress. The more you try to recall something, the more frustrated and agitated you will get. First, take a few deep breaths. Then jog your memory by sorting through related information in your head. Visualize the coworker's name, the last time you saw him with his wife, their car, their home, etc.

If, after a minute, this doesn't work, distract and calm yourself by thinking about another topic. For instance, I like golf, so I'll focus on my favorite course—the sand traps, the greens. While I'm doing this, the information I need often bubbles up in my mind.

Problem: **You spend hours memorizing a presentation or studying for a test, then you can't remember key information the next day.**

Solution: Last-minute memorizing isn't effective. You need to give your brain time to digest information. Don't spend more than 50 minutes at a time trying to learn anything. Take a 10-minute break and then review your notes.

I practice the "Rule of 1s"—I review material after one hour, one day, one week, one month, etc., to log it into my long-term memory.

Problem: **You need to remember a specific errand to do later in the day.**

Scientists refer to this as "prospective memory" because you are trying to recall a specific time in the future, not in the past. Even people who have excellent memories find this difficult without a small, external reminder.

Solution: If I need to remember that I have clothes in the dryer, I'll leave the light on in the laundry room. If I have to return books to the library, I'll leave my library card sticking out of my wallet or my books on the front seat of the car.

Problem: **You misplaced your keys or the TV remote.**

Solution: You sometimes can jog your memory by recalling where you last saw the missing object and retracing your steps—but an object is usually misplaced because you weren't paying attention, so you are unlikely to recall where you left it. Create a forget-me-not spot—for example, a hook for your keys or on top of the TV for the remote—and get in the habit of using that spot.

Problem: **You forget a particular set of numbers, such as your bank ATM code.**

Solution: Your brain isn't built to remember abstract information such as numbers or names. What it remembers best are vivid images. The more you can associate information with pictures in your mind that are meaningful to you, the more powerful your memory.

Example: If you're trying to remember your bank code—6052—associate each two-digit sequence with a person, place or action. I might connect "60" with Babe Ruth hitting 60 home runs in a single season…and "52" with the pop group, the B-52s, singing their hit song, "Love Shack." So my ATM code is an unforgettable visual image—Babe Ruth trotting around the bases as the B-52s sing.

Problem: **You're at a business convention and want to remember the names of a dozen people you have met.**

Solution: I use a powerful technique called the "Roman Room Method." You associate bits of information with images in your house. So if I'm trying to remember the names of a dozen acquaintances, I might visualize my office, going around the room, assigning each name to an easily retrievable mental hook.

Example: Let's say I want to remember a woman whose last name is Penny. My hook for her might be the closet door in my office and her emerging from the closet. This often is enough to trigger the name. If I find that association is not strong enough, I add one element to the mental picture. It may be a particular characteristic—her hair color, nose, the way she gestures. In this case, I see her coming out of the closet with her pockets overflowing with pennies. I might "hook" another person to my computer, another to the bookcase, a third to a painting.

You can link different rooms with different categories of information. For instance, I might use triggers in my office to remember business contacts and triggers in the kids' playroom to remember people with whom I discuss parenting.

Helpful: Once you use a particular room, don't use it again for a few days or weeks. Otherwise, previous associations can interfere with new ones.

■ ■ ■ ■

How to Keep Your Memory Strong

Using all five senses to help you remember tasks and learn new things will keep your memory strong.

In addition to visualizing an object or event, imagine how it would smell, taste and feel.

Example: To remember to bring dessert to an event, imagine eating it—with all the sensations—earlier in the day.

Also: Relax—memory gets overwhelmed when the body is stressed.

And: If you cannot remember someone's name, try to recall where you were, or with whom, when you last saw the person, and the name may come to you.

Douglas Mason, PsyD, clinical neuropsychologist, Clermont, FL.

Elderly May Be Taking Unsafe Meds

Philip Wang, MD, DrPH, psychiatrist and epidemiologist, Brigham and Women's Hospital, and assistant professor of psychiatry, medicine and health-care policy, Harvard Medical School, both in Boston.
The New England Journal of Medicine.

Older antipsychotic medications appear to be no safer than newer antipsychotic drugs in elderly people, and should not be used to replace the newer drugs without careful consideration, according to a study.

THE STUDY

In this study, Dr. Philip Wang, a psychiatrist and epidemiologist at Brigham and Women's Hospital and an assistant professor of psychiatry, medicine and health-care policy at Harvard Medical School, and his colleagues set out to define the short-term risk of death among elderly patients taking the older, or conventional, antipsychotic medications. The older medications used in the study included Thorazine and Haldol, while the newer, or second generation, drugs included Abilify and Clozaril.

The researchers looked at nearly 23,000 patients age 65 or older who began taking antipsychotic medications between 1994 and 2003.

In the first 180 days of use, 17.9% of the patients on conventional antipsychotics died compared with 14.6% of those taking the newer medications. This translates into a 37% higher risk of death for those patients prescribed the older medications.

The greatest increase in the risk of death for the people taking conventional antipsychotic medications occurred in the first 40 days after beginning therapy. During this period, the risk was 56% higher.

BACKGROUND

The issue of replacing one generation of drugs for another has become a concern since the US Food and Drug Administration (FDA) started requiring newer antipsychotic drugs to carry a "black-box" warning. The warning states that these medications nearly double the risk of death among older patients compared with a placebo.

Older drugs do not carry such a warning—but probably only because the FDA didn't have the necessary data, Wang says.

The elderly are just more vulnerable, and clearly, there's a susceptibility to antipsychotics that was never picked up in trials.

Philip Wang, MD, DrPH

Some experts have worried that clinicians are interpreting the absence of data as an absence of risk, and are prescribing older drugs because they think they are safer.

"If they're switching because they think there's no risk because the FDA didn't include older drugs in the advisory, then that's not a good switch," Wang says. "If they're going to switch, they should do so fully informed.

"The older drugs have at least a comparable risk—and maybe higher—but they don't have a black-box warning," he adds.

Antipsychotic medications are widely used in the elderly population for a variety of conditions, including dementia, delirium, psychosis and agitation. The researchers note that although more than 25% of Medicare beneficiaries in nursing homes have such prescriptions, many of the drugs that are widely used for elderly patients have not been well studied in that population.

"Very often, the information on the benefits and the risks of drugs in the elderly is just taken from trials of younger adults," Wang says. "The elderly are just more vulnerable, and clearly, there's a susceptibility to these medications that was never picked up in trials."

The study sheds no light on what the best medications are for the elderly, only on what issues need to be kept in mind, Wang says.

"Clinicians are in a tough spot," he says. "They have to be very cautious and thoughtful and do a good job of balancing what they think the benefits will be against the risks. If they approach this as if there were no risk to the drugs, that's problematic."

info For more information on the black-box warning on antipsychotics, go to the US Food and Drug Administration Web site at *www. fda.gov/cder/drug/advisory/antipsychotics.htm.*

■ ■ ■ ■

What Makes Us Forget?

A number of environmental and health factors can contribute to short- and long-term memory loss. *Among the most common…*

●**Prescription drugs** can adversely affect memory. If you are taking any medications, ask your doctor whether memory loss is a known side effect.

●**Low thyroid function** can also cause poor memory and concentration. With a simple blood test, your doctor can check thyroid levels. If they are low (hypothyroidism), he/she can prescribe medication.

●**Toxic metals,** such as lead and mercury, can lead to brain degeneration. A holistic doctor can test your urine for levels of these metals and recommend treatment, such as chelation therapy, if necessary.

Mark Stengler, ND, naturopathic physician, La Jolla Whole Health Clinic, La Jolla, CA.

■ ■ ■ ■

Beware of this Common Antihistamine

The drug *diphenhydramine*, sold as Benadryl, and also an ingredient in Excedrin PM, Nytol, Sleep-Eze, Sominex, Tylenol PM and Unisom, has been shown to cause altered attention levels, disorganized speech, changes in consciousness and alertness, behavioral disturbances and dizziness in people age 70 and older. It may also cause urinary retention, which can lead to urinary tract infections.

Diphenhydramine acts by blocking the neurotransmitter *acetylcholine.* If you notice these adverse effects while taking diphenhydramine, ask your doctor about other, safer medications or alternative treatments.

Joseph V. Agostini, MD, assistant professor of medicine, geriatrics section, Yale University School of Medicine, New Haven, CT.

Aging May Cause People to Say Things They Don't Mean

William von Hippel, PhD, associate professor of psychology, University of New South Wales, Sydney, Australia.
Adam Gazzaley, MD, PhD, assistant professor of neurology and physiology, University of California, San Francisco.
Psychology and Aging.
Nature Neuroscience online.

Scientists have discovered the physiological mechanisms that cause absent-minded and rude behavior to increase with age.

STUDY # 1:
AGING OR RUDENESS?

The first study, led by William von Hippel, associate professor of psychology at the University of New South Wales in Sydney, Australia, attempted to figure out why some older people speak with what appears to be a complete lack of tact.

In von Hippel's study, 41 people who were between the ages of 18 and 25, and 39 people who were between the ages of 65 and 93 participated in psychological testing.

The study participants were asked how likely they would be to share personal information or ask people for personal information in public situations.

According to von Hippel, the older participants were approximately 20% more likely to ask personal questions in public compared with the younger people. In fact, some of the older adults were twice as likely to ask personal questions in public. He suspects that this behavior may be caused by age-related losses in inhibitory ability.

We all think inappropriate things. Perhaps aging just leads us to say more of them, and perhaps we shouldn't be faulted for that.

William von Hippel, PhD

"The normal aging process leads to changes in the brain that have social consequences. These brain changes often do not affect intelligence, but they can affect other aspects of mental functioning, like inhibition. Thus, even older adults who are as sharp as a tack may say things that embarrass or upset us, without intending to do so," explains von Hippel.

"We all think inappropriate things, and we can't be faulted for that. Perhaps aging just leads us to say more of them, and so perhaps we shouldn't be faulted for that, either," he adds.

STUDY #2:
RECALLING WHAT'S IMPORTANT

The second study, led by Dr. Adam Gazzaley, assistant professor of neurology and physiology at the University of California, San Francisco, used *functional magnetic resonance imaging* (fMRI), a sophisticated brain-scanning technology, to compare the recall abilities of older people with that of younger people. Gazzaley and his team found that people do not lose their recall ability as they age, but rather they lose the ability to filter out irrelevant information.

Gazzaley and his colleagues compared 17 young adults between 19 and 30 years old with 16 older adults between 60 and 77 years old. All of the study participants were shown pictures of faces and pictures of nature scenes as they underwent fMRI to see which parts of their brains were active during the task.

Sometimes, the participants were asked to remember the faces and not the scenes, and other times they were asked to remember the opposite information.

When recalling the nature scenes, an area in the left brain was activated in both groups. When instructed to ignore the nature scenes, activity in that area of the brain was reduced in the younger participants, but remained active for most of the older participants. This suggests that older people are less able to suppress irrelevant information, according to Gazzaley.

"Although older people were able to focus on what was important, they were also still focusing on the irrelevant, and that was causing them to remember less well," says Gazzaley.

A CLUE

The good news from Gazzaley's study is that these changes were not universal. Some older folks didn't have trouble suppressing irrelevant information.

"There was a subpopulation that was able to remember and didn't have suppression deficiency. These people were able to perform like younger subjects," Gazzaley says.

That means "that somewhere in here is a clue to successful aging," he adds.

info To learn more about the aging brain, read the article from the University of Southern California Health Magazine at *www.usc.edu/hsc/info/pr/hmm/01spring/brain.html.*

■ ■ ■ ■

Older and Wiser

Older people get along better with others than younger people do. They are also more likely to avoid conflict by waiting for things to improve…younger people are more likely to engage in yelling and name-calling.

Kira S. Birditt, PhD, research fellow, Institute for Social Research, University of Michigan, Ann Arbor.

■ ■ ■ ■

Personality Traits Change with Age

Conscientiousness (carrying out tasks dutifully and meticulously) improves as people grow older. Agreeableness (warmth, generosity and helpfulness) improves most during the 30s and 40s (and remains at that level). Neuroticism (worry and a sense of instability) and extroversion (the need for social support) decreases with age for women but not for men. Openness to new experiences declines as people get older, but only slightly.

Sanjay Srivastava, PhD, professor, department of psychology, University of Oregon, Eugene.

Promising News for Parkinson's Patients

Stanley Fahn, MD, H. Houston Merritt professor of neurology and director, Center for Parkinson's Disease and Other Movement Disorders, Columbia University, New York City. He is also scientific director, Parkinson's Disease Foundation, past president, American Academy of Neurology and founder of the Movement Disorder Society.

There is no preventive or cure for Parkinson's disease, but research is now making advances in both areas.

Renowned neuroscientists, doctors and other health-care workers joined Parkinson's patients and family members at the World Parkinson Congress in Washington, DC, to discuss innovative therapies that show promise in controlling symptoms as well as restoring motor function.

Research reported at the Congress...

COENZYME Q10

New finding: A small trial funded by the National Institutes of Health (NIH) found that taking 1,200 milligrams (mg) of *coenzyme Q10* (a natural nutrient that is present in all human cells) daily may slow the progression of early-stage Parkinson's disease.

More study is needed to confirm that CoQ10 does indeed slow the progression of the disease. In addition, because the dosage of CoQ10 that was studied was found to be only mildly effective, additional research is also needed to determine whether a higher dose (2,400 mg daily) works better.

Implication: Parkinson's patients who are eager to try all possible therapies should ask their doctors about taking 1,200 mg of CoQ10 daily. No side effects have been shown at this dosage.

DOPAMINE AGONISTS

Levodopa, also known as *L-dopa*, (Larodopa), is the gold standard in treating Parkinson's. However, many patients taking levodopa eventually develop uncontrolled flailing movements—a condition called *dyskinesia*—and motor fluctuations, in which medication levels in the brain drop and Parkinson's symptoms return.

Some doctors prefer to hold off prescribing levodopa in favor of a *dopamine agonist*, a drug that mimics the effects of dopamine, a chemical in the brain that allows the muscles of the body to make fluid movements. Dopamine agonists reduce Parkinson's-related disabilities—and work even better when combined with levodopa.

Dopamine agonists that have been approved by the US Food and Drug Administration (FDA) are *bromocriptine* (Parlodel), *pergolide* (Permax), *pramipexole* (Mirapex), *ropinirole* (Requip) and *apomorphine* (Apokyn). *Rotigotine*, the only dopamine agonist offered in patch form, is available in Europe. The FDA could approve this drug soon. The patch may be desirable for patients who have trouble swallowing or who want the convenience of using a patch once a day.

New finding: In a two-year study involving 186 early-stage Parkinson's patients, brain scans of those taking ropinirole or levodopa suggest that dopamine agonists may slow the decline of Parkinson's disease symptoms. Levodopa was found to worsen the disease, although patients' symptoms improved.

Implication: Because medications may interfere with brain scan results, more study is needed to confirm these findings. Ropinirole should be considered as treatment. Among the most likely candidates are younger patients who experience motor fluctuations and dyskinesia from levodopa.

Important: Ropinirole has been shown to cause side effects, such as sleepiness, nausea, hallucinations and, in rare cases, odd behavior, including compulsive shopping and gambling.

MINOCYCLINE AND CREATINE

New finding: In an NIH-sponsored clinical trial, 200 Parkinson's patients who did not yet require medication were randomly assigned to receive 200 mg daily of the antibiotic *minocycline*, 10 grams (g) daily of *creatine* (a nutritional supplement used to increase lean body mass and strength) or a placebo for 12 months.

Minocycline was chosen because of its anti-inflammatory effects. Inflammation has been detected in the brains of Parkinson's patients. Creatine is an energy booster, and decreased energy utilization is a problem in Parkinson's disease. Minocycline and creatine were found to be potentially beneficial.

Implication: More study is needed before minocycline or creatine can be prescribed as a treatment for Parkinson's disease.

DEEP BRAIN STIMULATION

New finding: An advanced surgical technique known as *deep brain stimulation* (DBS) has been shown to provide significant benefit to moderate and advanced Parkinson's patients for up to four years after the onset of treatment.

With DBS, a surgeon implants an electrode inside the brain to stimulate specific brain sites that control movement. The electrode is connected to a palm-sized pacemaker that is implanted beneath the skin just below the clavicle. By stimulating key parts of the brain, the pacemaker helps alleviate motor symptoms, such as tremor.

Serious complications from DBS, such as stroke, occur in fewer than 2% of patients. More common side effects include speech impairment, personality and/or mood change, depression and a decline in cognitive function in older patients.

Implication: DBS is particularly helpful for people who respond to levodopa but experience dyskinesia and wearing off of the drug. DBS is covered by Medicare and many other forms of health insurance.

info For more information on Parkinson's disease, go to the World Parkinson Congress Web site, *www.worldpdcongress.org.*

■■■■

What Is Parkinson's Disease?

Parkinson's disease, the second most common degenerative brain disease (after Alzheimer's), affects 1 million Americans and typically begins between the ages of 50 and 79. It occurs when *neurons*, or nerve cells, that control movement start to die off for unknown reasons. The result is a shortage of the brain-signaling chemical *dopamine*, which triggers the muscles that allow fluid body movements, such as lifting an arm or walking. The decline in dopamine levels leads to tremor, slowness of movement, stiffness of the limbs and trunk, difficulty walking and lack of facial expression.

Younger Look, No Face-Lift!

David Colbert, MD, FAAD, founder, New York Dermatology Group, a private dermatological practice and research facility, New York City. His patients include many people in the film and television industry.

Not long ago, men and women who wanted a more youthful appearance assumed that they would have to have a face-lift. A face-lift smooths sagging skin by pulling it up and tightening it, but the surgery doesn't give the skin itself a younger look.

Cosmetic dermatologists, on the other hand, have a number of options to create younger-looking skin by getting rid of many lines and age spots. Some of these techniques make it possible to "plump" the face to reverse the sunken look that age can cause. These techniques are all non-surgical and safe.

FILLERS

Fillers are materials that create volume to make up for the tablespoons of facial fat people lose as they age. The filler is injected directly into deep wrinkles to plump them. The materials are effective for many people older than age 60, assuming that their skin is reasonably taut. Fillers can decrease facial lines and wrinkles, treat frown lines between the eyes and also plump hollow cheeks and thinning lips.

Although there are a number of fillers, Restylane is one of the most popular, along with Perlane (a thicker form of Restylane), which is used for deeper wrinkles.

Procedures take approximately one hour. The results are immediate and can last from three to six months, after which the body absorbs the material. The procedure can be a bit uncomfortable, but the only side effects are a few hours of slight puffiness in the area and sometimes small, barely visible lumps that disappear within a few days to a few weeks. Approved by the US Food and Drug Administration (FDA), Restylane is a bioengineered, nonanimal, stabilized *hyaluronic acid*. It is almost identical to a substance found naturally in the body, making it safe to have repeat procedures.

I like to combine Restylane treatments with Botox. Although many people associate Botox skin injections with the "frozen" look sometimes seen on the faces of film stars, I prefer to use it more judiciously to relax muscles and give the face a destressed look.

Note: I do not recommend silicone injections to smooth the skin. Unlike other fillers, silicone is permanent, meaning that you are stuck with the result and your face may not age well around it.

Cost: Restylane and Perlane cost approximately $750* for the first syringe. There may be a discount for additional syringes used during the same treatment. Most people need more than one syringe. Botox costs $400 to $600 for a single area of the face treated, also with some discount for each additional area treated.

A patient's own fat is a good filler, as well, because it gives the face an especially soft, natural look. For such fat transfer, the person's own fat is taken from another area of the body, usually the thighs or buttocks. Because this requires a microliposuction procedure, exceptionally thin people are not candidates. Once the fat is harvested, it is frozen and remains usable for three years.

Fat transfer requires several treatments during a few months. Although this procedure hasn't been in use long enough for us to definitively say how long the results last, we are finding it to be semipermanent. And unlike synthetic fillers, natural fat tends to build up and stay—eventually eliminating the need for more injections.

You may experience some bruising and swelling for a week or so after the procedure, and there is a slight risk of infection. While this is a more expensive treatment (the total cost is approximately $5,000), it is cost-effective because it lasts so long.

*All costs are approximate and are not covered by insurance.

PEELS

Peels are available in gentle, medium and strong intensities. All peels chemically remove skin on the face and/or hands, which exposes the under layer—new skin that has been sheltered from the sun and other elements, and therefore, looks better. The difference among peels is how deeply they penetrate.

•**Gentle peels** affect only the top layer and diminish fine lines and fade age spots. Ideally, you would get gentle peels approximately once a month. Many spas offer these, but technicians there may not have adequate training and use weaker chemicals than dermatologists. You can resume normal activities immediately after gentle peels.

•**Medium peels** go deeper and more effectively remove age spots and fine lines as well as improve skin color and texture. They require two or three sessions for three to five weeks. You can resume normal activities immediately afterward. Results last approximately one year.

•**Deep (or strong) peels.** The strongest peel—either a *phenol* or a *trichloroacetic acid* (TCA) peel—penetrates deep into the skin. It dramatically rids the face of moderately deep lines and age spots in just one treatment. Often, just specific wrinkled or discolored areas of the face are deep-peeled.

This peel is relatively painful because it destroys the upper layer of skin and results in temporary blisters and scabbing. There is some risk of infection, so meticulous post-procedure care is necessary. People who have darker skin are not candidates because these peels lighten the skin and therefore, would create too much contrast with the neck. Also, anyone who has taken the drug Accutane within the last year is not a candidate because during this period, the skin is too sensitive for a deep peel. The recovery process takes at least three weeks.

Cost: Gentle peels run from $200 to $400 each…medium peels, from $200 to $1,200, depending on how much of the face is peeled… phenol or TCA peels, up to $4,000, also depending on the amount of skin treated.

LASER AND PHOTO REJUVENATION

Laser treatment tones the skin and improves skin texture.

Photo rejuvenation uses pulsed light to eliminate age spots and undesirable pigmentation.

Laser therapy also stimulates the production of *collagen*, the natural substance in the skin that helps keep it plump and unlined. This stimulation continues for several months after the treatment, giving ever-improving results. These treatments are painless, and one to three treatments can achieve desirable results.

For skin that appears leathery and discolored by sun exposure, a topical photosensitizing solution called Levulan is applied one hour before the light-based therapy session begins. Levulan allows the light to go deeper into the skin, thereby enhancing the effect of the treatment. We have not found any risks or side effects for laser or photo rejuvenation treatments.

Cost: Laser and photo rejuvenation treatments run from $200 to $1,200 depending on how much skin is treated. Adding Levulan brings the cost to $500 to $1,500.

■ ■ ■ ■

Before You Consider Plastic Surgery...

The growing demand for plastic surgery is attracting many new practitioners.

Trap: In most states, it's legal for any medical doctor (MD) to perform plastic surgery—including those whose training is in a different field and who have no experience in it.

Safety: Check a doctor's experience and credentials before committing to a procedure. Get references from other patients, and verify the doctor's certifications through the American Board of Medical Specialties, *www.abms.org.*

Steven G. Wallach, MD, FACS, plastic surgeon, New York City.

■ ■ ■ ■

How to Keep Your Skin from Wrinkling

To prevent lines and wrinkles as you get older, try the following healthy suggestions...

●**Avoid the sun**—the number-one cause of wrinkling. Use a sunscreen that has a minimum SPF of 15 daily. If you must spend time in the sun, use sunscreen that has a minimum SPF of 30.

●**Don't smoke.** Smoking cigarettes is the number-two cause of wrinkling.

●**Don't drink a lot of alcohol.** Alcohol dehydrates the skin and can cause broken or distended capillaries on the nose and face.

●**Get plenty of exercise.** It promotes healthy blood circulation and stimulates hormones that help build muscle, which indirectly improves the appearance of the skin.

●**Hydrate.** Drink plenty of water to keep skin hydrated from the inside out. Keep skin topically hydrated by using a good moisturizer.

Tom Diaz, MD, medical director, Lifestyle Center, The Diaz Clinic, Irving, TX.

———————————————

Yes, You Can Improve Your Hearing Now!

Anand Devaiah, MD, FACS, assistant professor, departments of otolaryngology–head and neck surgery and neurological surgery, Boston University School of Medicine. He is a spokesperson for the American Academy of Otolaryngology–Head and Neck Surgery, *www.entnet.org.*

One-third of Americans older than age 60—and half of those older than 75—have some degree of hearing loss. Although a number of factors can contribute to the risk of hearing impairment (including hereditary factors), the most common cause is simply age—and the cumulative effect of years of exposure to noise.

The good news: Cochlear implants and recent advances in hearing aids now make it possible for people who have severe or profound hearing loss to significantly improve their ability to hear conversation and other sounds.

Basics: Sound is picked up by the ear and transmitted to the brain through a complex pathway. Sound vibrations are collected by the outer ear, pass through the ear canal and cause the eardrum to vibrate. This, in turn, causes the vibration of three small middle ear bones. These bones ultimately connect to an opening in the *cochlea*, the part of the ear that turns the vibration of sound into nerve impulses. These impulses then travel through the auditory nerve to eventually reach the brain.

AS HEARING STARTS TO FADE

The first thing people usually notice is difficulty hearing what other people are saying…

- **Mild hearing loss.** It's difficult to hear other people in a noisy environment like a restaurant or at a party.

- **Moderate hearing loss.** Normal conversation becomes hard to hear even in a quiet room, and virtually impossible in a noisy room.

- **Severe hearing loss.** People can hear only shouted conversations.

- **Profound hearing loss.** The final stage before deafness, where even shouted words often go unheard.

WHEN TO SEE THE DOCTOR

You should see a doctor *immediately* if you experience sudden hearing loss—especially if the loss occurs in one ear only. This could be a sign of *idiopathic sensorineural* hearing loss. Nobody knows why it occurs, but doctors have found that treating patients using steroids promptly—ideally within the first 72 hours after the onset of symptoms—can restore hearing to normal or near-normal levels.

Caution: If steroid treatment doesn't start within two weeks, the hearing loss can be permanent.

Gradual, age-related hearing damage typically occurs in both ears and is not a medical emergency. If you're experiencing noticeable hearing loss, however, you should still be checked as soon as possible by an *otolaryngologist* (ear, nose and throat specialist) who can determine exactly how much hearing loss has occurred…look for underlying medical problems that might contribute to the hearing loss…and prescribe treatment—including a hearing aid, if necessary.

Schedule an appointment with an otolaryngologist if you…

- **Notice that it's harder to hear** when you are on the telephone.

- **Have trouble hearing conversation** if there's background noise.

- **Often ask people to repeat themselves.**

- **Hear a persistent ringing,** humming or buzzing sound in your ears (a condition known as *tinnitus*).

- **Notice changes in balance** associated with a change in your hearing—balance and hearing are both functions of the ear.

YOUR CHECKUP

Your otolaryngologist will take a full history of your symptoms and any factors that might put you at risk for hearing loss. An *audiogram* will be obtained to test how well you hear sounds over a wide range of frequencies.

The audiogram gives the single best picture of how well your auditory nerve and the rest of your sound-conducting system are functioning. It will show if your hearing follows a pattern consistent with age-related hearing loss or noise exposure, or indicates that there is some other condition, such as an inner ear disturbance or something that is preventing the proper movement of one or more of the three bones of the middle ear.

Expect an ear, head and neck exam, which will help check for underlying conditions that may be causing or related to your hearing loss. *Potential causes of hearing loss include…*

- **Ear infections,** with the acute and chronic effects of such infections.

- **Holes in the eardrum.**

- **Otosclerosis,** a condition in which a bone in the middle ear becomes fixed in place and may need to be replaced or freed with surgery.

- **Autoimmune diseases,** such as lupus and rheumatoid arthritis.

- **Ménière's disease,** an inner ear ailment marked by symptoms such as dizziness and fluctuating hearing loss.

SELECTING A HEARING AID

Once your doctor has determined the nature and degree of your hearing loss, the next step is to discuss different treatment options. The majority of people who have a hearing loss can be treated using hearing aids, but depending on the nature of your problem, you may require medical or surgical therapy.

Today's hearing aids are complex devices that can be customized to your own hearing profile, amplifying certain frequencies and not others. When properly prescribed and fitted, they can significantly improve the hearing abilities of most people who have a hearing loss.

Your level of hearing loss will dictate what type of hearing aid you should have. It is critically important to get a comfortable, well-designed, custom-molded hearing aid, not a one-size-fits-all model. Both analog and digital models (some of which are programmable for multiple environments) are available. With programmable models, you can boost different frequencies to hear best when you're talking in a crowded restaurant or when you're talking on the phone.

Cost: Can vary from $600 to $3,000. Some insurance plans cover the cost of hearing aids, others subsidize the cost.

Each individual type of hearing aid serves different needs. After you've settled on a model, your otolaryngologist will take a mold of your ear, fit the device, tune it to complement your existing hearing and show you how to care for it.

More than 90% of the people who get fitted with a hearing aid find that it helps restore hearing function.

After getting your hearing aid, it is important to follow up with your hearing professional, especially your audiologist, to ensure that the device continues to suit your needs and that you continue to use it properly. Because the standard hearing aid sits in the ear canal, it can keep ear wax from naturally making its way out of the ear, and you may require periodic removal of the wax.

COCHLEAR IMPLANTATION

For some causes of profound hearing loss, a possible treatment is cochlear implantation. This procedure is used in both adults and children and is a great benefit to some people. Every patient must be carefully evaluated on a case-by-case basis, since not everyone will benefit from such a device.

A cochlear implant is made up of three parts: (1) a small microphone that picks up sounds around the user. These sounds are then transmitted to (2) a speech processor, worn on the belt or carried in the user's pocket, which converts the sound into electrical signals that are then transmitted to (3) an electrical receiver (that has been surgically implanted under the skin behind the user's ear) that has an electrode going into the cochlea. The signals from the electrode are ultimately picked up by the auditory nerve and ascend along the complex pathways to the brain. The user "hears" sound once the device is activated and programmed to best suit that person. The quality and intelligibility of the sound varies from person to person.

Cost: Approximately $60,000, including post-operative training. Insurance coverage varies.

2

Asthma & Allergies

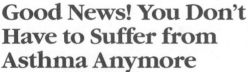

Good News! You Don't Have to Suffer from Asthma Anymore

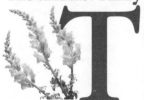 There is a huge difference in how well asthmatics believe their symptoms are being controlled and how well they are actually managing their disease, according to experts.

"We have known for a long time that asthma can be controlled better, that it is not being controlled as well as it can be, and that we ought to do something about it," explains Dr. Norman Edelman, a professor of medicine at the State University of New York at Stony Brook and a medical consultant to the American Lung Association. Improving symptom control means that asthmatics must first recognize that they are not being controlled as well as they could be.

POLL RESULTS

A recent poll taken by the Asthma and Allergy Foundation of America (AAFA) found that 88% of nearly 600 adult asthmatics reported managing their symptoms well.

However, in that same group, 61% said they have had to catch their breath while running up the stairs, 48% said their asthma symptoms have woken them and 50% have had to stop exercising in the middle of their regimens.

Among 118 respondents whose children have asthma, 89% felt their children's symptoms were being well-controlled, yet half of the children had missed days of school and/or work. In addition, half were unable to complete their exercise programs and 45% were awakened because of asthma symptoms.

PERCEPTION VS. REALITY

"This was an interesting study of perception versus reality," says Mike Tringale, AAFA's director of communications. "These people have learned to live with compromised lives."

Norman Edelman, MD, professor of medicine, State University of New York at Stony Brook, and medical consultant, American Lung Association.

Mike Tringale, director of communications, Asthma and Allergy Foundation of America.

He adds, "Now, however, because of better understanding of the disease, better preventive education and better medicines, most people with asthma don't have to have any symptoms."

Poorly managed asthma can lead to numerous health problems, including weight gain from not exercising. "Weight gain is terrible for asthma, because it exacerbates the symptoms," he says.

There are also more subtle psychological changes. "People's personalities are affected. Even though you are going about your daily activities, like going to work, you are still disabled because you are not functioning at your maximum. It changes who you are," Edelman says.

CLOSING THE KNOWLEDGE GAP

To close the knowledge gap, both the American Lung Association and AAFA have started programs to alert people who have asthma that most can control their symptoms more effectively.

Asthmatics have learned to live with compromised lives.

Mike Tringale

The American Lung Association introduced a five-question test on its Web site for asthmatics older than age 12. The questions ask how often asthma symptoms keep them awake at night, cause shortness of breath and prevent them from completing work at school or in the office.

"Approximately 100,000 people have taken the test online, and two-thirds of them have found that they don't have their asthma under control," says Edelman.

The test's success has spurred the Association to develop another quiz designed for children under age 12, to be answered by their parents.

The AAFA's program, called *Sleep Work Play*, helps asthma patients better recognize their symptoms so they can talk to their doctors about controlling them more effectively.

AAFA's program includes a Web site questionnaire that asks asthma patients about their sleep, work and play habits. It also encourages users to take the completed questionnaire to their doctor to discuss how to better manage their asthma symptoms.

"People haven't been talking in the same language. Doctors don't probe deeply enough into patients' symptoms; parents don't question their kids," says Tringale.

info For adults, the asthma control questionnaire can be found at the American Lung Association Web site at *www.asthmacontrol.com*. The kids' quiz is at the Asthma and Allergy Foundation of America at *www.sleepworkplay.com*. Click on "sleeplearnplay."

■ ■ ■ ■

What Is Asthma?

Asthma, a chronic lung disease, affects more than 17 million Americans, according to the American Academy of Allergy, Asthma & Immunology. It is marked by an inflammation of the airways that makes it difficult for air to move in and out of the lungs. Asthmatics often experience a cough, shortness of breath and difficulty breathing during an attack.

Outrageous! Insurers Put Asthmatics at Risk

Nancy Sander, president and founder, Allergy and Asthma Network/Mothers of Asthmatics.

Jennifer Kim, MD, attending physician, division of allergy, Children's Memorial Hospital, and clinical instructor of pediatrics, Feinberg School of Medicine, Northwestern University, both in Chicago.

Michael Blaiss, MD, immediate past president, American College of Allergy, Asthma and Immunology, and clinical professor of pediatrics, University of Tennessee Health Sciences, Memphis.

American College of Allergy, Asthma and Immunology annual meeting, Anaheim, CA.

Preferred drug lists and preauthorization policies, which are designed to hold down the cost of medical care, may delay—or even prevent—people who have asthma from getting the most effective treatment.

Even more alarming, some drug companies are reimbursing pharmacies or home health-care providers for unapproved medications in nebulizer form (a fine spray or vapor) that can actually worsen asthma symptoms.

These findings come from two studies by the Allergy and Asthma Network/Mothers of Asthmatics (AANMA).

THE FIRST STUDY

The first study gathered information from 19 Medicaid patients and 24 health-care providers about the medications they use and prescribe. Nancy Sander, lead author of both studies and president and founder of AANMA, and her colleagues conducted two focus groups—one for patients and one for health-care providers—in Atlanta; Birmingham, Alabama; and San Antonio, Texas.

Both patients and providers said that preauthorization policies and preferred drug lists limit their access to effective asthma treatment. These procedures result in "undue suffering, poorly controlled symptoms, missed work and school days, delays in obtaining prescriptions and emergency department visits," both groups said.

Dr. Jennifer Kim, an allergist at Children's Memorial Hospital in Chicago, says that preferred drug lists and preauthorization policies, such as those established by Medicaid, can definitely be a problem. "For a group of people who already have poor access to health care, this only puts up more barriers and more hoops for them to jump through to get the treatment they need," she says.

The medications Kim has the most trouble obtaining for her patients are nonsedating antihistamines and Xolair (omalizumab), an injectable medication that is used to treat severe asthma, she says.

"The problem with preferred drug lists is that it's all about the dollar. It's not a list that's preferred by physicians or by patients" based on what works best, says Sander.

THE SECOND STUDY

The second—and more alarming—study detailed reports of the improper substitution of nebulizer medications. Sander and her team found that, without the knowledge of the patient or doctor, some nonapproved compounded medications are being used instead of the nebulizer medications approved by the US Food and Drug Administration (FDA). These compounded medications do not offer the same quality control that FDA-approved medications do.

"We don't know the true strength of these medications," says Dr. Michael Blaiss, the immediate past president of the American College of Allergy, Asthma and Immunology. "There can be contaminants, such as fungi or bacteria, in these medications and one can get infections. We're talking about something that children and adults with severe lung problems are inhaling. This can really be a dangerous thing for patients."

Most of these compounded medications are approved in other forms, such as a powder or tablet, according to Blaiss, but not in the nebulized form. "These medications have to be aerosolized at a certain particle size, and if they're not, they won't reach the right portion of the airways to be effective," says Sander.

WHAT PATIENTS CAN DO

While the FDA and individual states investigate, there are steps asthmatics can take to protect themselves, Sander says. FDA-approved medications come in plastic vials, on which all the information is embossed. Medications that come with a paper label have probably been compounded, she says. Medications should also arrive in sealed, foil containers with the prescribing information enclosed. Patients who receive medication that is loosely arranged in the box should check with their doctor or AANMA.

For people who already have poor access to health care, preauthorization policies only put up more hoops for them to jump through.

Jennifer Kim, MD

If any patients think they may have received improperly compounded medication, they can also call the AANMA at 800-878-4403 or 866-227-2934.

info The Allergy and Asthma Network/Mothers of Asthmatics Web site has more information and pictures of what approved and unapproved medications look like at *www.aanma.org/chasm*. Click on "Are There Fakes and Frauds in Your Nebulizer?"

■ ■ ■ ■

Common Painkillers May Trigger Asthma

Aspirin and some related painkillers may trigger asthma attacks in as many as 20% of people who have the condition, reports a new study. Many painkillers, including *nonsteroidal anti-inflammatory drugs* (NSAIDs) such as ibuprofen, can cause attacks—but the fewest were caused by acetaminophen (found in Tylenol and Panadol), which caused a reaction among 7% of those studied.

Advice: Asthmatics should make acetaminophen their first choice for an over-the-counter pain reliever—but consult their doctors about it and be prepared in case a reaction occurs.

Christine Jenkins, MD, head, asthma group, Woolcock Institute of Medical Research, Royal Prince Alfred Hospital, Camperdown, Australia.

Asthmatics Need 'Action' From Their Doctors

Michael A. Kaliner, MD, Institute for Asthma & Allergy.
Loren Yamamoto, MD, professor of pediatrics, University of Hawaii, Honolulu.
International Conference of the American Thoracic Society, San Diego.

Many asthmatics stop taking their medicine or skip doses, and those who do take their medication rarely discuss the side effects with a doctor, according to a large international survey.

The problem may be due to poor doctor–patient communication.

SURVEY RESULTS

The findings, from the Global Asthma Physician and Patient (GAPP) survey, involved nearly 3,500 adults in 16 countries. The results point out just how serious the communication gaps between doctor and patient can be.

An overwhelming majority of asthma patients—73%—said they never or rarely discuss medication side effects with their physicians.

Although nearly 20% said they are not aware of short-term side effects of medication, only 5% of the physicians who prescribe these drugs said that they think patients don't know about these possible side effects.

"The data in the United States show that doctors don't seem to be spending as much time as they should with asthma patients," says survey team member Dr. Michael A. Kaliner, of the Institute for Asthma & Allergy.

Because asthma is a chronic disease, successfully controlling it takes commitment by both patients and their health-care providers, he says. However, when physicians are under pressure to see many patients in a relatively short time period, as is the case in some health maintenance organizations (HMOs), conversations about asthma care may be rushed or incomplete, he notes.

ACTION PLANS

National guidelines for asthma management call for treatment plans that are written, discussed and provided by the doctor in partnership with the patient. However, some studies have shown that these written plans are often absent.

> *Doctors don't seem to be spending as much time as they should with asthma patients.*
>
> *Michael A. Kaliner, MD*

In one study of more than 500 asthma patients who came to the emergency room, less than 10% had action plans for dealing with their asthma. "We gave them the plans once they came to the emergency department," notes one of the lead investigators, Dr. Loren Yamamoto, professor of pediatrics at the University of Hawaii.

However, doing this was so time-consuming that an extra staff person was needed, Yamamoto says. After the study was completed, that staff member could no longer be funded.

■ ■ ■ ■

Chlorine Could Be a Culprit

In a recent study, 60% of the people swimming in highly chlorinated pools experienced the temporary constriction of airways known as exercise-induced asthma. Of those who swam in water with half as much chlorine, only 20% had breathing difficulties.

Self-defense: Swim in outdoor pools—indoor pools have limited ventilation. Check that the pool's chlorine level is below five parts per million (ppm). At public pools, ask the facility's maintenance person what the water's ppm is. For home pools, investigate alternatives to chlorine, such as ultraviolet filtration systems, which are becoming popular in Europe and at some universities in the United States.

Martin P. Schwellnus, MD, PhD, department of human biology, University of Cape Town, South Africa.

Cat Allergens Have 9 Lives, Too

Jared W. Allen, PhD, postdoctoral researcher, David Geffen School of Medicine, University of California at Los Angeles.

David Mendelson, MD, associate professor of radiology, Mount Sinai Medical Center, New York City.

Radiological Society of North America annual meeting, Chicago.

A cat and its dander can trouble people who have asthma long after the animal has left the room, according to a new study.

Cat allergens, in fact, can hamper the lung function of asthmatics who are allergic to cats for up to 22 hours after exposure, says Jared W. Allen, a postdoctoral researcher at the David Geffen School of Medicine at the University of California, Los Angeles.

"Cat allergens can be smaller particles than normal allergens, such as pollen or flowers, and [they can] reach deeper into the airway of the lungs," Allen explains.

THE STUDY

Allen started this study after noticing that asthmatics often complain of symptoms even days after exposure to the triggers—such as cats or cat hair—that had spurred the attack.

Conventional lung-function tests may come up normal, he says, so his team decided to do more sophisticated testing that can measure the amount of air that is trapped deep in the lung.

"The amount of air trapped in the lung correlates with airway reactivity—how sensitive your airways are," he says. "The more air that is trapped, the more symptoms you will have."

His team performed a test called *high-resolution computed tomography* (HRCT) to examine the functioning of the small airways deep in the lungs to detect the extent of impairment caused by exposure to the allergen.

Allen's team first induced an asthma attack in 10 people who had known allergies to cats, and then performed a HRCT. The next day, they exposed these individuals to cats, and took another scan six hours later. The researchers performed yet another scan 22 hours after that cat exposure, during another induced asthma attack.

Even after the outward symptoms (such as difficulty breathing) abated, all 10 people continued to experience a decrease in lung function, the testing showed.

CONCLUSIONS

"Our conclusions are that there is a significant response in the small airways of the lung that can persist for up to 22 hours," Allen says. "And the patient's airways could be hypersensitive to additional challenges."

So, if exposure to cat allergens has left a person with symptoms, and then he/she is exposed again, he may be even more sensitive the second time, Allen explains. If that second exposure occurs within 22 hours, he says, the second attack could be worse than the first.

The findings may help explain why some people who have allergies and asthma seem to still have symptoms when traditional tests come out normal, says Dr. David Mendelson, an associate professor of radiology at Mount Sinai Medical Center in New York City.

"To me, the provocative thing is that [Allen] used these newer techniques, and you can see a positive result [for airway problems] when you have no other objective evidence of a patient's complaint," Mendelson says.

info To learn more about indoor allergens, visit the American Academy of Allergy, Asthma & Immunology at *www.aaaai.org/patients*. Click on "AAAAI Tips Brochures" under "Featured Resources." Then scroll down to the article on "Indoor allergens."

■ ■ ■ ■

Important for Asthmatics— Read Labels!

People who have asthma are especially sensitive to *sulfites*, a type of preservative typically found in bottled wines. Sulfites can also be found in processed foods, such as dried fruits, molasses, condiments, sauces and soup mixes, dehydrated and prepeeled raw potatoes, baked goods and jellies.

Self-defense: Read food labels and avoid products that contain sulfur, sulfites, bisulfites or metabisulfites.

Mayo Clinic Health Letter.

Inhaled Corticosteroids Get Mixed Reviews in Kids' Asthma Studies

Hans Bisgaard, MD, head, Danish Pediatric Asthma Centre, and professor of pediatrics, Copenhagen University Hospital, Denmark.

Theresa Guilbert, MD, assistant professor of pediatrics, Arizona Respiratory Center, University of Arizona, Tucson.

Diane Gold, MD, MPH, associate professor of medicine, Harvard Medical School and Brigham and Women's Hospital, both in Boston.

The New England Journal of Medicine.

Two new studies report mixed results on the short-term benefit of inhaled corticosteroids for the treatment of asthma in infants and young children.

THE FIRST STUDY

Scientists had theorized that using inhaled corticosteroids to control the airway inflammation that causes asthma symptoms might not only prevent the disease from getting worse, but also might prevent damage to the lungs. For such therapy to be effective, it would need to be initiated in the first year of life, when the lungs are still developing and the damage from asthma begins.

The first study, which tested this theory, included 411 one-month-old infants who were not necessarily diagnosed with asthma. When the subjects experienced their first episode of wheezing, they were randomly assigned to receive either a two-week course of the inhaled corticosteroid *budesonide* or an inhaled placebo. Parents in both groups were also instructed to give fast-acting asthma-relief medication as needed. Intermittent treatment when wheezing occurred continued for three years.

The corticosteroid group reported that 83% of their days were symptom-free, while the placebo group had 82% symptom-free days. In total, 24% of the infants in the treatment group had persistent wheezing, compared with 21% in the placebo group.

"Intermittent inhaled corticosteroid therapy had no effect on the progression from episodic to persistent wheezing, and no short-term benefit during episodes of wheezing in the first three years of life," says study author Dr. Hans Bisgaard, a professor of pediatrics at Copenhagen University Hospital and head of the Danish Pediatric Asthma Centre.

Bisgaard says he was very surprised by the results and adds, "The findings may serve as a warning to treatment practices extrapolated from adult studies, and it emphasizes the need to provide evidence on medicine in children."

THE SECOND STUDY

In contrast to Bisgaard's research, a second study found that inhaled corticosteroid therapy improved symptom control. However, it found no long-term benefits from these medications.

The study looked at 285 two- and three-year-olds at very high risk for asthma. The children were randomly chosen to receive continuous treatment with the inhaled corticosteroid *fluticasone propionate* or an inhaled placebo. The youngsters took the medications twice daily for two years, and the researchers followed-up for another year when they were off the medications.

During the treatment years, the proportion of episode-free days was 93% for the treatment group and 88% for the placebo group. During the observation year, the proportion of episode-free days was 87% for the former treatment group and 86% for the placebo group.

The most significant side effect from the long-term use of inhaled corticosteroids was an apparently slower growth rate—the placebo group was 1.1 centimeter (cm) taller than the treatment group. However, during the observation year that difference began to even out and was only 0.7 cm at the end of the study.

"This high-risk group did respond nicely to inhaled [cortico]steroids while they were on them. But starting them early didn't prevent anything," says study author Dr. Theresa Guilbert, an assistant professor of pediatrics at the Arizona Respiratory Center at the University of Arizona in Tucson.

EXPLAINING THE DIFFERENCES

One possible reason the Guilbert study found symptom relief while the Bisgaard study didn't is the difference in the study populations, according to Dr. Diane Gold, an associate professor of medicine at Harvard Medical School and Brigham and Women's Hospital, both in Boston.

The Bisgaard study included a much more diverse group of children, including youngsters who may not go on to have asthma. In addition, many of these children were exposed to maternal or environmental smoke in the home, which could adversely affect any treatment plan.

Also, asthma is notoriously difficult to diagnose in children younger than two, and wheezing can be a sign of any of a number of viral infections that typically don't respond to inhaled corticosteroids.

"Both studies together strengthen the evidence that treatment with inhaled corticosteroids doesn't alter the natural course of asthma," says Gold. However, "That doesn't mean that [they] shouldn't be used very selectively with young kids who are having frequent symptoms," she adds.

Both Gold and Guilbert emphasize that clinicians should follow the US National Asthma Education and Prevention Program Guidelines and use their clinical judgment about the need for inhaled corticosteroids. Guilbert adds that she would encourage physicians to step down the dose once asthma control has been achieved.

info To learn more about asthma and various ways to prevent flare-ups, visit the National Heart, Lung, and Blood Institute at *www.nhlbi.nih.gov/health/dci/Diseases/Asthma/Asthma_WhatIs.html.*

Beware: Deadly Asthma Inhaler

Shelley Salpeter, MD, clinical professor of medicine, Stanford University, and physician, Santa Clara Valley Medical Center, San Jose, CA.
Jeffrey Glassroth, MD, professor of medicine, Tufts University, Boston.
Annals of Internal Medicine.

Fueling an ongoing controversy, a recent data review suggests that the *long-acting beta-agonist bronchodilator* inhalers, a popular class of asthma medications, may be dangerous.

These drugs, which are designed to help relax airway muscles and improve breathing, include Serevent and Advair. As a group, they are expected to gross nearly $7 billion in consumer sales this year.

THE STUDY

Dr. Shelley Salpeter, a clinical professor of medicine at Stanford University, and his colleagues launched a broad review, or *meta-analysis*, examining the results of 19 asthma drug studies that involved nearly 34,000 patients.

They found that people who used long-acting beta-agonists had a 2.6 times greater risk of asthma-related hospitalization, a 1.8 times greater risk of life-threatening complications and a 3.5 times greater risk of death compared with those taking a placebo.

The findings suggest that *salmeterol* (Serevent) could be responsible for 4,000 of the annual 5,000 asthma deaths in the United States, according to the study authors. However, the researchers caution that the very small number of deaths that were recorded in the studies limits the "reliability" of these numbers.

"The take-home message is that long-acting beta-agonists worsen asthma control and increase the risk for moderate asthma exacerbations, life-threatening asthma exacerbations and asthma deaths," Salpeter says. "These can occur without any warning, [such as] increased symptoms, which make them especially dangerous," he adds. "These agents should not be used."

ANOTHER OPINION

However, not all of the experts agree. Dr. Jeffrey Glassroth, professor of medicine at Tufts

University in Boston, says that while they have some risks, long-acting beta-agonists can still "be helpful to some people." If the drugs weren't used, "We might prevent some adverse reactions, but we might create as many—or even more—problems in our asthmatic population," Glassroth says.

"What I would like to see is more rigorous adherence to the current guidelines that suggest they aren't first-line therapy. There are other things to be used first, and for many patients, that may be all they need," he says.

It is not known why these drugs can be dangerous for some people and not others, Glassroth says, although research suggesting that African-Americans are at greater risk indicate that genetic factors may play a role.

info Learn more about asthma drugs from the US National Institutes of Health's MedlinePlus Web site at *www.medlineplus.gov.* Click on "Drugs & Supplements," and find "Bronchodilators, Adrenergic (Inhalation)" in the alphabetical listing.

Kids' Asthma Linked to Moms' Nutrition

Carlos Camargo, MD, DrPH, associate professor of medicine and epidemiology, Harvard Medical School, Boston.

Joel Liem, MD, research fellow in pediatric allergy and clinical immunology, University of Manitoba, Winnipeg, Canada.

Anita Kozyrskyj, PhD, associate professor of pharmacy and medicine, University of Manitoba, Winnipeg, Canada.

Bruce Bender, PhD, head of pediatric behavioral health, National Jewish Medical and Research Center, Denver.

Researchers have found evidence that asthma in children is linked to maternal nutrition and stress.

STUDY #1:
VITAMIN D

In one study, expectant mothers who took high doses of vitamin D reduced their child's risk for asthma.

Vitamin D deficiency is common in areas where asthma is also widespread, raising the suspicion that the two are connected, says Dr. Carlos Camargo, senior author of the study and an associate professor of medicine and epidemiology at Harvard Medical School in Boston.

Camargo and his team followed 1,300 mother-child pairs for more than three years. By the time the children were two years old, there was already a clear association between a higher vitamin D intake during pregnancy and a lower risk of wheezing and asthma in the children, he says. The link after three years was even stronger, Camargo adds.

Results of previous studies have suggested that vitamin D may have an effect on a fetus's developing immune system.

"Doctors should understand that vitamin D insufficiency is real," Camargo says. "It's important to get [vitamin D] from diet or supplements, and the way to do that is through fortified milk, fish and supplements."

STUDY #2:
ASTHMA AND PREMATURITY

A Canadian study found that pregnant women who have asthma are more likely to have premature and low-birth-weight babies.

This survey of 13,980 children who were born in Manitoba found that mothers who had asthma were, on average, 2.77 times more likely to have a baby born at less than 28 weeks' gestation and 3.04 times more likely to have a baby born at less than 32 weeks' gestation than a nonasthmatic mother.

"Maternal asthma is a risk factor for prematurity and low birth weight in babies, and physicians and other health-care professionals need to assess present and past asthma, even up to five years prior, in order to properly assess risk for premature labor," says lead author Dr. Joel Liem, a research fellow in pediatric allergy and clinical immunology at the University of Manitoba.

STUDY #3:
ASTHMA AND STRESS

Another research group at the University of Manitoba found that children were 1.3 times more likely to develop asthma if their mothers experienced stress (defined as visiting a doctor for depression or anxiety or getting a prescription to treat one or both of these conditions). "The highest risk was in children with repeat exposure to mother's stress," says Anita Kozyrskyj, lead author of the study and associate professor of pharmacy and medicine at the University.

Kozyrskyj could only speculate on the possible mechanisms behind this association. "It may be related to the fact that stress alters Mom's behavior, and there is some evidence that stress in the first year of life can cause some changes to the gastrointestinal system," she says.

MORE STUDIES

Another recent study found that children and parents of children are overreporting how much asthma medication the child is taking. By one measure, only one-third of the medicine was actually being used.

"Most patients don't follow daily treatment regimens no matter how good their doctors are," says Bruce Bender, lead author and head of pediatric behavioral health at the National Jewish Medical and Research Center in Denver. "That disconnect is huge, and it's a large factor in how well we control asthma in kids and adults."

Another study conducted at the VA Greater Los Angeles Healthcare System found that patients who had intermittent (as opposed to persistent) asthma accounted for nearly half of all asthma-related emergency department visits.

Natural Relief for Allergies and Asthma

Richard Firshein, DO, director of Firshein Center for Comprehensive Medicine, which specializes in treating allergies and asthma, New York City. An asthmatic himself, he is author of *The Nutraceutical Revolution* (Riverhead) and *Reversing Asthma* (Warner).

Millions of Americans have asthma and allergies, often triggered by such airborne substances as mold, dust mites or pollen. The immune system identifies these normally harmless substances as dangerous and releases inflammatory chemicals that cause sneezing, wheezing, congestion and other symptoms.

The drugs used for these conditions—antihistamines, inhaled corticosteroids, etc.—curtail symptoms but frequently cause side effects.

Better approach: Studies have shown that many over-the-counter (OTC) supplements act as natural antihistamines/anti-inflammatories that can prevent or reduce allergy or asthma flare-ups—without side effects. Patients who use nutritional supplements often are able to stop taking asthma and allergy drugs or significantly reduce the dosages. You can take one or all of the supplements below daily, but always check with your doctor first.

QUERCETIN

Quercetin is a member of a class of nutrients known as *bioflavonoids*. It is a powerful anti-inflammatory that helps prevent the lungs, nasal passages and eyes from swelling after allergen exposure. It also inhibits the release of *histamine*, a chemical that triggers allergy and asthma flare-ups.

Quercetin works better for prevention than short-term treatment. It usually takes several weeks to become effective.

What I recommend to my patients: 300 milligrams (mg) twice daily. If your symptoms are severe, increase the amount to 1,000 mg twice daily until symptoms abate. Then switch back to a maintenance dose of 300 mg twice daily.

VITAMIN C

This potent antioxidant has a mild antihistamine effect.

What I recommend to my patients: 500 to 1,000 mg daily. Vitamin C may cause diarrhea in some people.

Divide the daily amount into two doses to reduce the risk of this side effect. Also, patients who have a history of kidney stones should talk to their doctors before taking vitamin C supplements.

NETTLES

A traditional herbal remedy for allergies, nettles inhibits the body's production of inflammatory *prostaglandins*. In one study of 69 allergy patients, 57% had significant improvement in symptoms after taking nettles. Nettles works quickly, often within hours, and can be taken during flare-ups.

What I recommend to my patients: 300 to 600 mg daily.

MAGNESIUM

This mineral is a natural bronchodilator that relaxes airway muscles and promotes better breathing. Supplementation with magnesium may be especially helpful if you're taking corticosteroids or other asthma drugs, which tend to reduce the amount of magnesium in the body.

What I recommend to my patients: 200 to 600 mg daily.

ALLERGY TESTS

Your doctor may recommend skin or blood tests to determine if your allergies are caused by dust mites, mold, pollen, etc. Once you know what you're allergic to, you can take steps to minimize exposure.

Example: If you're allergic to dust mites, you can buy mattress and pillow casings that are impervious to allergens…and use a vacuum with a high-efficiency particulate air (HEPA) filter, which reduces the allergens in the air.

■ ■ ■ ■

Surprising Symptoms Caused by Allergies

Allergies can cause any part of the body to become swollen or inflamed. They can also make a person feel lethargic or cranky…have mood changes, joint pain, an irritable bowel or intestinal cramps. Look for triggers—a specific place or time when symptoms occur, such as at work, after consuming certain foods or beverages or after exposure to inhalants, such as pollen. If you can't figure out the triggers on your own, see an allergist.

Thomas Brunoski, MD, a specialist in food and environmental allergies, Westport, CT.

90% of All Sinusitis Diagnoses Are Wrong!

Alan Hirsch, MD, founder and neurological director, The Smell & Taste Treatment and Research Foundation, and author of *What Your Doctor May Not Tell You About Sinusitis.* Warner.

As many as 45 million cases of sinusitis are diagnosed each year—and approximately nine times out of 10, that diagnosis is incorrect.

Sinusitis, also called a sinus infection, is a bacterial infection of the sinus linings. Infection causes the linings to swell and interferes with the normal drainage of mucus. This results in congestion, headache, reduced sense of smell and/or taste, tenderness around the eyes, cheeks, nose and/or forehead and other symptoms.

The majority of patients who think (or have been told) that they have sinusitis actually have other conditions—allergies, a cold or migraine headaches. Errors in diagnosing sinusitis are a leading cause of unnecessary treatments, including the use of antibiotics and even surgery.

CAUSES AND DIAGNOSIS

There are many small sinus cavities—over the eyes, along and behind the nose, above the teeth, etc. These cavities have tiny holes (ostia) that drain into the nose. Anything that interferes with normal drainage causes mucus to accumulate. This includes colds, allergies and other conditions that trigger congestion.

Many people have anatomical abnormalities, such as a deviated septum, that inhibit drainage. When the mucus builds up, it provides a rich medium for bacterial growth and infection.

Most cases of sinusitis are acute, lasting one to two weeks, and get better on their own without medical treatment. Less often, sinusitis is chronic, lasting three months or more. Patients who get four or more cases of acute sinusitis annually are also considered to have the chronic form. Chronic sinusitis may clear up without treatment, but this happens less often than with the acute form.

Most people who have sinusitis have symptoms that include a greenish nasal discharge, a fever of more than 100°F, swollen lymph nodes and tenderness over the sinuses.

The only sure way to diagnose sinusitis is with a sinus puncture. The patient is given a local anesthetic. A needle is guided through a nostril into a sinus cavity to extract mucus. The mucus is then examined in a laboratory for signs of bacterial infection. Other sinusitis tests include computed tomography (CT) and magnetic resonance imaging (MRI) scans, though these aren't as accurate as the sinus puncture.

TREATMENT AND PREVENTION

Doctors routinely prescribe oral antibiotics to patients who appear to have sinusitis, but participants in studies who are given no treatment recover just as quickly as those who are given antibiotics.

The only effective treatments for sinusitis are intravenous antibiotics given for three days to one week in the hospital...or surgery to restore normal drainage in the sinus cavities. Few patients really need these treatments because true sinusitis is rare.

Most patients can control sinus discomfort, regardless of the underlying cause, and lower the risk of infection by reducing or eliminating congestion. *Best approaches...*

●**Drink water—at least eight glasses each day.** It thins mucus in the sinuses and promotes normal drainage. This is especially important if you have a cold or an allergy flare-up.

●**Don't take over-the-counter (OTC) antihistamines or decongestants.** They dry mucus and impede normal drainage.

●**Ask your doctor about *sumatriptan*** (Imitrex). This medication, typically prescribed for migraines, can relieve sinusitus symptoms, postnasal drip, nasal congestion, a sense of fullness or pressure in the face, etc. This drug is effective in approximately 75% of cases.

●**Irrigate with a *neti* pot.** Available in natural-health stores, a neti pot looks like a small teapot. It is used to flush a saline solution through the nose, nasal passages and sinuses.

Flushing these areas once or twice daily when you're congested can improve drainage and reduce symptoms—or prevent sinusitis when you have a cold or allergies.

■■■■

How to Use a Neti Pot

Mix approximately one-third teaspoon of salt and a pinch of baking powder in one cup of lukewarm water. Pour the solution into the neti pot.

Rotate and tip your head over a sink, and pour the solution into one nostril. Keep pouring until it flows out of the other nostril.

Spit out any fluid that enters the mouth. Repeat on the other side.

■■■■

Best Way to Ease Allergies

Breakfast in bed may help alleviate allergy symptoms. People who have allergies are sensitive to temperature changes. That's why they cough and sneeze when they leave a warm bed. Drinking hot tea in bed warms the body and prevents this reaction. Caffeinated or decaffeinated tea increases the speed of nasal *cilia*, tiny hairs in the mucus membranes, to rid the nose of allergy-triggering dust that has accumulated during sleep.

Helpful: Fill a thermos with hot tea at night and drink a cup in the morning before getting out of bed.

Murray Grossan, MD, otolaryngologist and head and neck surgeon, Cedars-Sinai Medical Center, Los Angeles. *www.ent-consult.com.*

How to Protect Against Killer Food Allergies

Steve L. Taylor, PhD, professor of food science and co-director, Food Allergy Research and Resource Program, University of Nebraska, Lincoln.

Many people who have food allergies experience mild symptoms, such as a rash, runny nose or itchy eyes, when they eat small amounts of a problem food. But they may still be at risk for a potentially deadly reaction.

In the US, food allergies cause up to 30,000 emergency room visits and 200 deaths annually due to *anaphylaxis*, an acute reaction that can cause respiratory distress and/or a heart *arrhythmia* (irregular heartbeat).

Recent development: The Food Allergen Labeling and Consumer Protection Act, which went into effect in January 2006, requires food manufacturers to list eight major allergens on their food labels to help people who have food allergies identify and avoid problem foods.

IS IT REALLY AN ALLERGY?

Not all reactions to food are due to allergies. Tens of millions of Americans have a food *intolerance*, such as a sensitivity to the lactose in milk. The most common symptom of a lactose intolerance is gastrointestinal discomfort, including diarrhea, cramping and flatulence.

Food allergies affect approximately 11 to 12 million Americans. When you have a food allergy, the immune system mistakenly identifies as harmful the various proteins—or even a single kind of protein—within one or more foods. This triggers a cascade of events that causes immune cells to respond to the "threat" by releasing large amounts of histamine and other chemicals that produce the allergic symptoms.

The most common food allergen is shellfish. Up to 2% of Americans are allergic to shrimp and/or other shellfish, such as lobster, crab and crayfish. This type of allergy is often ignored—primarily because most people tend to eat shellfish far less often than other allergenic foods, such as eggs, peanuts and fish.

TESTING FOR ALLERGIES

A food allergy usually can be diagnosed by taking a thorough medical history. *The doctor will want to know...*

•**When do symptoms occur?** Food allergies typically cause symptoms within a few minutes to several hours after exposure. Symptoms include stomach cramping, hives, lip swelling, runny nose, congestion and asthma. If you have a food intolerance, symptoms may not occur until the next day.

•**How much did you eat?** *Any* exposure can trigger symptoms in people who are allergic to certain foods. For some patients, 1 milligram (mg) —an amount that's almost impossible to see— will provoke an allergic response. A reaction can even be triggered by kissing (see article on page 37) or sharing utensils with someone who has eaten a substance to which you are allergic. A skin reaction can occur from touching the substance.

Unlike an allergy, if you have a food intolerance, symptoms are usually linked to the amount consumed. Someone who is sensitive to milk, for example, can often drink a small amount without having a reaction.

Two tests can identify most food allergies. *They are...*

•**Skin prick.** Extracts of suspected foods are pricked into the skin using a needle. The appearance of a rash within a few hours—or even a few minutes—indicates a food allergy.

Caution: The skin-prick test isn't advisable for patients who have severe allergies. The tiny amounts of food used in the test could trigger a life-threatening reaction.

•**Radioallergosorbent test (RAST).** This blood test detects antibodies to specific food proteins. The test occasionally produces false positives—indicating an allergy where none is present. It is often combined with the skin-prick test for more accurate results.

TREATMENT

People who have a history of serious food reactions *must* carry an EpiPen. Available by prescription, an EpiPen is a self-injector that delivers a dose of *epinephrine*, which stimulates the heart and respiration and helps counteract deadly anaphylaxis.

Important: Use the EpiPen immediately if you experience difficulty breathing or throat constriction. Even if you take the shot promptly, get to an emergency room as soon as possible for follow-up treatments.

Also helpful: Take an antihistamine, such as Benadryl, according to label instructions. It can lessen the severity of symptoms while you get to an emergency room.

New development: Omalizumab (Xolair), a medication currently used for asthma, appears to significantly blunt reactions in food-allergy patients who receive a monthly injection of the drug. In an early study, patients who reacted to trace amounts of peanuts were able to eat eight to 10 nuts without experiencing problems. Further studies must be completed to determine whether the US Food and Drug Administration (FDA) deems it an effective—and safe—therapy for food allergies.

AVOIDING PROBLEM FOODS

Because there isn't a cure for food allergies —and even trace amounts of a protein can trigger reactions—strict avoidance of the problem food is the best defense...

•**Always read food labels**—even if you've safely eaten that product in the past. Manufacturers frequently change or add ingredients.

•**Ask about any "hidden" ingredients in medications.** Some prescription and over-the-counter (OTC) drugs, as well as vitamins and supplements, may contain milk proteins or other common food allergens. This information should be on the label, but check with your doctor or pharmacist before taking any medication or supplement.

●**Talk to the chef or restaurant manager** when eating out. The waiter or waitress doesn't always have accurate information about food ingredients and preparation. Ask to speak to the chef or manager instead and tell him/her what you're allergic to. Explain that any contact with the offending food can be *life-threatening*.

If you're allergic to shellfish, for example, tell the chef or manager that you can't eat a hamburger that was cooked on the same grill that was used to cook shrimp.

Other hidden sources of food allergens: Cooking oils that are used to cook different foods…knives and cutting boards that aren't washed between uses.

●**Wear a medical alert bracelet/necklace.** Anaphylaxis can cause a loss of consciousness within minutes. A medical alert bracelet/necklace lets medical personnel know that you require urgent treatment for your allergy.

■ ■ ■ ■

Treat Food Allergies with Bacteria!

Food allergies may soon be treated using the bacteria *Listeria*. Animal studies have shown that allergies to peanuts, milk and wheat improved 20-fold when subjects were given a shot of the offending food combined with heat-killed Listeria. Human trials are being planned.

Dale T. Umetsu, MD, PhD, professor of pediatrics, Children's Hospital Boston.

Kissing and Peanuts Can Be Deadly Combo

Scott Sicherer, MD, associate professor of pediatrics, Mount Sinai School of Medicine, New York City.
American Academy of Allergy, Asthma & Immunology annual meeting, Miami.

People who are allergic to peanuts might be taking a big risk if they kiss someone who has just eaten a peanut product—even if that person has brushed his or her teeth, according to research by the American Academy of Allergy, Asthma & Immunology.

STUDY: PEANUTS AND KISSING

For this study, researchers wanted to determine how much peanut allergen lingered in saliva after eating a meal, and after brushing teeth.

The 10 people in the study ate two tablespoons of peanut butter in a sandwich, and their saliva was then collected and tested. It was tested again after they cleaned their teeth.

The peanut allergen remained in the saliva immediately after the meal, and even after teeth were cleaned or rinsed. One hour after eating, the allergen level in six of the seven subjects was undetectable.

The study authors suggest that people wait several hours after eating an allergen before kissing anyone.

The possibility of having a severe allergic reaction after kissing someone who has eaten peanuts was highlighted in the case of a 15-year-old Quebec girl who died after kissing her boyfriend. However, the coroner later determined that the cause of death was a severe asthma attack, and not a peanut-contaminated kiss.

STUDY: TEENAGERS AND ALLERGIES

Another study found that teens took risks with their food allergies.

"Teenagers are at high risk of dying from food anaphylaxis, and we wanted to see why," says study senior author Dr. Scott Sicherer, an associate professor of pediatrics at Mount Sinai School of Medicine in New York City. "Is it because they think they are invincible or because they are forgetful?"

Researchers asked 174 participants, ages 13 to 21, to fill out questionnaires. In total, 75% of the individuals had a peanut allergy or two or more allergies; 82% had had *anaphylaxis*, a severe allergic reaction that can cause death; and 52% had had more than three such reactions during their lifetime.

Overall, 74% of respondents said they always carry *epinephrine*, the standard antidote for anaphylaxis. But the percentage varied greatly depending on what activity they were participating in—94% said they carried epinephrine when traveling, but only 43% said they carried it when playing sports.

In addition, 75% said they always read food labels. However, 42% admitted they would eat a food that had a label indicating that it "may contain" an allergen.

Teenagers are at high risk of dying from anaphylaxis. Is it because they think they are invincible or because they are forgetful?

Scott Sicherer, MD

Only 60% of teens told friends about their food allergy. And although 68% felt that educating their friends would make life easier, most did not want to undertake it themselves.

MORE STUDIES ON ALLERGIES

Additional research found that adults who had a severe allergic reaction to food and were prescribed *epinephrine auto injectors* (EAIs) were not properly trained in using the device and had not received adequate follow-up from a healthcare professional.

Other researchers found no evidence indicating that mothers who ate peanuts while pregnant or breast-feeding increased the risk of their children developing a peanut allergy.

info Learn more about teens and food allergies from the Food Allergy and Anaphylaxis Network at *www.fanteen.org.*

■ ■ ■ ■

Some Children May Outgrow Their Nut Allergy

Approximately 9% of children who have tree nut allergies will outgrow them, a new study suggests. Children who are allergic to peanuts (a ground nut) have a 20% chance of outgrowing their allergy.

Previously, it was believed that allergies to tree nuts—which include cashews, almonds, walnuts, hazelnuts, macadamia nuts, pecans, pistachios and pine nuts—lasted a lifetime. In their study of 278 people ranging from three to 21 years of age, researchers at Johns Hopkins University School of Medicine in Baltimore also found that even some children who have had a previous, especially severe allergic reaction to tree nuts can outgrow their allergy. However, children who are allergic to multiple types of tree nuts are unlikely to outgrow their allergy, the research team says.

Based on their results, the study authors recommend that children who have tree nut allergies be reevaluated periodically by an allergist/immunologist.

info The Nemours Foundation has more information about nut and peanut allergies at *http://kidshealth.org/kid.* Click on "Staying Healthy," and scroll down to "Nut and Peanut Allergy" under the "Fabulous Food" section.

American Academy of Allergy, Asthma & Immunology.

Astounding! 70% Have 14k Mystery Rash

Mayo Clinic news release.

Gold is among the leading causes of a skin condition called *allergic contact dermatitis.* According to experts at the Mayo Clinic, allergic contact dermatitis is a skin inflammation that is characterized by swollen, reddened and itchy skin. It is caused by direct contact with an allergen.

TESTING

The Mayo team analyzed results from contact dermatitis testing that was conducted on 3,854 patients. Each patient was tested using an average of 69 allergens. Of the patients studied, 69% had at least one positive reaction and 50% had two or more positive reactions.

The top 10 contact dermatitis allergens were…

•**Nickel,** frequently used in jewelry and clasps or buttons on clothing.

•**Gold,** commonly used in jewelry.

•**Balsam of Peru,** a fragrance derived from a tree resin. It is used in perfumes as well as in skin lotions.

•**Thimerosal,** a mercury compound used in vaccines and local antiseptics.

•**Neomycin sulfate,** a topical antibiotic, common in first-aid creams and ointments. It also can be found in cosmetics, deodorants, soap and pet food.

•**Fragrance mix,** a group of the eight most common fragrance allergens that are found in foods, cosmetic products, insecticides, antiseptics, soaps, perfumes and dental products.

•**Formaldehyde,** a preservative that is used in paints, medications, fabric finishes, paper products, household cleaners and cosmetics.

•**Cobalt chloride,** a metal that is found in medical products, hair dye, antiperspirant and metal-plated objects, such as snaps, buttons and tools. Also found in cobalt blue pigment.

•**Bacitracin,** a topical antibiotic.

•**Quaternium 15,** a preservative that can be found in cosmetic products, such as self-tanners, shampoo, nail polish and sunscreen, as well as in industrial products, such as polishes, paints and waxes.

The study also confirmed that patch testing using a standard contact dermatitis series of substances is useful for identifying common contact allergens.

Avoiding allergens is the chief treatment for contact dermatitis. In some cases, corticosteroid creams can be used to treat rashes caused by contact dermatitis.

info The American Academy of Dermatology has more information about allergic contact dermatitis at *www.aad.org.*

▪ ▪ ▪ ▪

Most Americans Test Positive For Allergens

The most common allergen is dust mites—27% of those tested responded positively to this allergen. Reacting to an allergen doesn't necessarily mean that you will develop allergies, but there is a strong correlation between the two.

Samuel Arbes, DDS, PhD, epidemiologist, National Institutes of Environmental Health Sciences.

3

Breast Cancer Treatments

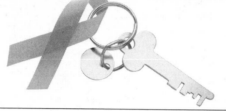

Benign Breast Lesions May Harbor Cancers

Breast lesions that are often deemed to be benign following a needle biopsy can still harbor adjacent cancers and should be removed anyway, United States researchers recommend.

"Our study shows that all papillary lesions of the breast should be surgically excised to avoid missing a cancer," says the lead author of the study, Dr. Cecilia L. Mercado, an assistant professor of radiology at New York University Medical Center.

Papillary lesions, which account for 1% to 3% of all lesions sampled by core needle biopsies, are benign growths in the duct of the breast. Current treatment for these lesions includes radiographic follow-up and surgical removal, depending on each doctor's recommendation.

While these lesions may be diagnosed as benign, they can harbor adjacent *atypical ductal*

hyperplasia (ADH) and *ductal carcinoma in situ* (DCIS)—cancerous cells that are confined to the lining of the milk ducts. Left untreated, both of these conditions put a woman at an increased risk for cancer in the future.

THE STUDY

For this study, the researchers analyzed the imaging and outcomes of 42 patients who had been diagnosed with benign papillary lesions after core needle biopsy. Of the 43 biopsies that were performed, 36 (84%) of the lesions were surgically removed and seven (16%) received long-term imaging follow-up.

As a result of surgical removal of the lesion and laboratory follow-up, the diagnoses of nine of the 42 patients (21.4%) were changed to ADH or DCIS. That percentage is much higher than what has been reported in previous research.

"This is one of the largest series and shows statistically significant findings. The results of our study revealed a considerable upgrade rate to either ADH or DCIS," Mercado says. "Therefore, all benign papillary lesions of the breast

Radiological Society of North America news release.

should be surgically excised, since a considerable number of atypical lesions and malignant lesions could be missed."

∎ ∎ ∎ ∎

Breast Asymmetry Linked to Cancer Risk

Researchers examined the mammograms of 252 women who later developed breast cancer and 252 women of the same age who did not develop the disease.

Result: The women who developed breast cancer had higher breast volume asymmetry (the difference in volume between the left and right breasts) than other women.

Theory: Estrogen, which has been linked to breast cancer, may also play a role in breast asymmetry.

Diane Scutt, PhD, director of research, School of Health Sciences, University of Liverpool, England.

Digital Test that's More Accurate than Mammogram For Most Women

Etta D. Pisano, MD, professor of radiology and biomedical engineering, University of North Carolina School of Medicine, Chapel Hill.

Rowan T. Chlebowski, MD, medical oncologist, Los Angeles BioMedical Research Institute, Torrance, CA.

Robert A. Smith, PhD, director, cancer screening, American Cancer Society.

The New England Journal of Medicine.

American College of Radiology Imaging Network.

Compared with standard mammograms, which are recorded on film, computer-based digital mammograms are more accurate for more than half of the women who get breast cancer screenings, a large study has discovered.

Women who have dense breast tissue, those who are younger than age 50 and those who are premenopausal would benefit from digital mammograms, the researchers say.

THE STUDY

In the study, lead author Dr. Etta D. Pisano, a professor of radiology and biomedical engineer-

ing at the University of North Carolina School of Medicine, and her colleagues evaluated data on 42,760 asymptomatic women who were screened for breast cancer using both digital and film mammography.

"Overall, film and digital mammography were equally accurate," Pisano says. "But for women with dense breasts, women under age 50 and women who were pre- and perimenopausal, digital was significantly better. The kinds of cancer that the digital [mammography] found and film missed were important cancers—the kind that kill women," she notes.

"For the 65% of women who had improved accuracy, they should get that kind of mammography," Pisano says. "But for other women, there is no benefit of digital over film, and it's more expensive."

THE TREND TOWARD DIGITAL

However, Pisano adds that although digital mammography makes up only approximately 8% of the market today, it will eventually replace film mammography. "There is a trend toward digital, mainly for the other advantages that it offers," she says. These advantages include the ease of storing and retrieving digital images, and the ability to make these images part of a patient's electronic medical record.

The cancer that the digital mammography found and film missed were the kind that kill women.

Etta D. Pisano, MD

Dr. Rowan T. Chlebowski, a medical oncologist at Los Angeles BioMedical Research Institute, says, "Even without a clinical benefit, digital would replace film. With the current mandate for electronic medical records, you are going to have a hard time getting a film mammogram into an electronic medical record.

"This study makes it more reasonable to go for the investment now, because you get an immediate clinical payoff," he adds.

DON'T WAIT

All the experts agree that women need to get screened for breast cancer, and not wait for digital screening if it is not available in their area.

"The finding that digital mammography is more accurate than film mammography in women under age 50 and women with medium and high breast density is an important finding that should lead to improvements in screening programs," says Robert A. Smith, director of cancer screening for the American Cancer Society.

However, although the availability of digital mammography screening is increasing, it is still limited, and it is unclear how soon—or even whether—it will entirely replace film mammography, he adds.

"The important thing is that women receive mammograms on a regular basis, regardless of which technology they use," Smith says.

"Younger women and women with denser breasts should not forego their regular mammograms if digital mammography is not available. While this study showed an advantage with digital imaging in these groups, it should be remembered that traditional film mammography also is effective," Smith adds.

Pisano agrees. "It is important that women get screened when they are supposed to be screened and not wait to get a digital [mammography]. If there is film available, it's better than nothing."

A Bad Sign: Breast Cancer Survivors Fail To Get Mammograms

Chyke A. Doubeni, MD, assistant professor of family medicine and community health, University of Massachusetts Medical School, Worcester.

Cheryl Perkins, MD, senior clinical advisor, Susan G. Komen Breast Cancer Foundation.

Cancer.

Breast cancer survivors usually get a mammogram immediately after their diagnosis and treatment, but become lax about later screenings, a recent study has found. Although they have a high risk of developing another malignancy, only one in three breast cancer survivors gets mammograms as recommended during the five years after their diagnosis, researchers report.

THE STUDY

When researchers reviewed mammography use in 797 women older than age 55 who had been treated for breast cancer, they found that in the first year after treatment, 80% of the women had gotten a mammogram. But only 63% of the women had gotten a mammogram in the fifth year after treatment began. Over the five-year study period, only one in three—33%—had gotten a mammogram every year, as recommended.

Overall, healthy women are not as faithful to mammograms as health-care professionals would like. One study found that while three-quarters of women older than 40 say they regularly have a mammogram, less than two-thirds actually do.

But, Dr. Chyke A. Doubeni, the study's lead author and an assistant professor of family medicine and community health at the University of Massachusetts Medical School in Worcester, thought that breast cancer survivors might be different.

"Some studies indicate that if you have a history of cancer, your awareness of your risk is much higher. So we would expect that most breast cancer survivors would get regular mammograms," he says.

Women who have had breast cancer have approximately three times the risk of getting cancer in the opposite breast, compared with women who have not had breast cancer, according to Doubeni.

INSURANCE IS NOT THE ONLY PROBLEM

Doubeni says his study uncovered another troubling finding—all of the women studied had access to health insurance. "Whether or not someone has insurance is an important factor in the use of mammograms," he says. "In this case, all the people we studied had health insurance."

Exactly why many of the women stopped getting regular mammograms was beyond the scope of the study, but Doubeni and other experts are making some educated guesses.

Over time, he says, many women, including breast cancer survivors, tend to get nonchalant about mammograms, perhaps because they forget to schedule the exam.

Survivors may not get regular mammograms due to miscommunication between a woman's oncologist and her internist or family practice doctor, with one doctor thinking the other one is reminding her to get this screening.

"At least one study...shows that the care of cancer survivors is really fragmented," Doubeni says, with several doctors involved but often no one with complete oversight.

Denial could also play a role, with the cancer survivors not wanting to think about the possibility of the disease recurring.

The findings are not a surprise to Dr. Cheryl Perkins, senior clinical advisor for the Susan G. Komen Breast Cancer Foundation in Dallas, and a breast cancer survivor herself. "We hear it a lot about mammography in general," she says, referring to women's tendency to not get regular mammograms.

Perkins speculates that "the longer you are cancer-free, the more 'normal' you feel, and then [you] begin to behave more like the general population."

Perkins believes that the fear of a recurrence keeps breast cancer survivors from getting mammograms. But she would tell them, "The earlier you detect anything that might recur, the better your chances to have a successful treatment the next time around."

info To get more information about mammograms, visit the American College of Radiology Web site at *www.radiologyinfo.org/content/mammogram.htm*.

Good News from a Harvard Doctor Who Survived the Disease

Carolyn M. Kaelin, MD, MPH, FACS, director of the Comprehensive Breast Health Center at Brigham and Women's Hospital, surgical oncologist at Dana Farber Cancer Institute, and assistant professor of surgery at Harvard Medical School, all in Boston. In 2003, Dr. Kaelin discovered she had breast cancer. She has since had three lumpectomies, a mastectomy, chemotherapy and reconstructive surgery. She is author of *Living Through Breast Cancer*. McGraw-Hill.

Last year, more than 275,000 American women were diagnosed with breast cancer. While the incidence of breast cancer has increased in the last decade, the death rate from the disease has declined. The vast majority of women who have breast cancer go on to lead full, normal lives.

Several recent studies highlight the latest breakthroughs in breast cancer treatment and prevention...

***New finding:* Standard treatments extend life even longer.** Two standard medical treatments for breast cancer are chemotherapy (medicines that kill cancer cells) and hormonal therapy (medicines that stop *estrogen* from stimulating cancer cells to reproduce). Scientists have known that these treatments can improve the survival rates of breast cancer patients at the five- and 10-year marks, but they didn't know whether the treatments could extend the life of a breast cancer survivor by more than that.

A recent study published in *The Lancet* found that women who have nonmetastatic breast cancer (the disease has not spread to other parts of the body) who receive chemotherapy and/or hormonal therapy after surgery outlive women who don't—beyond the 10-year mark. After 15 years, the survival rate for women who had chemotherapy and *tamoxifen*, an antiestrogen drug, was 85.3% for women ages 50 to 69 and 88.4% for those younger than age 50, versus a 75% survival rate for women who did not have chemotherapy or hormonal therapy.

***New finding:* Herceptin reduces recurrence.** Up to 20% of women who have breast cancer have cells that contain an overabundance of the growth-related protein *HER2*. This substance makes their tumors particularly fast-growing and deadly. The drug *herceptin* has been developed to block HER2, slowing the duplication of cancer cells. Previous studies have shown that herceptin improves survival rates in HER2-positive women who have early-stage breast cancer (confined to the breast and adjacent lymph nodes) and metastatic breast cancer.

A study reported at a recent American Society of Clinical Oncology meeting confirms the benefits of herceptin. HER2-positive women who were given herceptin after surgery, along with standard chemotherapy, had a 52% lower rate of tumor recurrence than women who weren't given the drug. Women who have invasive breast cancer routinely have tumor cells tested for HER2.

***New finding:* Exercise fights breast cancer.** Previous research showed that physical activity—a 30-minute walk, five days a week—can help prevent breast cancer, cutting risk by 20%. A study published in *The Journal of the American Medical Association* shows that exercise helps prevent a recurrence. Researchers at Harvard Medical School looked at 3,000 women who had been diagnosed with breast cancer, matching their levels of physical activity against recurrence over 10 years. They found that women who walked three to five hours a week at a moderate pace of two to three miles an hour cut their risk of recurrence in half.

They also found that exercise improved the overall chance of survival. After 10 years, 92% of the women who walked three to five hours per week were alive, versus 86% of those who walked less than one hour per week.

Exercise may cut the risk of cancer in many different ways, including decreasing levels of circulating estrogen, a cancer-promoting hormone, and decreasing *leptin*, a molecule associated with cellular proliferation in breast tissue.

Related finding: Exercise after chemotherapy boosts the activity of infection-fighting *T cells*, perhaps helping the immune system recover from the damage caused by the powerful anticancer drugs, according to researchers at Penn State University. For those who feel particularly fatigued, walking for five minutes several times a day is an option.

***New finding:* A low-fat diet may help.** In another study reported at the annual meeting of the American Society of Clinical Oncology, scientists at the University of California at Los Angeles followed more than 2,000 postmenopausal women diagnosed with breast cancer who were treated with surgery, hormonal therapy and, in some cases, chemotherapy. The women went on one of two low-fat diets—one diet had about 30% of calories from fat, the other, 20%. (The typical American diet is 40% to 45% of calories from fat.) Over five years, the women consuming the lower level of dietary fat had a significantly lower level of recurrence—9.8%, compared with 12.4% for the group consuming more fat.

This study, which was widely reported in the media, is provocative but not definitive. There are what scientists call "confounding factors" in the data—factors other than a low-fat diet that may account for the results. The most important of these is that the women on the lowest-fat diet lost an average of four pounds. That is very unusual for women being treated for breast cancer—they usually gain five to 30 pounds. Did the low-fat diet prevent recurrence—or did the weight loss? Also, because the women ate less fat, they may have been eating more fruits and vegetables, which contain anticancer nutrients.

What it means: Women who have been treated for breast cancer do not necessarily need a low-fat diet, but they should be thoughtful about what they eat and maintain a healthy weight.

Study Supports Surgery for Metastatic Breast Cancer

Elisabetta Rapiti, MD, MPH, senior researcher, Geneva Cancer Registry, University of Geneva, Switzerland.
Lori J. Goldstein, MD, director, breast evaluation center, and leader, breast cancer research program, Fox Chase Cancer Center, Philadelphia.
Journal of Clinical Oncology.

Typically, women who are diagnosed with advanced breast cancer that has *metastasized* (spread to other parts of the body) are given chemotherapy or hormone treatment rather than surgery. Many doctors believe that surgery offers no survival advantage for these patients, and may even worsen outcomes. But a recent Swiss study refutes that belief.

THE STUDY

In the study, researchers used the Geneva Cancer Registry to analyze detailed information on 5,000 cases of invasive breast cancer that had been diagnosed since 1970. Of the 300 women who had metastatic disease, more than half (58%) did not have surgery for their primary breast cancer. The remaining 42% had either a mastectomy or some type of lesser surgery to remove the tumor.

The researchers found that the women who underwent surgery and had negative surgical margins—indicating that the surgeon had removed all of the cancer—were 40% more likely to be alive five years after their diagnosis than the women who did not have surgery.

This means that 27% of the women who had surgery and had negative margins were likely to still be alive five years after the operation.

In comparison, 16% of the women who had surgery but had positive margins were still alive five years later; and 12% of those who did not have surgery had a five-year survival rate.

The women whose cancer had spread to the bone (rather than the brain or the liver—other common sites) and had surgery were even more likely—80% more likely—to be alive five years later than those who did not have surgery.

SURPRISING FINDINGS

"This is the first study to find such a marked improvement in survival at five years in women with metastatic breast cancer who have had surgical removal of the primary tumor," says study author Dr. Elisabetta Rapiti, senior researcher at the Geneva Cancer Registry at the University of Geneva. Another study found similar effects, but only followed-up the women for three years.

"These findings will be a surprise for many clinicians, as almost all national and international guidelines on the treatment of metastatic breast cancer either do not include surgery of the primary tumor, or even recommend against it," says Rapiti.

"Many clinicians, in fact, believe that in such [metastatic breast cancer] cases, surgery of the primary tumor can accelerate the progression of the metastases," she says.

For women, "This research already certainly reaffirms that [surgery] is not associated with a more rapid progression of the metastases or worse outcome," Rapiti adds.

MORE STUDIES NEEDED

Dr. Lori J. Goldstein, director of the breast evaluation center and leader of the breast cancer research program at Fox Chase Cancer Center in Philadelphia, doesn't think this retrospective study is enough to change standard treatment

"*Retrospective* studies are very useful in generating hypotheses," she says. However, what's needed are *prospective* studies, such as a randomized, controlled clinical trial, in which some women would be assigned to a surgery group

and others to a treatment group, and then the results would be compared over time.

Rapiti agrees, saying that larger studies are needed, comparing those who have surgery with those who do not.

"It would be naive to assume surgery will benefit all women with metastatic disease," Goldstein says.

Radiation Improves Breast Cancer Survival Rates

Sarah Darby, PhD, professor of medical statistics, Clinical Trial Service Unit, University of Oxford, England.
B. Jay Brooks, Jr., MD, chairman, hematology/oncology, Ochsner Clinic Foundation, Baton Rouge, LA.
The Lancet.

Women who receive radiation after a lumpectomy for breast cancer have better long-term survival odds than those who forego this treatment, a British study has found.

THE STUDY

The study revisited information on 42,000 women who had participated in 78 randomized trials around the world comparing different breast cancer treatments. The analysis was conducted by the Early Breast Cancer Trialists' Collaborative Group.

The risk of having a local recurrence was 7% for women who had radiation versus 26% for women who did not. All of the women had first had breast-conserving surgery.

At the 15-year mark, 30.5% of the women who had had radiation died versus 35.9% of the women who had not undergone radiation.

Radiation also reduced the risk of a local recurrence and improved the long-term survival for women whose cancer had spread to the lymph nodes in the armpit. The five-year risk of a local recurrence after mastectomy and surgery to the armpit was 6% for the women who had radiation versus 23% for those who did not. The 15-year death rate was 54.7% for those who had radiation and 60.1% for those who did not.

DEFINITIVE ANSWERS

Lumpectomy, or breast-conserving surgery, removes the tumor plus a margin of normal tissue around it, and can be performed if the cancer has not spread widely. Unfortunately, the procedure sometimes leaves some rogue cancer cells behind, which can result in a recurrence. Therefore, women who have the option of a lumpectomy often choose a mastectomy (removal of the entire breast) out of fear of such a recurrence—although the odds of survival are the same between the two procedures.

It is now clear that radiotherapy saves lives in women…even if they have already had a mastectomy.

Sarah Darby, PhD

Previous research had shown that administering radiation after surgery reduces the risk of a local recurrence. However, it had been unclear if longer term, 15-year survival rates were affected by radiation treatments soon after surgery.

For some women, the current research may offer some clarity. "The findings fit in well with previous research, and provide definite answers where previously there was uncertainty," explains study coauthor Sarah Darby, a professor of medical statistics at the University of Oxford's Clinical Trial Service Unit in the United Kingdom.

"It is now clear that radiotherapy saves lives in women who have had breast-conserving surgery and in women whose cancer has substantial spread to the armpit, even if they have already had a mastectomy," Darby says.

According to the authors, it probably makes little sense to offer radiation to women who have already been cancer-free for several years. It might be worth considering, however, in women who had lumpectomy for breast cancer or mastectomy for cancer that had spread to the lymph nodes within the past year or so.

TREATMENT

"It's important to treat breast cancer thoroughly from the beginning," notes Dr. B. Jay Brooks, Jr., who is chairman of hematology/oncology at the Ochsner Clinic Foundation in Baton Rouge, Louisiana. "If not, it increases the risk of local failure and, if that happens, it puts a woman at high risk of that cancer becoming metastatic."

Brooks stresses that radiation is not the only advance for women who have breast cancer. Hormone therapy, such as tamoxifen and aro-

matase inhibitors, are also radically decreasing risk, he says.

info To learn more about radiation after lumpectomy, visit the American Cancer Society Web site at *www.cancer.org*.

Drug that Blocks More Breast Cancer Recurrences

Heikki Joensuu, MD, physician, Helsinki University Central Hospital, Helsinki, Finland.
Mark Pegram, MD, director, women's cancer program, Jonsson Comprehensive Cancer Center, David Geffen School of Medicine, University of California at Los Angeles.
The New England Journal of Medicine.

A new head-to-head study has found that the chemotherapy drug *docetaxel* (Taxotere) is more effective than *vinorelbine* (Navelbine) in helping extend patient survival after breast cancer surgery. The Finnish study also found that patients who received infusions of *trastuzumab* (Herceptin) were less likely to get recurrences than those who received a placebo.

THE STUDY

For this study, Dr. Heikki Joensuu, a physician at Helsinki University Central Hospital, and his colleagues randomly assigned more than 1,000 women who had breast cancer to receive three cycles of either docetaxel or vinorelbine, followed by three cycles of other cancer drugs. They wanted to determine which regimen was best for recurrence-free survival.

"There were 42% fewer breast cancer recurrences during the first three years of follow-up among women treated with docetaxel as compared to those who received vinorelbine," says Joensuu. However, docetaxel was associated with more adverse side effects, such as allergic reactions, swelling and fever.

In another part of the study, a subgroup of 232 women who had more aggressive cancers were assigned either to receive nine weeks of Herceptin infusions or a placebo.

The women who got Herceptin experienced 58% fewer cancer recurrences during the three-year follow-up than those who did not get the drug, the researchers report.

FINDING THE OPTIMAL DURATION

According to Joensuu, this study supports previous research. "A few prior studies have shown that administration of adjuvant [Herceptin] for one year reduces the rate of breast cancer recurrence by approximately 50%" in women who have aggressive cancers, he says.

However, in this study the Herceptin was administered for only nine weeks, which could explain why it was not linked to an increased risk of cardiac failure, as it was in previous research.

"We don't know the optimal duration of [Herceptin]—is nine weeks as good as one year?" asks Dr. Mark Pegram, director of the women's cancer program at the Jonsson Comprehensive Cancer Center, part of the David Geffen School of Medicine at the University of California at Los Angeles.

If the nine-week regimen turns out to be ideal, Pegram says, "it could be very good news for patients," sparing them time and much expense.

Death rates from breast cancer have decreased in recent years, partly because of postoperative chemotherapy. Experts are continually testing new regimens to determine which drugs best reduce the risk of recurrence.

New Breast Cancer Drug Safer than Tamoxifen

Leslie Ford, MD, associate director for clinical research, Division of Cancer Prevention, National Cancer Institute.

B. Jay Brooks, Jr., MD, chairman, hematology/oncology, Ochsner Clinic Foundation, Baton Rouge, LA.

Lawrence Wickerham, MD, associate chairman, National Surgical and Adjuvant Breast and Bowel Project and protocol officer, Study of Tamoxifen and Raloxifene (STAR).

Len Lichtenfeld, MD, deputy chief medical officer, American Cancer Society.

Victor Vogel, MD, MHS, FACP, protocol chairman, Study of Tamoxifen and Raloxifene (STAR).

The osteoporosis drug *raloxifene* (Evista) is equivalent to tamoxifen in its ability to reduce breast cancer risk in high-risk postmenopausal women, and has fewer side effects, according to a recent study.

THE STUDY

The clinical trial, called the Study of Tamoxifen and Raloxifene (STAR), was initiated in 1999 and involves almost 20,000 women, making it one of the largest breast-cancer prevention trials ever conducted.

The participants, all of whom were postmenopausal and at a heightened risk for breast cancer, were randomly assigned to receive either 60 milligrams (mg) of raloxifene or 20 mg of tamoxifen daily for approximately four years.

> *We now have two medicines that can be given to high-risk women to decrease their chances of developing breast cancer.*
>
> B. Jay Brooks, Jr., MD

Both drugs reduced the risk of developing invasive breast cancer by approximately 50%, the researchers report. However, the women taking raloxifene had 36% fewer uterine cancers and 29% fewer blood clots than the women taking tamoxifen. The risks of stroke, heart attack and bone fracture were the same in each group. In addition, the study found that, unlike tamoxifen, raloxifene did not increase the risk of developing cataracts.

GOOD NEWS

"This is good news for women," says Dr. Leslie Ford, associate director for clinical research in the Division of Cancer Prevention at the National Cancer Institute. "We think that this gives women a real choice for addressing two of the leading causes of morbidity and mortality as they age—breast cancer and fractures."

"We now have two medicines that can be given to high-risk women to decrease their chances of developing breast cancer," explains Dr. B. Jay Brooks, Jr., chairman of hematology/oncology at the Ochsner Clinic Foundation in Baton Rouge, Louisiana. The bottom line, he says, is to make sure women understand that there are options for reducing breast cancer risk.

"We can predict which women are at a high risk for developing the disease and we can do something about that. Not enough women and physicians understand that," Brooks adds.

TAMOXIFEN VS. RALOXIFENE: NO CLEAR ANSWER

The US Food and Drug Administration (FDA) approved tamoxifen in 1998 to reduce the odds of high-risk women getting breast cancer. "This was a major step in our battle against breast cancer. However, even with cutting breast cancer risk in half, [tamoxifen] got little use because of the rare but serious side effects that we knew occurred," Ford says.

"Evista is as good as tamoxifen in preventing invasive breast cancer and it has fewer side effects. I think we'll see a shift over to the use of Evista," Brooks says.

Dr. Lawrence Wickerham, associate chairman of the National Surgical and Adjuvant Breast and Bowel Project and STAR protocol officer, concurs. "We believe that raloxifene is the winner of this trial," he says.

However, despite these positive results, raloxifene was not effective against *in situ* (noninvasive) breast cancers. Tamoxifen had previously been shown to reduce the incidence of these types of breast cancers by half.

"There's an important caveat," says Dr. Len Lichtenfeld, deputy chief medical officer of the American Cancer Society. "Taking away the increased risk of uterine cancer and blood clots from tamoxifen comes at a price. The outcome of the study is not as clear-cut as we might have hoped for," he adds.

In addition, tamoxifen is the only drug currently approved for breast cancer risk-reduction in premenopausal women—and it will probably stay that way, according to Dr. Victor Vogel, STAR protocol chairman. "We anticipate that if [Eli] Lilly gets approval [for raloxifene], the indication will only be for postmenopausal women, so tamoxifen will remain the drug of choice for reducing risk in premenopausal women," he says.

Trial participants who were taking raloxifene will continue to receive the drug until they have completed five years of treatment. Women in the trial who were taking tamoxifen can continue or can choose to get raloxifene instead.

Raloxifene is currently approved only to prevent or treat osteoporosis. An estimated 500,000 postmenopausal American women are taking the drug for this use.

info For more information on the STAR trial, visit the National Cancer Institute at *www.cancer.gov/star.*

Preventive Mastectomy Brings Women Relief

Ann Geiger, PhD, associate professor of public health sciences, Wake Forest University Baptist Medical Center School of Medicine, Winston-Salem, NC.
Julia Smith, MD, PhD, director, Breast Cancer Screening and Prevention Program, New York University (NYU) Cancer Institute, and director, Lynne Cohen Breast Cancer Preventive Care Program, NYU Cancer Institute and Bellevue Hospital, New York City.
Journal of Clinical Oncology.

Most breast cancer patients who choose to have their unaffected breast removed along with the diseased one say they don't regret their decision, a recent study has found. Furthermore, their quality of life equals that of women who chose not to have a preventive mastectomy, according to researchers. The women who chose the preventive mastectomy were also found to be a little less concerned about the cancer recurring.

THE STUDY

A research team surveyed 580 women who had been diagnosed with breast cancer between 1979 and 1999. In total, 519 underwent a preventive mastectomy on the unaffected breast.

Women who have preventive mastectomy don't appear to suffer any ill psychological effects.

Ann Geiger, PhD

The women answered questions about their quality of life, body image, sexual satisfaction, concern about breast cancer recurrence, depression and perception of their own health.

Of those who chose preventive mastectomy, 86.5% said they were satisfied with their decision, and 76.3% reported "high contentment" with their quality of life.

Of the 61 women who did not have a preventive mastectomy, a similar number (75.4%) reported high contentment with their quality of life.

Approximately half of the women who had the preventive mastectomy remained concerned about the possibility of a recurrence, compared with 75% of those who left the healthy breast alone. While preventive procedures reduce the risk of recurrent cancer by up to 95%, a risk always remains because it is impossible to remove all breast tissue, the researchers say.

IMPLICATIONS

"Overall, we think these are reassuring results, in that women who have preventive mastectomy don't appear to suffer any ill psychological effects compared to those who just had the breast cancer treated," says Ann Geiger, lead author of the study and an associate professor of public health sciences at Wake Forest University Baptist Medical Center School of Medicine in Winston-Salem, NC.

This latest study adds to scientists' knowledge about preventive mastectomies, an area that has garnered little research, Geiger says. "Most research has been done on bilateral preventive mastectomy—when no cancer is present," she says, but the woman is at high risk due to a strong family history of the disease.

NO SURPRISE

The study results come as no surprise to Dr. Julia Smith, director of New York University Cancer Institute's Breast Cancer Screening and Prevention Program and director of the Lynne Cohen Breast Cancer Preventive Care Program at the NYU Cancer Institute and Bellevue Hospital in New York City. "It's totally consistent with our experience with patients," she says of the survey findings.

Making the decision is not easy, she adds, whatever the woman's medical history. "These are very important decisions," Smith says, and it's crucial that women go to a center that is known for its high-risk assessment programs. "If women go to these programs, and they get their own individual risk profile assessed, then they can understand, with the help of a good medical oncologist and his or her team, what the risks and benefits of this preventive surgery are for them," she says.

The key to making this decision is asking, "Given the risks and the benefits, what will allow this woman to live her life fully?" Smith says.

info For more information on breast cancer, visit the Susan G. Komen Breast Cancer Foundation at *www.komen.org.*

Study Proves Tamoxifen Prevents and Treats Breast Cancer

Bernard Fisher, MD, founding member and director, National Surgical Adjuvant Breast and Bowel Project, Pittsburgh.

Claudine Isaacs, MD, director, Clinical Breast Cancer Program, and associate professor of medicine and oncology, Lombardi Comprehensive Cancer Center, Georgetown University, Washington, DC.
Journal of the National Cancer Institute.
Cancer Biology and Therapy.

The final results of a 13-year study confirm that *tamoxifen*, a drug long used to *treat* breast cancer, can also *prevent* the malignancy in healthy women who are at high risk for the disease.

"This study proves the principle that prevention is a legitimate kind of approach to treating breast cancer, and justifies the continuing research to find [preventive] drugs with less side effects and better risk reduction," says lead researcher Dr. Bernard Fisher, a founding member and director of the National Surgical Adjuvant Breast and Bowel Project (NSABP).

Tamoxifen is one of a class of drugs called *selective estrogen receptor modulators* (SERMs). These drugs work by attaching to the molecule in breast cancer cells that normally reacts with estrogen, stopping the cancer cells' growth and limiting its spread, according to the American Cancer Society.

THE STUDY

The NSABP study tracked the outcomes of more than 13,000 healthy women at high risk for breast cancer. Participants took either 20 milligrams (mg) of tamoxifen or a placebo every day for five years.

Researchers wanted to learn if the drug that is so effective in preventing breast cancer recurrence could also be used to prevent the disease from developing in high-risk women. The study was *double-blind*, meaning that neither the study participants nor their doctors knew who was getting the medication.

After six years, researchers found that the incidence of invasive breast cancer was nearly 50% lower among women who took tamoxifen —a result so dramatic that researchers lifted the double-blind aspect of the study to allow those women on the placebo to take tamoxifen. Approximately one-third of that group opted to take the drug.

Prevention is a legitimate approach to treating breast cancer.

Bernard Fisher, MD

After following the majority of the women for another seven years, the researchers found that the rates of invasive breast cancer continued to be much lower for the women who took tamoxifen. The rate of invasive breast cancer over the course of the study was 43% lower in the tamoxifen group than in the placebo group—there were 42.5 cases per 1,000 women in the placebo group compared with 24.8 cases per 1,000 women in the tamoxifen group.

Also significantly lower was the incidence of noninvasive cancers, such as *ductal breast cancer in situ* (DCIS), which was 37% lower among the women who took tamoxifen compared with those who took the placebo.

"This is the only proven prevention method for breast cancer," Fisher says.

BENEFITS OF THE STUDY

Dr. Claudine Isaacs, director of the Clinical Breast Cancer Program at Georgetown University's Lombardi Comprehensive Cancer Center, says this study is significant because it was placebo-controlled, had a very large group of participants and focused on prevention.

"Because it is focused on prevention, they did a very careful assessment of the side-effect profile," she says. Tamoxifen's side effects included a 32% decrease in bone fractures over seven years of follow-up, but an increase in the risk of uterine cancer, stroke, pulmonary embolism and cataracts.

Isaacs says doctors can use a well-validated risk–benefit model that includes a woman's age,

medical and family histories as well as other factors to help decide whether tamoxifen might be right for her.

"A clinician should go through the risk–benefit ratio with a patient, and if the benefits outweigh the risks, he can tell her she should consider [tamoxifen]," Isaacs says, adding that it is very much a personal choice.

RELUCTANCE

While researchers estimate that approximately 25% of all American women between 35 and 70 years of age, or 2.5 million women, are at high risk for breast cancer and could be helped by using tamoxifen, many are reluctant to take this drug to help prevent the disease.

In a study conducted at the University of California at Davis, researchers told 255 women that they were eligible for preventive tamoxifen therapy if their estimated risk for breast cancer was 1.66 or above. The estimated average five-year risk among the women in the study was 2.8.

But after an educational session explaining tamoxifen's potential risks and benefits, only 45 of the women—just 17.6%—said that they would be inclined to take the drug on a regular basis to help prevent breast tumors.

Study author Dr. Joy Melnikow, a professor of family and community medicine at UC Davis, says it seemed that the women in the study had seen friends get breast cancer and survive, and weren't as afraid of the disease as one would think. "They didn't see it as a death sentence," she says.

OTHER RESEARCH

In other recent research on tamoxifen, Swedish researchers found that breast cancer survivors who took tamoxifen for five years, rather than two, were not only at a decreased risk of developing cancer in the other breast, but were also at a lower risk of death from all causes, including heart disease.

Trials are now under way involving drugs that might carry fewer side effects than tamoxifen and further reduce breast cancer risk, Fisher says. *Raloxifene* (Evista), a drug originally developed to treat osteoporosis, is just one of these candidate drugs, he notes.

info For a breast cancer risk assessment tool, visit the National Cancer Institute Web site, *http://bcra.nci.nih.gov.*

▪▪▪▪

Acrylamide Role in Breast Cancer Refuted

Breast cancer is not linked to *acrylamide*, commonly found in potato chips, bread, coffee, cereal and other fried, baked or roasted high-carbohydrate foods. Acrylamide is currently classified as a probable human carcinogen because, in high doses, it has been found to cause cancer in laboratory animals.

Recent finding: Women who consumed large amounts of foods that contain acrylamide did not increase their risk of developing breast cancer.

Important: Additional studies are needed to determine if acrylamide causes other cancers.

Lorelei Mucci, MPH, instructor in medicine, Harvard School of Public Health, Boston.

Long-Term Estrogen Therapy Linked to Breast Cancer

Wendy Y. Chen, MD, MPH, Brigham and Women's Hospital and Dana Farber Cancer Institute, both in Boston.
Jennifer Wu, MD, obstetrician/gynecologist, Lenox Hill Hospital, New York City.
Archives of Internal Medicine.

Postmenopausal women who have had a hysterectomy and have used estrogen therapy for 15 years or more appear to be at a higher risk of breast cancer, according to a recent study.

THE LATEST STUDY

For the study, Dr. Wendy Y. Chen, lead researcher of the new study, who works at Brigham and Women's Hospital and the Dana Farber Cancer Institute, both in Boston, and her colleagues collected data on 28,835 women who were part of the Nurses' Health Study. Of the 934 women who developed invasive breast cancer during the study period, 226 had never used hormones and 708 were using estrogen at the time.

Chen's team believes that the effect of estrogen is cumulative. "We found that there was a 42% increased risk for all types of breast cancer for women who had used estrogen alone for 20 or more years," she says. However, for the type of breast cancer that is hormone sensitive, there was a 48% increased risk after 15 years of estrogen use, she reports.

Past studies that looked at estrogen taken along with the hormone progestin have linked this combination to an increased risk of breast cancer among postmenopausal women. However, results recently released from the Women's Health Initiative (WHI), a large clinical trial of hormone therapy, found no significant connection between estrogen therapy alone and breast cancer in women who took the hormone for seven years.

DECISIONS

Given these findings, women need to consider whether they want to use estrogen—which is typically used to ease menopausal symptoms such as hot flashes, vaginal dryness and loss of energy—over an extended period, Chen says. "Estrogen only causes cancer after prolonged exposure. For women who use estrogen alone, and have been on it for more than 10 years, they would want to consider how much longer they want to remain on estrogen," she says.

> *Patients must understand that the benefits of estrogen come with certain risks.*
>
> *Jennifer Wu, MD*

For women taking estrogen for less than 15 years, studies have not shown a significant increase in risk, Chen says. "But after 15 years, women should speak to their physicians about the benefits of being on estrogen and how that would be weighted against the risks."

Women who decide to stay on estrogen should have regular mammograms, Chen advises.

GUIDELINES MAKE SENSE

Dr. Jennifer Wu, an obstetrician/gynecologist at Lenox Hill Hospital in New York City, thinks these findings support the current guidelines for estrogen use. "The current recommendation for estrogen therapy is to use the lowest effective dose for the shortest duration of time," Wu says. "Patients must understand that the benefits of estrogen come with certain risks."

4

Cancer Breakthroughs

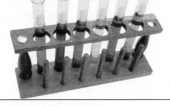

Are Experts Overselling Genetic Cancer Risk?

Looking for genes that could boost a person's risk of cancer is not likely to reap great rewards, according to new research. While vast sums of money and resources are being invested in the search for common, inherited genetic variants that increase susceptibility to cancer, scientists now say that such genes probably don't exist. And if they do, they probably won't have much effect on the incidence of cancer, according to Dr. Stuart Baker, from the US National Cancer Institute, and Dr. Jaakko Kaprio, from the University of Helsinki, Finland.

STUDYING THE STUDIES

The experts point to studies suggesting that the environment, diet and lifestyle have a much larger effect on the incidence of cancer than genetics. Those studies have found changes in cancer rates within one or two generations, which is just too quick to be related to the introduction of new genes, Baker and Kaprio note.

The idea that your genetic makeup is going to be the main factor that determines your susceptibility to cancer has been oversold, explains Dr. Michael Thun, vice president of epidemiology and surveillance research at the American Cancer Society. "The things we know that are bad for you are bad for you in so many different ways that they won't become OK just because you're less susceptible to one or another disease," he says. Most of the genetic changes that cause cancer happen during your lifetime, not at birth, he adds.

A pivotal study of cancer in twins also suggests that genes are not the key culprits in this disease. Looking at the data from identical and non-identical twins, that study found that genetic susceptibility had only a small-to-moderate effect on the incidence of cancer.

Baker and Kaprio both believe that studies that have shown a strong association between

Michael Thun, MD, vice president, epidemiology and surveillance research, American Cancer Society. *British Medical Journal.*

specific genes and a higher risk for cancer may be biased.

However, they note that certain genes may increase the risk for very specific types of cancer—for example, the BRCA1 and BRCA2 genes, which doctors know are strongly linked to breast cancer. But genes that encourage cancer in general are less likely, they say.

Still, "research on what the genetic changes are that give rise to a cancer is already profoundly important," Thun says. "The age of the human genome is here. The understanding of genes will transform the way we think about many diseases, and is already transforming the way we understand cancers."

info For more information on cancer genetics, go to the Web site of the National Cancer Institute at *www.nci.nih.gov/cancerinfo/prevention-genetics-causes/genetics*.

Vaccines Help 40% of Cancer Patients

Michael Morse, MD, associate professor of medicine, division of medical oncology, Duke University Medical Center, Durham, NC, and editor of *Handbook of Cancer Vaccines*. Humana. He has published more than 150 scientific papers, book chapters and abstracts on immunotherapy and has developed several cancer vaccinations.

Until recently, cancer treatment was limited to three options—surgery, chemotherapy and/or radiation.

Now: Cancer vaccines are a promising new treatment for virtually all types of malignancies.

To find out more, we spoke with Dr. Michael Morse, a medical oncologist and leading authority on cancer vaccines…

●**Is the idea of cancer vaccines new?** Not at all. In the 1700s, it was observed that people who had tumors occasionally improved after they experienced an infection. Then, more than a century ago, a New York surgeon named William Coley identified a patient who had an incurable sarcoma (cancer of the bone, muscle or other supportive tissue) but who experienced a significant reduction of the sarcoma after contracting a skin infection.

Coley then tried treating some patients by injecting them—and their tumors—with a fluid in which two types of bacteria were grown. This was called *Coley toxin*, which artificially induced inflammation in cancer patients and resulted in an improvement in 40% of patients and a cure in 10%. This treatment, *nonspecific immunotherapy*, activates the immune system in a general way.

In the last 20 years, immunotherapy for cancer, using vaccines to activate the immune system in a specific way, has become an important field of cancer research.

●**How do cancer vaccines work?** Cancer vaccines aren't like vaccines for viral diseases, such as influenza. Although they don't currently prevent cancer, we do hope that one day they will. Rather, they use various methods to stimulate the cells of the immune system to attack cancer cells.

A cancer vaccine uses an *antigen*, a protein-based derivative from a tumor. Once inside the body, the antigen is taken up by *dendritic cells*, sentinel-like immune cells that break up the antigen and represent it in a form that T-cells can recognize. These T-cells are stimulated by the dendritic cells to then divide into large numbers and to acquire the capacity to recognize and destroy harmful tumor cells.

Our goal is to trigger the immune system to produce an abundance of these "smart" T-cells that can work to eliminate the malignancy.

●**What kinds of cancer can vaccines fight?** Virtually every type of cancer has been studied in a clinical trial, including brain cancer. Many of these trials have involved patients whose cancer has *metastasized*, or spread to other parts of the body.

Vaccines are also being used in *adjuvant* settings—in a person who has had a tumor and has a high risk of a recurrence. For example, a patient who has been surgically treated for breast cancer may subsequently receive chemotherapy, hormonal therapy *and* a cancer vaccine in a clinical trial to discover whether immunotherapy helps make the other two treatments more successful in preventing a recurrence. Many of these adjuvant studies are focused on melanoma, a deadly skin cancer, because it is thought to be more susceptible to the immune system's attack.

●How successful are cancer vaccines? Studies show that 3% to 5% of solid tumors, such as those found in the lung, breast or prostate, shrink after using a cancer vaccine. In nonsolid, or *hematological*, cancers, such as leukemias and lymphomas, the response rate is slightly higher, because of the unique antigens in these types of cancers.

These success rates may sound low, but there's reason to be optimistic. Many studies report that a patient whose immune system is successfully activated by the vaccine either lives longer or experiences slower growth of the cancer than someone whose immune system is not successfully activated.

A recent study of the vaccine *Theratope*, used for breast cancer, did not show a positive result overall but it did show a benefit in a subgroup of women who were on hormone therapy, mostly the drug *tamoxifen* (Nolvadex). The median overall survival for patients on hormone therapy who also received Theratope was 36.5 months, compared with 30.7 months for those who also received the control vaccine. Further clinical trials will focus on the effectiveness of cancer vaccines in these and other subgroups. Before long, we may learn the best way to give dozens of specifically targeted vaccines to help many kinds of patients.

Researchers also have reason for cautious optimism because these vaccines do work—they generate T-cells that recognize and fight cancer. Before cancer vaccinations, there were fewer such T-cells. Even when tumors do not significantly shrink, cancer patients who have an immune response to vaccines have had longer periods before the cancer worsened and they survived longer than the non-vaccine patients.

●Are cancer vaccines toxic? No, not in the way that chemotherapy can be toxic. Using a vaccine to stimulate the immune system might be thought of as a "natural" way to treat cancer. It does not have the same side effects as those caused by chemotherapy and radiation, but it can cause fevers, allergic reactions and autoimmune disorders. Cancer patients consider vaccines nontoxic, and that's one reason why they are so excited about the prospect of this treatment.

●How can people who have cancer find out about the availability of the vaccines?

Cancer vaccines are being tested but are not yet available as part of the standard treatment regimen offered by cancer specialists.

However, there are more than 150 ongoing clinical trials involving cancer vaccines. Talk to your oncologist about cancer vaccines to see if this treatment might be available and right for you.

ⓘinfo For more information on clinical trials for cancer vaccines, contact the National Cancer Institute at 800-422-6237, *www.cancer.gov/clinicaltrials.*

What Every Man Needs to Know About Prostate Cancer Screening

J. Stephen Jones, MD, vice-chair, Glickman Urological Institute, The Cleveland Clinic Foundation, and author of *The Complete Prostate Book: What Every Man Needs to Know* and *Overcoming Impotence.* Prometheus.

Since its introduction 20 years ago, the *prostate-specific antigen* (PSA) blood test has become a key tool for screening men for prostate cancer.

Until the PSA test, men received only a *digital rectal exam* (DRE), in which the doctor inserts a gloved, lubricated finger into the rectum to feel the prostate for lumps and thickenings that suggest a tumor.

The PSA test became popular because it can help detect some prostate cancers earlier than the DRE alone. An elevated PSA level doesn't necessarily mean that cancer is present, but it can indicate the need for a biopsy.

Yet now, after years of use, experts disagree about whether men should receive routine PSA testing. Some medical groups, such as the American Urological Society and the American Cancer Society, advocate annual screening for all men age 50 and older—and starting at age 40 or 45 for men at high risk (African-Americans and men who have a family history of the disease). Other groups, including the American Medical Association, advise doctors to spell out the risks and benefits of PSA testing and let the patients decide. Unfortunately, few men have all the facts about PSA testing. *What men need to know…*

INTERPRETING TEST RESULTS

PSA is produced by the walnut-sized prostate gland. When cancer is present, the prostate secretes more PSA than usual. But cancer isn't the only reason for increased PSA levels. Infection or the enlargement of the prostate that accompanies aging, known as *benign prostatic hyperplasia* (BPH), can also raise PSA levels. Even ejaculation within 48 hours of the test can affect PSA. Therefore, PSA levels can be difficult to interpret.

What is a "normal" PSA level? Until the last several years, it was defined as below 4.0 nanograms/milliliter (ng/mL), but newer data on prostate cancer have made it clear that a man's risk often rises at lower PSA levels. Many experts now say that 2.5 or below is normal for men in their 40s…up to 3.5 is normal for men in their 50s…up to 4.5 is normal for men in their 60s…and up to 6.5 is normal for men 70 and older. PSA levels naturally rise with age, even in the absence of cancer.

Another way of looking at PSA is by using percentages—one-third of men who have a PSA level between 2 and 4 have prostate cancer…44% have prostate cancer when their PSA level is 4.1 to 7…and one-half have the disease at a PSA level of 7.1 to 10. Above 10, the chance that a man has prostate cancer rises to two-thirds.

WHAT'S WRONG WITH THE PSA?

If screening using the PSA test (followed by other tests, such as biopsy, when indicated) catches most cancers—and early detection is generally desirable—why do many experts question whether men should have the PSA test?

The answer is not simple. Most prostate tumors grow very slowly—if at all—and are best left alone because they are unlikely to lead to death. Other prostate cancers need aggressive treatment to keep them from spreading. In these cases, early detection can mean the difference between life and death.

How can you tell the difference? You can't with certainty. That's why a substantial number of prostate cancers will be treated even though they are not life threatening. Treatment generally means surgery to remove the prostate and/or radiation to kill the tumor. These treatments carry significant risks for impotence and urinary incontinence.

Proponents of PSA testing point out that prostate cancer deaths have declined in the years since the test has been widely used. However, PSA skeptics say that this trend could also be the result of better treatment, not just better diagnosis.

IMPROVING ACCURACY

In recent years, several variations of the PSA test have been used to improve its accuracy and limit the number of men who are advised to get a biopsy. *They are…*

●**Free vs. bound PSA.** The majority of PSA floats through the bloodstream bound to protein molecules, while a smaller portion of PSA is *free*. Evidence has shown that when PSA is produced by cancer, higher levels than usual are in the bound form and a smaller proportion is free. Less free PSA (15% or below) means a greater chance that it's cancer. This test is recommended for men who have abnormal results from the standard PSA test.

●**PSA velocity.** The rate at which PSA changes between three or more annual readings is a significant predictor of cancer. The PSA level should not increase more than 0.75 per year, according to the National Cancer Care Network, a consortium of cancer specialists. The group recommends a biopsy if levels rise faster.

●**PSA density.** The larger a noncancerous prostate, the more PSA it will normally produce. So density—the amount of PSA divided by the size of the gland—may indicate whether prostate cancer is present. High density—that is, a big number in a man who has a small prostate—means a greater risk. A range of 0.10 to 0.15 and above indicates increased risk.

Drawback: Measuring the prostate requires rectal ultrasound, a procedure that involves placing a thumb-sized probe into the rectum.

WHAT TO EXPECT FROM A BIOPSY

If your PSA results are abnormal, the next step is a biopsy. Some men get a biopsy as soon as possible, while others wait several months and repeat the PSA test. The second PSA test results are different enough to warrant a third PSA test in less than 20% of cases, but it is often worth waiting and repeating the test.

Important: If your doctor suspects a prostate infection (from a clinical exam and bacterial culture), he/she should prescribe a course of antibiotics before repeating the PSA test.

If a biopsy is indicated, your doctor will refer you to a surgeon, who will perform the procedure.

What the biopsy involves: While you lie on your side, the surgeon inserts an ultrasound probe through your rectum. A needle-like device is guided through a hole in the probe to take tiny prostate tissue samples that will be examined under a microscope. An estimated 40% of surgeons take only six tissue samples, which allows cancer to be missed 30% to 50% of the time. That's why it's crucial for the surgeon to take at least 12 tissue samples, which decreases the false-negative rate to less than 20%.

Important: Injecting local anesthesia into nerves at the base of the prostate makes the procedure less painful. Not all surgeons are familiar with this technique. Before the biopsy, make sure that local anesthesia is available.

Following the biopsy, there may be slight soreness in the area around the rectum for a few days.

The risk for infection from the biopsy is 1%. To minimize this risk, surgeons should give an antibiotic beforehand.

How to Choose the Very Best Treatment

J. Stephen Jones, MD, vice-chair, Glickman Urological Institute, The Cleveland Clinic Foundation, and author of *The Complete Prostate Book: What Every Man Needs to Know* and *Overcoming Impotence.* Prometheus.

Most of the 230,000 prostate cancers that are diagnosed in the US each year are found when the malignancy is still confined to the prostate. Choosing a treatment at this stage is not simple.

Active treatment—surgery and/or radiation—is highly effective, but side effects, including impotence and urinary incontinence, are common. A majority of men who undergo treatment will develop impotence either immediately or within five years.

On the other hand, treatment may not even be required. While some prostate cancers are indeed dangerous and must be treated quickly and aggressively, others cause no harm. Unfortunately, it's impossible to say with certainty whether treatment—or no treatment—is more desirable.

WATCHFUL WAITING

The most misunderstood option in treating prostate cancer is "watchful waiting." Many men believe that it means "doing nothing." It does not. Watchful waiting means following the cancer very closely. It aims to minimize unnecessary treatment of tumors that cause no trouble, while also taking precautions to avoid giving an aggressive cancer a dangerous head start.

The most obvious candidates for watchful waiting are men whose age (typically 70 and older) and other illnesses (heart disease, for example) make it unlikely that they will live long enough to have any ill effects from the prostate malignancy. But refinements in diagnosis have made watchful waiting a reasonable choice for some younger men as well—if it's done properly. *Here's how...*

•**Fully evaluate the tumor.** Watchful waiting should be considered only for a tumor that appears unlikely to grow quickly. The key measure to look at is the *Gleason score*, which refers to the tumor "grade" (how abnormal the cells are and how likely they are to spread). Grades are assigned to the two areas of the prostate that have the highest and second-highest concentrations of cancer cells. The Gleason score (a number from 2 to 10) is expressed as the sum of the two grades (for example, $3 + 4 = 7$). The lower the score, the better.

Prostate-specific antigen (PSA), the protein produced in excess by prostate tumors, also may be considered. When the PSA is less than 10, watchful waiting may be a possibility. If it is greater than 20, few doctors would advocate it. A PSA between 10 and 20 falls in a gray zone.

•**Repeat the biopsy within one year.** If the cancer has gotten worse (a PSA or Gleason score that is significantly higher) within one year of the first biopsy, it will probably continue to worsen. How often to biopsy after that depends on age and other factors. A 55-year-old man may want to have a biopsy each year, to discover quickly if treatment is needed. A 75-year-old that has a low-grade tumor may not want to have a third biopsy for years. In both cases, a rectal exam and PSA testing should be done at least every year.

SURGERY AND RADIATION

The most common treatments for localized prostate cancer—surgery and radiation—are comparably effective. Using either procedure, the cancer usually doesn't come back. They both carry similar (and substantial) risks of impotence and urinary incontinence.

●**Surgery** involves removal of the entire prostate (*prostatectomy*). Technical advances have improved *nerve-sparing surgery*, which aims to protect potency and reduce incontinence risk by leaving the nerve bundle next to the prostate intact. This is only possible for some tumors and is not always successful in preserving function.

With *laparoscopic surgery*, the entire prostate is removed, but the operation is done through a thin tube, or laparoscope. It's less invasive than conventional surgery and involves less blood loss.

Men seem to recover faster when they undergo laparoscopic surgery (approximately three weeks versus six weeks for standard prostatectomy), and some reports suggest that there's a better chance of preserving potency—but neither has been definitively shown.

Latest development: Using *robotic laparoscopic surgery*, the surgeon views the operating field on a screen and manipulates surgical instruments that have precision controls. It takes years of training and experience to become truly adept at robotic laparoscopic surgery—there are few such experts nationwide. But most surgeons that are skilled in conventional prostatectomy can quickly master the robotic technique. It appears to be as effective as other types of surgery, but studies are ongoing.

●**Radiation therapy** includes *external beam therapy* (the oldest type, which focuses intense energy on the tumor from a number of angles to destroy it, while limiting exposure of normal tissues). In *brachytherapy*, "seeds," or tiny pellets of radioactive material, are implanted within the prostate itself to deliver radiation to the tumor.

Latest development: *Intensity-modulated radiation therapy* (IMRT) finely adjusts an external radiation beam to conform to the shape of the tumor. And seeds can now be targeted more precisely using ultrasound imaging. Side effects include irritation to the bladder or rectum.

AN IMPROVED ALTERNATIVE

●**Cryotherapy,** which involves freezing the prostate to destroy it, is an alternative to surgery. Although this procedure was developed decades ago, only recent advances have made it a reasonable option.

The tissue-freezing instrument (cryoprobe) is smaller than previously (the diameter of pencil lead rather than a pencil), and the temperature can be adjusted more precisely, which reduces damage to other tissues.

Cryotherapy is far less invasive than surgery, and recovery is much shorter—only a week or two. Studies show that five- to seven-year survival and cancer control after cryotherapy are comparable with that offered by surgery or radiation. Cryotherapy is less likely to cause lasting urinary incontinence than other procedures.

A Better Way to Gauge Prostate Cancer Risk?

Ian M. Thompson, MD, professor and chairman, department of urology, University of Texas Health Science Center, San Antonio.
Robert A. Smith, PhD, director of cancer screening, American Cancer Society.
Journal of the National Cancer Institute.

A team of researchers has developed a prostate cancer "risk calculator" that they say is better than the *prostate-specific antigen* (PSA) blood test alone. The calculator adds age, race, family history, prior biopsy findings and *digital rectal exam* (DRE) results to PSA levels to assess a man's risk of prostate cancer.

THE STUDY

Study author Dr. Ian M. Thompson, professor and chairman of the department of urology at the University of Texas Health Science Center in San Antonio, and his colleagues collected data from more than 5,500 healthy men older than age 55 who had participated in a large-scale prostate cancer prevention trial.

During the study, all of the men underwent annual PSA and DRE testing, as well as at least one prostate biopsy. After seven years, nearly 22% of the men went on to develop prostate cancer, and 5% developed high-grade disease.

> *PSA is a very important predictor of cancer, but it is only one part of the picture.*
>
> Ian M. Thompson, MD

At the end of the study, the researchers used statistical risk models to analyze all of the accumulated data—biopsy reports, patient age, race, family history of prostate cancer and previous biopsy results, as well as PSA levels and DRE findings.

Thompson's team found that a family history of prostate cancer or an abnormal result on the PSA or DRE test were strongly associated with an increased risk of prostate cancer. A prior negative biopsy result was associated with a decreased risk for the disease.

By compiling such patient variables together, the researchers say they were able to develop a prostate cancer risk calculator that is more accurate than looking at PSA levels alone. "PSA is a very important predictor of cancer, but it is only one part of the picture," explains Thompson. Too often, PSA levels are interpreted as black-and-white indicators of either "normal" or "elevated" risk status. The truth is that rising PSA levels reflect a more graduated increase in cancer risk, he adds.

IMPLICATIONS

"This study provides a way to integrate other important risk factors to allow men and their doctors to better understand their risk and make a more intelligent decision whether to proceed with further testing," says Thompson.

But Dr. H. Ballentine Carter, of the Johns Hopkins School of Medicine, cautions that the calculator's current design fails to distinguish between slow-growing cancers and more life-threatening varieties, which, he says, could lead to a rash of unnecessary biopsies.

Robert A. Smith, director of cancer screening at the American Cancer Society, says the new model has its pros and cons. "It does not distinguish between significant and not-significant disease. The calculator provides *some* help but not enough," he says.

"But it also allows an individual to take his PSA level and actually interpret it in the context of some other information based on the experience of a large number of men, [so he can] understand what the likelihood is that he has prostate cancer. So, I think it could actually be useful," Smith concludes.

info You can find out more about the Prostate Cancer Risk Calculator at *www.compass. fhcrc.org/edrnnci/bin/calculator/main.asp.*

■ ■ ■ ■

Prostate Cancer Facts

According to the American Cancer Society (ACS), prostate cancer is the second-leading cancer killer of men. An estimated one in six men will receive a prostate cancer diagnosis in his lifetime, and more than 30,000 Americans die of the disease each year.

The ACS now recommends an annual prostate-specific antigen (PSA) blood test as well as a digital rectal exam (DRE) for healthy men older than 50. The organization advises that men at higher risk—such as African-Americans and patients who have a history of prostate cancer in their family—begin such testing at age 45.

Radiation Therapy Helps 94% of Younger Men Who Have Prostate Cancer

Andre Konski, MD, clinical research director, radiation oncology department, Fox Chase Cancer Center, Philadelphia.
Durado Brooks, MD, director of prostate cancer, American Cancer Society.
Cancer.
The New York Times.

A radiation treatment that is commonly used to treat prostate cancer in men older than 55 is equally effective in younger men, according to the results of a preliminary study.

THE STUDY

In the study, Dr. Andre Konski, clinical research director of the radiation oncology department at the Fox Chase Cancer Center in

Philadelphia, and his colleagues studied 84 men who underwent *external beam radiation* treatment for prostate cancer five years before.

They compared the outcomes of patients younger than 55 with those 60 to 69 years of age and with those 70 and older. All of the men were in similar stages of the disease.

At the five-year mark, Konski's team found no statistically significant difference in the health status of the men in the three groups. In all, 94% of the men in the youngest group were still alive, compared with 95% of the men 60 to 69 years old and 87% of those 70 and older.

In addition, between 96% and 98% of the patients that were alive showed no signs that the prostate cancer had spread.

LOOKING AT THE RESULTS

Konski cautions that the results do not address the outcomes of younger patients who have more aggressive forms of prostate cancer. And, he adds, the study does not prove that radiation is better than other treatments.

However, the results do refute the common assumption that because their cancer tends to be more aggressive, younger patients need more aggressive treatment, such as removal of the prostate. This study suggests that "when you have a younger man who has an earlier-stage disease, he would do as well [on radiation therapy] as an older man does," Konski says.

"Patients need to factor in all risks and benefits, but external radiation should be given as a viable option for patients to consider," he adds.

Dr. Durado Brooks, director of prostate cancer for American Cancer Society, feels that the follow-up period of five years is too short to draw any conclusions. He notes that it can take a long time for prostate cancer to recur, "and while a five-year follow-up study is encouraging, it's by no means definitive."

Brooks is not sure that this study will lead to any changes in how prostate cancer is treated. "We don't have enough definitive information to say this is the treatment you should choose," he says.

ANOTHER PROSTATE STUDY

In a related study, researchers in Iceland report finding a variant gene that has strong links to prostate cancer.

Geneticists at DeCode Genetics say the gene is carried by approximately 13% of men of European ancestry and may raise a man's risk of developing prostate cancer by approximately 60%. The gene variant probably accounts for 8% of all cases of the disease, they say.

The gene is also twice as common in African-American men as in Caucasian men, helping to explain "a significant part" of why prostate cancer is more prevalent in African-Americans, DeCode's chief executive officer, Dr. Kari Stefansson, says.

info The Prostate Cancer Foundation can provide more information about prostate cancer at *www.prostatecancerfoundation.org*.

■ ■ ■ ■

Radiation Lowers Recurrence Rates

Advanced prostate cancer patients who received radiation within 16 weeks of surgery had a 50% lower risk of recurrence for 10 years than men who did not receive radiation.

Bonus: After five years, long-term side effects, including urinary dysfunction, were the same for patients who received radiation and those who did not.

Gregory Swanson, MD, associate professor of radiation oncology and urology, University of Texas Health Science Center, San Antonio.

The Best Ways to Help People Who Have Cancer

Lori Hope, a three-year lung cancer survivor and author of *Help Me Live: 20 Things People with Cancer Want You to Know.* Celestial Arts. She is managing editor of *Bay Area BusinessWoman News*, has produced more than 20 documentaries and has won two Emmy awards. *www.lorihope.com*.

One in two men and one in three women will get cancer during their lifetimes, according to the American Cancer Society. The advent of new treatments has allowed many cancer patients to live relatively normal lives, and approximately 9 million Americans survive cancer.

When someone has cancer, friends and family members want to help and give support, but sometimes they unknowingly say things that may be disturbing.

There are many ways to express concern and love when someone has cancer or any serious illness…and just as many ways to make someone cringe. *Here's what cancer survivors wish people would do…*

BE PRESENT

People may disappear or withdraw when a loved one gets sick. Some are afraid of saying or doing the wrong thing. Others are geared toward fixing problems and get frustrated when they can't help. Still others have experienced their own cancer tragedies and don't feel strong enough to face the emotional turmoil again.

Although it's uncomfortable to confront a person's outpourings of fear and grief, make the effort. Cancer patients need to cry and release their pain. One of the greatest acts of love is to be with him/her, to listen as he shares his fears.

If you live far away, call or write. Let him know that he's loved…that he matters…and that your heart is with him.

If you simply can't be there, try to explain why the situation is too difficult for you.

GIVE HOPE

People often talk about their own experiences when they meet a person who has cancer. Their intention may be to show empathy or unload their own burdens, but the stories can hurt more than help.

Example: When people heard about my diagnosis, many said things like, *Lung cancer— that's really bad.* A waiter at an Italian restaurant even told me that his wife died of the same cancer. He shared all the gruesome details—about the surgery, how the cancer returned and how she died. It brought back all of my own terror.

People who have cancer don't need to be reminded that they could die—they live with that fear every day. They would rather hear stories of hope and success.

Better: When I told my cousin about my diagnosis, she related a story about one of her professors who had had the same cancer 20 years before—and who is still alive and healthy.

When I told my best friend, with whom I have always taken an annual vacation, she said that we would still be vacationing together when we were old ladies. That's the type of encouragement people who have cancer need to hear.

ASK PERMISSION

Few of us ask permission before sharing our feelings or advice, but asking permission is important when you are talking to someone who has a life-threatening illness. That's when people are at their weakest and most vulnerable.

People say things like, *You really should try this immune-boosting herb* or *You should ask your doctor about this new treatment I read about.* The word *should* suggests that the person who has cancer would be remiss not to take your advice.

Instead, ask him if he is interested in your advice or information or wants to hear your stories. Back off if he says *no. Possible ways to ask…*

I have been looking into this type of cancer. Would you like to hear some of the treatment options I've read about?

A friend told me about an herb that might help. Would you like to hear about it?

LAUGH

We all tend to be overly serious when we're around people who have serious illnesses. That's appropriate sometimes, but not all the time. People who have cancer may want to forget the pain and just laugh and be happy.

I interviewed a woman who received a cancer diagnosis on a Friday. She had all weekend to worry before she saw her doctor again on Monday, so to make herself feel better, she went to a video store and rented a bunch of comedies.

Going through cancer is not all about fear. There's always room for humor and joy.

DON'T HARP ON POSITIVE THINKING

It's normal to be angry, depressed or sad when you have cancer. No one feels positive all the time. Nevertheless, friends and family members often nag cancer patients about the importance of positive thinking and tune them out when they express worries, pessimism or fear.

The implication is that the cancer is somehow the patient's fault or that he can somehow control the outcome.

There is a myth that some people have a "cancer personality." There's no truth to this—and it implicitly blames the patient for causing the disease.

It is important to understand that people who have cancer need to allow themselves to feel everything. They shouldn't have to hide their true emotions. It's okay to feel rotten sometimes.

SPARE THE PLATITUDES

Platitudes are reassuring words that are usually said without much thought or understanding.

Everyone who has cancer has heard things like, *You never know how much time any of us has—you could go outside tomorrow and get hit by a truck.*

One woman I talked to had heard this cliché at least 10 times from people she knew—even from her doctor. Her comment? *Okay, so then in addition to the fact that I could die from cancer, I might also get hit by a truck.* That isn't very comforting.

No one who has had cancer sees it as "a gift." Cancer patients don't want to hear how lucky they are or what they can learn from the experience. They just want to get better.

Silence and compassion are more helpful than empty words.

■ ■ ■ ■

Better Cancer Pain Relief

Cancer patients who had *breakthrough* pain (sudden moderate to severe pain that is not controlled by regular drug therapy) experienced 33% greater relief within 15 minutes of dissolving a lozenge containing the painkiller *fentanyl* (Actiq) in their mouths compared with oral morphine, which they usually used.

Theory: The fentanyl lozenge dissolves fast, allowing it to be absorbed more quickly than oral pain medication.

Giovambattista Zeppetella, MD, medical director of St. Clare Hospice, Hastingwood, England.

Fiber May Not Really Fight Colon Cancer

Yikyung Park, ScD, visiting fellow, National Cancer Institute.
John A. Baron, MD, professor of medicine, Dartmouth Medical School, Lebanon, NH.
The Journal of the American Medical Association.

Research examining the results of 13 studies that included more than 725,000 people found that a high intake of dietary fiber does not reduce the risk of colon cancer. This is the largest study to date, and unlike previous studies, took into account other risk factors that could affect the outcome.

OTHER RISK FACTORS CHANGE CONCLUSIONS

A first look at the combined data found a 16% lower incidence of colon cancer in the people who had the highest fiber intake. But when the researchers adjusted the figures to take into account other risk factors—such as multivitamin use, folate intake, red meat consumption and milk and alcohol intake—they found that there was no relationship between dietary fiber intake and colon cancer risk.

PROBLEMS WITH PREVIOUS STUDIES

"In general, most previous studies have been inconsistent," says Yikyung Park, who led the study while at the Harvard School of Public Health and who is now a visiting fellow at the National Cancer Institute.

Dr. John A. Baron, professor of medicine at Dartmouth Medical School, says the real problem in reaching a definitive conclusion is that "fiber" is a vague term. "Fiber is just a word," he says. "It's like saying, 'taking a pill' or 'driving a vehicle.' It's such a broad term that it is not helpful."

Fibers often are characterized by the foods that contain them—cereal fiber, vegetable fiber, fruit fiber, Baron says. But there can be great differences between fibers within those families. Some fibers are soluble, some insoluble—insoluble fiber is believed to have the protective effect—and studies generally do not distinguish between the two, he explains.

"Doing research in this area is difficult, and part of the problem has been people making too-optimistic or too-rapid decisions based on studies that have not been definitive," he adds.

Fiber is just a word. It's such a broad term that it is not helpful.

John A. Baron, MD

This report is certainly not the last word on the issue, Park says. "This is still a very active area of research. Clearly, more studies are needed."

FIBER STILL HAS BENEFITS

There are still good reasons why people should consume dietary fiber, Park says. "There are studies showing that dietary fiber reduces the risk of other diseases, such as heart disease and diabetes, so people should continue to eat dietary fiber," she says.

Diabetics More Likely to Get Colon Cancer

Donald Garrow, MD, clinical instructor, masters in clinical research fellow, Medical University of South Carolina, Charleston.

Kevin Adgent, MD, physician, Wilmington, NC.

American College of Gastroenterology annual scientific meeting, Honolulu.

A recent study has found that people who have diabetes are more vulnerable to colon cancer.

THE STUDY

Dr. Donald Garrow, a clinical instructor and a masters in clinical research fellow at the Medical University of South Carolina, Charleston, and his team analyzed data on more than 226,000 Americans that was collected as part of the National Health Interview Survey.

Most diabetics surveyed in the study had obesity-linked type 2 diabetes, in which the body becomes insensitive to insulin. After compensating for factors that affect colon cancer risk—including age, gender, alcohol and tobacco use, and exercise—the researchers found that diabetics were 1.4 times more likely to develop colon cancer than nondiabetics.

Other studies have found the same association, Garrow says, but he believes his study is the largest cross-sectional survey to date. Exactly why diabetics have a greater risk of developing colon cancer isn't clear, Garrow says. One theory is that elevated insulin levels in diabetics' blood cause cells in the colon's mucosal lining to develop into cancer cells, he explains.

IMPLICATIONS

Dr. Kevin Adgent, an internist in Wilmington, North Carolina, praises the study's large sample size, and says the findings "make me more aware of getting my diabetic patients screened properly."

Garrow says the study underscores the importance of diabetics following colon cancer screening guidelines. The American Cancer Society now recommends that beginning at age 50, men and women at average risk for colon cancer should be screened using the *fecal occult blood test* (FOBT), sigmoidoscopy and colonoscopy, and/or double barium enema.

info To learn more about diabetes, visit the American Diabetes Association at *www.diabetes.org*.

■ ■ ■ ■

Help for the Medical Test No One Wants to Talk About

Here's a topic that most people do not like to discuss—colonoscopies. I had my first one recently.*

I expected the test to be horrible, but it wasn't at all. The preparation the night before, however, is another story. Sadly, many people avoid the test because of that, but there are ways to make it less onerous.

For advice, I spoke with two of our favorite advisers—Bruce Yaffe, MD, a New York City internist who specializes in digestive diseases, and Andrew Rubman, ND, director of the Southbury Clinic for Traditional Medicines in Connecticut.

Ask your physician about the different types of purgatives for cleansing the bowel. *Phospho-soda* is the easiest. Most people need only two doses

---

*Current screening guidelines recommend colonoscopies beginning at age 50—earlier if you have inflammatory bowel disease or a family history of colon cancer. Check with your doctor.

—approximately 3 ounces. *Halflytely* and other preparations require drinking approximately a half-gallon of foulish-tasting liquid.

Phospho-soda tastes like liquid salt. *To make it more tolerable…*

●**Chew ice or very minty gum,** such as Dentyne Ice, to numb your mouth.

●**Mix the solution with a teaspoon of vanilla extract** and a glass of ice-cold ginger ale or other clear beverage.

●**Hold your nose** as you swallow.

Phospho-soda also is available in pill form (Visicol). Bowel preparation requires 28 pills and approximately nine glasses of fluid. It is best for people who can't tolerate the liquid form.

Caution: Phospho-soda should not be used by anyone older than age 65 or anyone who has heart or kidney problems, diabetes or other conditions that complicate his/her general health.

It usually takes a few hours for the bowels to start moving—it took less than two hours for me. Expect 10 to 20 bowel movements over a five-hour period. Lemonade-colored fluid coming out signals a well-cleaned colon. Particles are okay. Ice-tea–colored or sludgy fluid will require further preparation.

Apply A+D ointment or Vaseline to ease soreness. Using baby wipes also can help soothe tenderness.

If you have experienced nausea during colonoscopy prep, ask your doctor about antinausea drugs, such as Reglan.

Natural option: Ginger. Take one or two 395-milligram (mg) capsules one hour before starting the prep. Dr. Rubman likes ginger from Eclectic Institute (800-332-4372, *www.eclecticherb.com*).

Yaffe lets patients have the nutritional drinks Ensure or Sustacal up to six hours before anesthesia, but nothing—not even water—after that.

Prep is easier if you start cleansing your system several days before the test. *Following is Dr. Rubman's advice…*

●**Avoid excess fluids at mealtime.** This keeps the stomach sufficiently acidic and aids digestion and elimination. Drink water when you are thirsty.

●**Take the dietary fiber *glucomannan*—** one 665-mg capsule twice daily—with a large glass of water 30 minutes before a meal.

●**Do not use herbal laxatives,** such as those containing *senna* or *cascara*. They can cause spasms and discolor the lining of the colon. Also avoid beets, nuts, seeds and strong teas and coffee.

To recover more quickly from anesthesia, Dr. Rubman suggests a 50-mg multi-B vitamin and an orally absorbable form of B-12, such as *hydroxycobalamin*. Take them twice a day for four days, starting two days before the test. Take the multi with meals, and hold B-12 in the mouth until dissolved, between meals. On the day of the procedure, take these immediately after the test.

Finally, bring an extra pair of underwear (accidents are possible). Expect to eat within 30 minutes of completing the procedure—but don't drive for four hours after anesthesia.

Approximately 90% of all colon cancer deaths can be prevented if diagnosed early through colonoscopy. Don't let its bad rep keep you from being checked.

Marjory Abrams, publisher, newsletters, Boardroom Inc., 281 Tresser Blvd., Stamford, CT 06901.

Colonoscopy Benefits Last Longer than Thought

Timothy R. Church, PhD, professor of environmental health sciences, University of Minnesota School of Public Health, Minneapolis.

Stephen Shibata, MD, director, gastrointestinal program, City of Hope Cancer Center, Duarte, CA.

Robert A. Smith, PhD, director of cancer screening, American Cancer Society.

The Journal of the American Medical Association.

For people who are younger than 80 years, the benefits of a colonoscopy might last more than 10 years—the period of time currently recommended before the procedure is repeated. However, this screening, which looks for colon polyps that could become cancerous over time, may provide only a minimal benefit to people who are age 80 or older.

THE FIRST STUDY

The first study, conducted by researchers at the University of Manitoba in Winnipeg, Canada, looked at data on nearly 35,000 Canadians whose colonoscopies found no polyps. During the next 10 years, the incidence of colon cancer in these individuals was 72% lower than in the general population, the researchers report. In addition, the decreased risk of colon cancer continued for more than 10 years.

Although the Canadian team did not call for a change in the recommended screening interval, the researchers did say that the "findings suggest that screening colonoscopies do not need to be performed at intervals shorter than 10 years."

THE SECOND STUDY

The second study, conducted at Virginia Mason Medical Center in Seattle, looked at colonoscopies that were performed on 1,244 people in three age groups—50 to 54; 75 to 79; and 80 and older.

The big issue is identifying those people in whom the benefit of colonoscopy outweighs the risk.

Robert A. Smith, PhD

The incidence of colon cancer was much higher in the oldest participants—14% for the 80-and-older group—compared with 3.2% for the 50-to-54-year-old group. However, the study found that colonoscopy does not significantly extend the life expectancy of people older than 80 years—it increased survival only by approximately 45 days for the oldest group, compared with more than 10 months for people ages 50 to 54.

The results "suggest that the benefit of screening colonoscopy in very elderly patients may be smaller than what is commonly believed," the researchers say. They add that the information might "help avoid its use in patients who are unlikely to benefit substantively."

LOOKING AT THE RESULTS

Both studies were observational, and neither is definitive, says Timothy R. Church, a professor of environmental health sciences at the University of Minnesota School of Public Health in Minneapolis.

He agrees that the Canadian study "doesn't give us any reason to change the currently recommended interval of 10 years. [However,] it does leave open the possibility that an even longer interval might be possible."

The Seattle study, he says, "raises a legitimate question: When should you no longer screen for colorectal cancer?"

The answer, of course, would involve more factors than just age, Church says. "The decision needs to be based not strictly on age, but on the health of the individual. Some older people are in good shape and will live for 20 years or more. Others have multiple health problems—their hearts or other organs may be failing. They are likely to die of something other than colorectal cancer, so we definitely need to take into account what a person's health status is before making a screening decision," he explains.

"For this age group we have to be extra careful," agrees Dr. Stephen Shibata, director of the gastrointestinal program at the City of Hope Cancer Center in Duarte, California. "We need to know what the patient's health is, what the patient wishes. The patient and the physician need to have a discussion before they [decide on] a procedure."

"The big issue is identifying those people in whom the benefit [of colonoscopy] outweighs the risk," says Robert A. Smith, director of cancer screening for the American Cancer Society.

Other, less uncomfortable screening techniques, such as *fecal occult blood tests* (FOBT) and flexible *sigmoidoscopy*, may also be effective, Church adds.

info You can learn more about colorectal cancer from the Centers for Disease Control and Prevention at *www.cdc.gov/colorectalcancer.*

Cholesterol Drugs Don't Prevent (or Cause) Colon Cancer

C. Michael White, PharmD, professor of pharmacology, University of Connecticut, Storrs.
Eric J. Jacobs, PhD, epidemiologist, American Cancer Society.
Journal of the National Cancer Institute.
The Journal of the American Medical Association.

Two major studies have shown that the cholesterol-lowering drugs called *statins* do not reduce the risk of colon cancer.

THE FIRST STUDY

One study looked at 27 trials that included nearly 87,000 people. The researchers found that there was no reduced incidence of colorectal cancers (as well as a variety of other cancers) in people who took statins compared with those who did not.

Expectations had been raised by previous studies, one of which found a 47% reduction in colon and rectal cancers in people who took statins for more than five years.

However, those studies "had a lot of methodological flaws," according to C. Michael White, a professor of pharmacology at the University of Connecticut, and the leader of the analysis.

"In our study, we did a meta-analysis of all of the trials, and were not able to show any reduction in cancer or in cancer deaths," White reports.

Most of the people in those trials were taking a single drug, *pravastatin* (Pravachol), "but when we looked at other statins, we couldn't come up with a mixture that suggested there might be a protective effect," he says.

THE SECOND STUDY

The second study also found no reduced incidence of colon cancer in the more than 130,000 people who took statins in the Cancer Prevention Study II Nutritional Cohort.

According to the study researchers, "Our results do not support the hypothesis that statins, as a class of drugs, strongly reduce the risk of colorectal cancer."

The two studies are "consistent and complementary," says Eric J. Jacobs, leader of the study as well as an epidemiologist at the American Cancer Society.

"They are consistent in that both show no effect on colon cancer risk. They are complementary in that the meta-analysis was able to look at varieties of statins, whereas our study was able to look at longer-term use," he explains.

THE GOOD NEWS

But the news isn't as bad as it might seem, White says. "The good news is that when statins first came out, people were worried that they might cause cancer," he says. "Now, we know the effect is pretty neutral."

And the reports provide no reason to stop taking statins, White says. "They still do miraculous things for people with heart disease," he says. "Just don't take them to reduce the risk of cancer. There are other things to do [for that], like not smoking and improvements in diet."

info Steps you can take to avoid colon cancer are described on the National Cancer Institute Web site at *www.cancer.gov/cancerinfo/ wyntk/colon-and-rectum.*

New Study Means Better Melanoma Treatments

Boris Bastian, MD, assistant professor of dermatology and pathology, University of California, San Francisco.
Paul Meltzer, MD, PhD, head, section of molecular genetics, cancer genetics branch, National Human Genome Research Institute.
The New England Journal of Medicine.

S cientists are learning that not all melanoma skin cancers are genetically alike. And that may have far-reaching implications for the treatment and prevention of this disease.

I'm somewhat optimistic now that we may turn the corner on melanoma therapy.

Paul Meltzer, MD, PhD

THE STUDY

Dr. Boris Bastian, assistant professor of dermatology and pathology at the University of California, San Francisco, and his colleagues divided 126 different melanomas into four groups based on the amount of exposure to ultraviolet (UV) light from the sun.

Thirty melanomas appeared on skin that showed signs of chronic sun damage, while 40 were on skin that didn't show signs of sun damage. Another 36 melanomas were on areas that are rarely exposed to sun, such as the palms and soles of the feet. The remaining 20 melanomas occurred on mucous membranes, such as those found in the mouth, nose and genital areas.

After comparing these four groups, the researchers found significant genetic differences that often correlated with the location of the melanoma on the body.

IMPLICATIONS

"Up to now, melanoma was regarded as one disease and was treated as such. But our study shows that there are marked genetic differences in melanoma cases. These are distinct diseases," says Bastian.

Dr. Paul Meltzer, head of the section of molecular genetics in the cancer genetics branch at the National Human Genome Research Institute, says this study "may have significant clinical implications in the long run, [and is] laying the groundwork for a better individualized and personalized cancer therapy. I'm somewhat optimistic now that we may turn the corner on melanoma therapy."

Both Bastian and Meltzer theorize that one reason current melanoma therapies are not as effective as doctors would like is that they are not targeting the right type of melanoma.

"These findings may be very important for designing targeted therapies for these various types," says Bastian.

■ ■ ■ ■

How to Protect Yourself

While researchers continue looking for better ways to treat melanoma—and possibly prevent it—there are steps everyone can take to help protect their skin.

Most importantly, people should try to stay out of the sun between 10 am and 4 pm. When outside, wear clothing that protects the skin, including a hat. Sit or stand in the shade whenever it is possible.

Sunscreen should protect against both UVA and UVB light, and should be used generously and frequently during sun exposure. Of course, using sunscreen doesn't mean it's okay to be out in the sun all day, every day. It's very important for parents to protect young children from the sun because some of the genetic alterations that occur in melanoma may begin to develop when people are young.

New Sunscreen Promises More Protection

Darrell S. Rigel, MD, clinical professor of dermatology, New York University, New York City.

Kimberly A. Rawlings, spokeswoman, US Food and Drug Administration.

Jeffrey C. Salomon, MD, assistant clinical professor of plastic surgery, Yale University School of Medicine, New Haven, CT.

A new sunscreen approved by the US Food and Drug Administration (FDA) promises protection for both ultraviolet A and B (UVA and UVB) rays.

However, that doesn't mean people can disregard the standard advice to avoid the sun, experts stress.

THE NEW PRODUCT

Anthelios SX, made by L'Oreal, is new in that it contains ecamsule (Mexoryl), an agent that shields the skin from short-wave UVA rays—something sunscreens previously available in the United States were unable to do.

According to experts, UVB exposure causes sunburn and some skin cancers, while UVA causes aging and some other skin cancers.

Most sunscreens contain two active ingredients—*avobenzone* and *octocrylene*. Anthelios SX contains those ingredients as well, in addition to *Mexoryl*, a compound that stabilizes the UVA protections and makes them last longer.

Sunscreens containing Mexoryl have been available in Europe, Asia and Canada since 1993.

"There was nothing like this in the US," says Dr. Darrell S. Rigel, a clinical professor of dermatology at New York University and advisor to L'Oreal. "Basically, it lasts longer and it gives better protection against UVA."

OLD RULES STILL APPLY

But a better sunscreen doesn't change the basic rules of skin protection. "No sunscreen completely protects people against UVA radiation," says FDA spokeswoman Kimberly A. Rawlings. "This product and other sunscreens that reduce UVA exposure should be used in conjunction with limiting time in the sun and wearing protective clothing. The FDA has not compared this product with other sunscreens capable of reducing UVA exposure."

Dr. Jeffrey C. Salomon, an assistant clinical professor of plastic surgery at Yale University School of Medicine, says, "It's best to use a sunblock that contains both physical as well as chemical blockers. A lot of sunscreens break down in the sun. That's the dirty little secret that no one talks about," he adds. "In most sunscreens, there are both chemical and physical sunblocks."

Sunblocks such as zinc oxide and titanium physically block the sun from coming in, Salomon says.

"Chemical sunblocks break down rapidly in the sun," he says. "You want a sunscreen that blocks both UVA and UVB, that has a high SPF and that is waterproof."

■ ■ ■ ■

Sunscreen Stats

Sunscreen manufacturers and the media provide so much information on sun-protection products, that it's difficult to separate fact from fiction. *Following are just a few facts to help sort it all out...*

•**Use sunscreen daily**—even on rainy days and in winter. Even brief sun exposure adds up over time.

•**UVA and UVB rays cause skin cancer and premature aging.** UVA tans your skin. UVB burns it. Both cause wrinkles. SPF sunscreen ratings do not refer to UVA rays, so be sure your sunscreen also includes UVA block, such as transparent minimum 6% zinc oxide.

•**Sunscreen that boasts higher numbers is not much more effective.** SPF 15 blocks 93% of UVB rays...SPF 30 blocks 97%. The difference matters most to people who tan or burn easily.

•**Use adequate amounts of sunscreen.** An 8-ounce bottle of SPF 15, if applied properly, is enough for a weekend at the beach.

•**Waterproof sunscreen protects you for approximately 80 minutes in the water.** So reapply it if you are in the water longer and also after you towel off.

David Herschthal, MD, dermatologist, Tamarac, FL. *www.drherschthal.com.*

Laser Surgery Works to Treat Liver Cancer

Charles Cha, MD, assistant professor of gastrointestinal surgery and surgical oncology, Yale University School of Medicine, New Haven, CT.
Ronald W. Busuttil, MD, Dumont Professor of Transplantation Surgery, and chief, division of liver and pancreas transplant, David Geffen School of Medicine, University of California at Los Angeles.
Radiological Society of North America annual meeting, Chicago.

Long-term research has found that laser surgery using magnetic resonance guidance is effective in treating cancerous liver tumors in some patients.

THE STUDY

In a 12-year study, 839 patients at the University of Frankfurt received *magnetic-resonance-guided, laser-induced thermotherapy* to treat liver tumors (metastates) that resulted from colorectal cancer. This procedure uses laser light to destroy tumor tissue.

Lead researcher Dr. Martin Mack, an associate professor in the University's department of diagnostic and interventional radiology, and colleagues treated 2,506 liver tumors (metastates) and tracked patient survival to evaluate the long-term results of the procedure.

For patients who received the laser technology, the average survival from the date of diagnosis was 3.8 years, which compared well with survival of 1.5 to 5.0 years for those receiving traditional surgery, say the researchers.

ADVANTAGES

According to Mack, laser ablation has many advantages over other treatments.

"Traditional surgical resection has higher morbidity and mortality rates than laser ablation," says Mack. "Laser treatment can be done on an outpatient basis under local anesthesia. Typically, the patient stays only a couple of hours in the hospital, instead of a couple of weeks [as is common] after surgical liver resection," he adds.

In addition, laser surgery can be used to treat tumors in both halves of the liver—often during the same procedure. This is practically impossible in traditional surgery, where only the left or right lobe is surgically excised, the researchers note.

Moreover, if new tumors are found during follow-up exams, it is easier to do another laser treatment than to subject the patient to another invasive surgery.

"Many surgeons are already performing local ablation instead of resection because they have already recognized the positive effect of it," Mack says.

"I believe that minimally invasive tumor ablation together with chemotherapy will play the most important role in the treatment of tumors in the years to come," he adds.

NOT READY FOR PRIME TIME?

Some experts, however, don't think this method is as good as the standard surgery for the treatment of liver cancer.

"I would be wary of making too much out of this new technology," says Dr. Charles Cha, an assistant professor of gastrointestinal surgery and surgical oncology at Yale University School of Medicine.

"The long-term survival presented by Mack's group is impressive and does demonstrate some promise for this new and experimental technology," Cha concedes, but the five-year survival rate after resection for metastatic colon cancer is relatively good—approximately 40%—and this study did not include a surgical arm to which the laser surgery could be compared.

"The conclusion that this technology is better than resection is a bit of a stretch," he says.

Dr. Ronald W. Busuttil, chief of the division of liver and pancreas transplant at the David Geffen School of Medicine at the University of California at Los Angeles, agrees. "For this technique to really come to the fore, it needs to be compared against surgery and radiofrequency ablation," he says. "It's interesting, but I don't know if it's ready for prime time."

The survival rates of two other types of treatments—cryotherapy and radiofrequency ablation—for metastatic colorectal cancer have not yet matched the results of surgery, which remains the gold standard, Cha says.

"Until more definitive evidence is available, patients should not consider this technology as a replacement for standard surgical therapy, but rather as an alternative if surgery is not possible," he says.

Busuttil notes that there are many other ways to treat liver tumors caused by colorectal cancer that do not include surgery.

Esophagus Cancer Rates Soar 600%

Rhonda F. Souza, MD, associate professor of medicine, division of gastroenterology, Dallas VA Medical Center and Harold C. Simmons Comprehensive Cancer Center, University of Texas Southwestern Medical Center at Dallas.

B. Jay Brooks, Jr., MD, chairman, hematology/oncology, Ochsner Clinic Foundation, Baton Rouge, LA.

CA: A Cancer Journal for Clinicians.

The incidence of a deadly form of esophagus cancer that is associated with *gastroesophageal reflux disease* (GERD) is rising at an alarming rate, experts say.

Approximately 90% of people who develop adenocarcinoma of the esophagus die within five years and, currently, there are few effective prevention, screening or treatment methods available.

MOST RAPIDLY INCREASING CANCER

"Of all the cancers that are increasing, this one is the most rapidly increasing. It way outpaces melanoma and prostate cancer," says Dr. Rhonda F. Souza, coauthor of the report and associate professor of medicine at the Dallas VA Medical Center and the Harold C. Simmons Comprehensive Cancer Center at the University of Texas Southwestern Medical Center at Dallas.

The incidence of esophageal adenocarcinomas has soared 600% since the 1970s. By contrast, the incidence of gastric cancers has been on the wane in most Western countries for the last 50 years.

Despite the startling increase, the actual number of adenocarcinomas of the esophagus is not huge—7,000 to 8,000 new cases per year in the United States. "Even though it's increased, it's still not as prevalent as colon cancer," Souza says.

MAJOR RISK FACTORS

Unlike colon cancer, however, there are no effective screening techniques for esophageal adenocarcinomas. The major risk factors for this type of cancer are GERD and *Barrett's esophagus*, a condition in which part of the esophagus lining is replaced by tissue that is similar to what is normally found in the intestine.

Each year, approximately one-half of 1% of the people who have Barrett's (one person in 200) will go on to develop adenocarcinoma of the esophagus.

> *Of all the cancers that are increasing, esophagus cancer is the most rapidly increasing.*
>
> Rhonda F. Souza, MD

"People who get this cancer are those who have GERD and, in the US, probably 60 million people have reflux and approximately 20% of those have reflux on a weekly basis. Those are the ones who'd be most at risk to get this cancer," Souza says. "If you have chronic reflux, you need to pay attention, and if you have reflux and you have trouble swallowing, weight loss or bleeding, you should see a doctor. Those are early-warning signs."

Obesity may also play a role in the disease. "No one is really sure," Souza says. "In the West, body mass index is increasing, and it's thought that by becoming obese, people are more predisposed to getting heartburn [GERD]."

"Probably the single most important thing we can do is lose weight, because increased abdominal weight tends to hold back the normal flow of food, and that's one thing that can create GERD," says Dr. B. Jay Brooks, Jr., chairman of hematology/oncology at the Ochsner Clinic Foundation in Baton Rouge, Louisiana.

There is some evidence that aspirin and other nonsteroidal anti-inflammatory drugs (NSAIDs) may help prevent esophagus cancer from developing in patients who have Barrett's esophagus. Souza and her coauthor, however, are not convinced that the benefits of taking these drugs outweigh the risks.

ENDOSCOPY AS SCREENING TOOL

For those at high risk—a white male age 65 to 74 years old who has longstanding heartburn, for example—Souza recommends seeing a physician and getting an endoscopy even in the absence of any alarm symptoms and, hopefully, before a tumor has developed.

"Endoscopically, we can see precursor lesions," Souza points out. If any abnormalities are found, patients can then enroll in a more formal surveillance program. "Your chances are better because it's at an earlier stage," she adds.

"If people have reflux symptoms, they really do need to see their doctors because, many times, an upper endoscopy can detect things very quickly. Then you can treat it aggressively to try to prevent the progression. It's not 100%, but it's the best that we have at this point," says Brooks.

info For more information on esophagus cancer, visit the American Cancer Society at *www.cancer.org*. Click on "Choose a cancer topic."

Better Screening Finds More Thyroid Cancers

Louise Davies, MD, Department of Veterans Affairs Medical Center, White River Junction, VT, and assistant professor of surgery, Dartmouth Medical School, Hanover, NH.

R. Michael Tuttle, MD, endocrinologist at Memorial Sloan-Kettering Cancer Center, New York City.
The Journal of the American Medical Association.

The increase in thyroid cancer cases in the United States is the result of better, high-tech diagnostic tests that are picking up minuscule tumors—most of which pose no long-term threat, according to a recent study.

THE NEW NUMBERS

The number of thyroid cancers in the US more than doubled from 3.6 per 100,000 in 1973 to 8.7 per 100,000 in 2002, according to the report. But that increase was not accompanied by a rise in deaths, which have remained stable at just 0.5 per 100,000, the researchers say.

THE NEW TECHNOLOGY

The study should help settle the controversy about rising thyroid cancer rates. Some investigators have attributed the increase to environmental radiation from sources such as nuclear power plants. However, the report suggests that the real reason for the higher rates may be "increased detection of subclinical disease."

"New tests are available to detect abnormalities that we never saw in the past," says the co-author of the national report, Dr. Louise Davies, an assistant professor of surgery at Dartmouth Medical School.

Ultrasound scans and needle biopsies can detect nodules as small as 2 millimeters (mm), one-quarter of the size of a pencil eraser. Before the new techniques were available, doctors were detecting much larger nodules—1.5 centimeters (cm) or larger, explains Davies. Nearly 50% of the tumors that were detected during this study were 1 cm or less, she notes.

NO THREAT?

Most cancers of that size grow so slowly that they pose no threat to life, Davies says. "People should know that nodules are common and that there is a lot more thyroid cancer out there than really matters," she says.

New tests are available to detect abnormalities that we never saw in the past.

Louise Davies, MD

As in prostate cancer, autopsies have shown that a fair number of people, perhaps 5%, had thyroid cancers that were not detected while they were alive.

"Some of these [thyroid and prostate tumors] are so small and grow so slowly that they would not be evident during the lifetime of the patient," says Dr. R. Michael Tuttle, an endocrinologist at Memorial Sloan-Kettering Cancer Center in New York City.

THE DILEMMA

Experts agree that the detection of such small cancers presents a dilemma for physicians. "We need to start considering how aggressively we should treat these tumors," Davies says. "I think it is something people are struggling with."

"We're always looking for the needle in the haystack," Tuttle says. "In the worst-case scenario, we end up overtreating a good number of patients." But overtreatment might be necessary because of the potential of missing the few small cancers that will grow aggressively and become

life-threatening, he says. Currently, there is no way to identify which thyroid growths can be safely left alone and which require surgery, Tuttle says.

Although the report highlights a dilemma for doctors, it does offer comfort to the public, Tuttle says. What's important for patients to know is that we don't have an epidemic of thyroid cancer, he says.

Located beneath the voice box, the thyroid is a butterfly-shaped gland that produces thyroid hormone, which the body uses to regulate growth and metabolism.

info For more information on thyroid cancer, visit the American Thyroid Association at *www.thyroid.org/patients/brochures.html.* Then scroll down to "Cancer of the Thyroid Brochure."

■ ■ ■ ■

Sweet Way to Combat Cancer

In a recent study, tumors grew more slowly in cancerous mice that were fed honey, royal jelly (produced by bees as food for larvae) or propolis (a substance used in the hive) than in mice who received no special food.

Nada Orsolic, PhD, assistant professor of animal physiology, faculty of science, University of Zagreb, Croatia.

Low-Fat Diet Lowers Cancer Recurrence Rates

Diana Dyer, RD, nutritionist, cancer survivor and author of *A Dietitian's Cancer Story.* Swan. Her Web site, *www.cancerrd.com,* provides links to cancer research organizations and anticancer menus.

For the first time, a randomized, placebo-controlled study—one of the highest standards of scientific research—has demonstrated that dietary changes can reduce cancer recurrence rates.

In this study, 2,437 women who had early-stage breast cancer were randomly chosen to follow a low-fat diet (33.3 grams [g] of fat daily) or a higher-fat diet (51.3 g daily). After five years, there was more than a 20% reduction in breast cancer recurrence in the low-fat group.

The study did not prove that a low-fat diet can reduce cancer in women who did not have a history of the disease. Nor did it look at other nutritional factors, such as the consumption of fiber, fruits and vegetables, etc.

But more and more oncologists are convinced that future studies will continue to demonstrate that good nutrition can help guard against most types of malignancies.

A CANCER-PROTECTION PLAN

Diana Dyer, a registered dietitian and three-time cancer survivor, has reviewed the latest studies and interviewed top researchers to create an anticancer nutrition plan.

Even if you consume ample amounts of fiber (25 to 30 g daily) and try to eat broccoli and other cruciferous vegetables as often as possible, you may be surprised to learn that there is much more you can do to curb your cancer risk.

PRODUCE: NINE A DAY

For years, US dietary guidelines recommended five daily servings of fruits and vegetables (one-half cup equals one serving). Now five to nine daily servings are recommended.

In addition to providing fiber, fruits and vegetables are the best sources of antioxidants and other plant chemicals that help prevent damage to a cell's DNA and fight the inflammation that causes normal cells to become cancerous.

What most people don't know: Only approximately 22% of Americans eat five servings of fruits and vegetables daily.

If you're getting only two daily servings but increase your intake to five daily servings, you could potentially cut your risk of some types of cancer, such as esophagus and colorectal, by 20% to 50%.

More daily servings provide even greater protection. *To maximize the cancer-fighting effect, eat produce that has the highest levels of antioxidants...*

•**Vegetables.** Kale, beets, red peppers, broccoli, spinach, sweet potatoes and corn. Try a stir-fry with olive oil and many of these veggies...or top a pizza with them.

•**Fruits.** All berries, including blueberries and strawberries, plums, oranges, red grapes and pink grapefruit.

FAT: IT MUST BE THE RIGHT KIND

The average American diet includes 33% fat. Excessive fat—especially the saturated fat found in lunch meats, prime rib and other red meats and full-fat dairy products, such as butter, milk, cheese and sour cream—produces carcinogens that increase cancer risk.

What most people don't know: To maximize the absorption of fat-soluble—and cancer-fighting—phytochemicals and nutrients found in vegetables and fruits, 16% to 18% of your diet should be from healthful fat, such as monounsaturated fat.

Helpful: To add healthful monounsaturated fat to your daily diet, use olive oil for salads, sautéing, etc.

Avoid saturated fat altogether, or follow these suggestions...

•**Buy only very lean meats.** Limit portion size to 2 to 3 ounces (approximately the size of a deck of cards) per meal.

•**Use reduced-fat or fat-free dairy items.**

•**Minimize the use of margarine** as well as shortening.

FISH: IT FIGHTS CANCER, TOO

The omega-3 fatty acids found in wild salmon, light tuna and other cold-water fish are known to protect the heart.

What most people don't know: Omega-3s interact with other molecules in the body to help reduce inflammatory changes that can promote cancer. Aim for two to three servings of fish weekly. Or use one to two tablespoons of ground flaxseed meal daily. It's high in *alpha-linolenic acid* (ALA), a beneficial type of omega-3.

Caution: Avoid blackened fish. High-heat cooking and grilling produce carcinogens that increase cancer risk. If you do grill, marinate fish or meats in vinegar, lime juice, teriyaki sauce or other marinades, and turn once a minute. This reduces the production of carcinogens by approximately 90%.

USE HERBS AND SPICES OFTEN

Garlic, anise and other herbs, as well as ginger and other spices used in cooking, contain high levels of anticancer phytochemicals. To increase flavor, add herbs and spices to your foods instead of salt, sugar or fat.

What most people don't know: Cutting or smashing fresh garlic 10 minutes before cooking preserves the high levels of its anticancer compounds.

SOY: A LITTLE GOES A LONG WAY

Soybeans contain many anticarcinogenic compounds, including the phytoestrogen *genistein*. Phytoestrogens are plant chemicals that mimic the effects of natural estrogen—and help prevent it from causing cancerous changes in cells in both women and men.

Just one daily serving of soy (one cup of soy milk, one-half cup of tofu, one-half cup of soybeans) may reduce the risk for some breast and prostate cancers.

What most people don't know: Soy foods, such as soybeans, tofu and tempeh, are also good sources of cancer-fighting omega-3s.

Caution: Soy foods may *increase* the risk for hormone-sensitive cancers, such as some breast or prostate malignancies—or reduce the effects of the anticancer drug *tamoxifen* (Nolvadex).

Patients diagnosed with or at risk for these types of cancers should ask their doctors or a registered dietitian whether soy foods are appropriate for them.

■■■■

Cancer-Fighting Food Combos

Many fruits and vegetables known for their cancer-fighting properties work even better when combined.

Broccoli and tomatoes: Broccoli contains *sulforaphane*; tomatoes contain *lycopene*. Eaten together, they maximize each other's ability to fight cancer.

Soy and tea (black or green): A diet high in soy and tea can lower the risk of prostate and breast cancers.

Selenium and sulforaphane: When combined, these can have a significant effect on the genes that control cancer development. Selenium can be found in poultry, tuna, eggs and sunflower seeds. Sulforaphane can be found in broccoli, cabbage and watercress.

Andrew L. Rubman, ND, medical director, Southbury Clinic for Traditional Medicines, Southbury, CT.

Relax! We Debunk the 7 Biggest Cancer Myths

Gregory Pennock, MD, medical director, clinical research, M.D. Anderson Cancer Center, Orlando, FL. *www.mdandersonorlando.org.*

Despite all of the medical information in the media, many people are still misinformed about the realities of cancer. These misconceptions can prevent people from getting appropriate treatment. *Here, the truth behind common myths about cancer...*

Myth: Cancer is usually fatal. In a recent American Cancer Society (ACS) survey, 68% of respondents said that they believe the risk of dying from cancer is increasing. Not true. Though the number of Americans diagnosed with cancer has increased (because the US population is increasing and getting older), the risk of dying from cancer has decreased due to early detection and improved treatment. More than half of the people diagnosed with cancer survive the disease—and for some cancers, such as lymphoma and leukemia, the cure rate is between 70% and 80%.

Cancer isn't a single disease. It includes many types of tumors, all of which behave differently. Some tumors, such as those in the breast, are very responsive to chemotherapy and other treatments. Lung tumors are more resistant to treatment. The likelihood of a cure depends not only on the type of tumor but how far advanced it is at the time of diagnosis.

Myth: Cancer runs in families. Only about 8% of cancers are genetically linked. These usually are cancers that occur in younger patients, such as sarcoma or early-onset colon cancer. The vast majority of cancers occur without a known cause or are related to lifestyle.

A family history does increase the risk for certain cancers. For example, if a woman has a first-degree relative (such as a mother or sister) who developed the BRCA1 form of breast cancer at an early age, her risk for getting that cancer is higher.

However, only approximately 10% to 20% of women who are diagnosed with breast cancer have a family history of the disease. That's why it's important for every woman to undergo regular mammograms and do breast self-exams on a regular basis.

Myth: **Stress causes cancer.** There's a long-standing belief that people who experience a lot of stress or lack a positive attitude are more prone to cancer. A survey of long-term breast cancer survivors in Canada found that 42% attributed their cancer to stress.

This causes many people who have cancer to blame themselves or feel that they always have to be upbeat to prevent a recurrence.

There's no evidence that stress or a negative attitude causes cancer. In a study reported in the journal *Cancer*, 8,500 people were scored on factors such as fatigue, irritability, etc. After following the participants for almost nine years, on average, researchers found no link between emotional distress and cancer risk.

However, positive thinking may play a role in recovery. Patients who have a positive attitude are more likely to do things that improve outcomes, such as follow medical instructions and maintain a healthy lifestyle.

Myth: **Surgery causes cancer to spread.** In the ACS survey, 41% of the respondents said they believe that cancer spreads through the body during surgery.

In reality, the risk of cancer spreading during surgery is close to zero. This myth probably started in the days before early detection. It was common for doctors to find advanced cancers during surgery—even in patients who may have had only mild symptoms. Patients and their families concluded that the surgery itself made the disease worse.

Some cancers in the abdomen or ovaries produce large amounts of malignant fluid. In those cases, it's theoretically possible for cancer cells to spread if the fluid leaks into the abdomen during surgery, but there is no actual evidence that that has happened.

Myth: **Injuries cause cancer.** More than one-third of the respondents in the ACS survey thought that injuries such as a bruised breast or a hard fall could cause cancer later in life.

These types of injuries don't cause cancer. What may happen is that people hurt a part of the body, see a doctor about the injury and then learn that they have a tumor—but the tumor was already there. The injury just triggered the discovery.

Only a few cancers are caused by certain types of injuries. A serious sunburn during childhood, for example, increases the risk of skin cancer later in life. Chronic reflux disease (heartburn) can burn the esophagus and increase the risk of esophageal cancer.

Myth: **It's okay to keep smoking after a lung cancer diagnosis.** Some people believe that because the damage is done, they don't have to quit smoking—but those who continue to smoke after a lung cancer diagnosis have significantly poorer outcomes than those who quit. There's also evidence that the chemicals in cigarette smoke interfere with radiation and chemotherapy. Lung cancer patients who quit smoking respond better to the treatments.

Important: Lung cancer is the leading cause of cancer deaths in men and women. Lung tissue gradually returns to normal when people quit smoking. Ten years after quitting, lung cancer risk is reduced to one-third of what it was.

Myth: **Cell phones cause brain cancer.** Large population studies have shown no evidence that cell phones cause any kind of cancer, including brain cancer.

Cell-phone use today is much higher than it was a decade ago. If there were any truth to the cancer/cell-phone link, we would be seeing an increased incidence of brain cancers by now, but that hasn't happened.

■ ■ ■ ■

Experimental Treatments Really Work!

Experimental cancer treatments are more beneficial than previously thought.

Recent study: Approximately 11%—and in some cases, 27%—of the patients in Phase 1 cancer trials responded positively. Previous reviews showed that only 4% to 6% benefited.

Christine Grady, RN, PhD, department of clinical bioethics, Warren Grant Magnuson Clinical Center, National Institutes of Health.

5

Diabetes Update

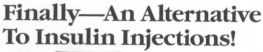

Finally—An Alternative To Insulin Injections!

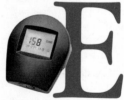

Exubera, the first inhaled insulin treatment for diabetes, has been approved by the US Food and Drug Administration (FDA), allowing millions of type 1 and type 2 diabetics the option of avoiding countless daily injections.

A NEW OPTION

Exubera is insulin that has been formulated into a dry powder that is inhaled into the lungs using a small, hand-held device. Like injected insulin, Exubera is administered before meals.

"This is the first new insulin delivery option introduced since the discovery of this drug in the 1920s," says Dr. Steve Galson, director of the FDA's Center for Drug Evaluation and Research. "There are more than 5 million Americans who take insulin injections every day, and Exubera may be an option for many of these patients. It will not replace all injectable insulin, but it's a highly innovative product that has the poten-

tial to improve the quality of life for millions of Americans with diabetes."

"This is highly positive," says Dr. Robert Rapaport, director of the division of pediatric endocrinology at Mount Sinai School of Medicine in New York City. "I think there will be some longstanding questions about its ultimate safety because it's the first inhaled medication that will be used like this. But, assuming the safety profile will be good, it will be a major advance."

Adds Dr. Stuart Weiss, a clinical assistant professor in the department of medicine at New York University School of Medicine, "There are still some questions as to lung function…and

Steven Galson, MD, director, Center for Drug Evaluation and Research, US Food and Drug Administration.

Robert Rapaport, MD, director, division of pediatric endocrinology, Mount Sinai School of Medicine, New York City.

Stuart Weiss, MD, clinical assistant professor, department of medicine (endocrinology), New York University School of Medicine, and endocrinologist, New York University Medical Center, New York City.

Robert Meyer, MD, director, Office of Drug Evaluation II, Division of Metabolic and Endocrine Drugs, Office of New Drugs, Center for Drug Evaluation and Research, US Food and Drug Administration.

smokers can't use it. There are all sorts of things to be concerned about." He believes that it's going to take a few years to see how safe it is.

SAFETY STUDIES

Studies on the safety and effectiveness of Exubera were conducted on more than 2,500 type 1 and type 2 diabetics. In fact, Pfizer Inc., the manufacturer of Exubera, apparently delayed the application for US approval for three years to finish safety studies.

"Because this is a new way to deliver insulin to patients, it has been extensively studied with respect to safety and efficacy," says Dr. Robert Meyer, director of the FDA Office of Drug Evaluation II, which oversees the Division of Metabolic and Endocrine Drugs.

"We have a large amount of data from the clinical trials speaking to the safety of this product overall, and its safety in the lungs as well. We feel that there is an extensive and reasonable safety database to allow us to make a determination of efficacy and safety for patients without underlying lung disease and who do not smoke," Meyer reports. "In addition, there are ongoing, continuing trials to monitor safety that will be reported after approval."

Exubera was found to reach peak concentrations more quickly than insulin delivered by injection. Patients who took Exubera achieved peak insulin concentration in 49 minutes, on average, compared with an average of 105 minutes when taking regular insulin, according to the FDA.

Like any insulin product, low blood sugar is a side effect of Exubera, and diabetics should carefully monitor their blood sugar regularly. Other side effects associated with Exubera in clinical trials included cough, shortness of breath, sore throat and dry mouth, the FDA reports.

A Medication Guide that contains FDA-approved information will accompany all Exubera prescriptions, the agency says.

NOT FOR EVERYONE

Exubera should not be used by smokers or by someone who quit smoking within the last six months. The drug is also not recommended for people who have asthma, bronchitis or emphysema. Baseline tests for lung function are recommended before beginning treatment, six months

after treatment begins and then repeated annually, according to the FDA.

Inhaled insulin is unlikely to completely replace injected insulin, but for many people, it may greatly improve glucose control.

"It's very hard to predict what the impact will be," Weiss says. "A lot of people who need to be on insulin are not on insulin. For that type 2 diabetic who is afraid of needles or will not take a shot, this is an ideal product."

Exubera is also unlikely to be the only inhaled insulin on the market for long. Eli Lilly and Co., Kos Pharmaceuticals Inc., MannKind Corp. and Novo Nordisk A/S all are developing their own versions.

■ ■ ■ ■

Inhaled Insulin Has Drawbacks

Exubera requires carrying a device the size of a flashlight, plus foil-wrapped insulin packets. Insulin shots are less cumbersome, quicker and virtually painless.

Other drawbacks: Long-term effects on the lungs are unknown…inhaled insulin often still requires a patient to take one or two injections of long-acting insulin each day…insurance coverage is uncertain.

Anne Peters, MD, professor of clinical medicine, Keck School of Medicine, University of Southern California, Los Angeles.

Double Trouble— Up to 30% May Have Both Type 1 and 2

Francine Kaufman, MD, pediatric endocrinologist, head of the Center for Diabetes and Endocrinology, Children's Hospital, Los Angeles, and past president, American Diabetes Association.

Stuart Weiss, MD, clinical assistant professor, department of medicine (endocrinology), New York University School of Medicine, and endocrinologist, New York University Medical Center, New York City.

Doctors are finding that an increasing number of patients who have symptoms of obesity-linked type 2 diabetes also have the more rare type 1 form of the disease.

"We call it 'double diabetes,' or hybrid diabetes," says Dr. Francine Kaufman, past president of the American Diabetes Association and head of the Center for Diabetes and Endocrinology at Children's Hospital, Los Angeles.

A GROWING NUMBER

Kaufman, a pediatric endocrinologist, says double diabetes is a phenomenon that's being increasingly recognized by doctors. In fact, recent reports suggest that up to 30% of newly diagnosed children have both type 1 and type 2.

"They may clinically look like they have type 2—be overweight and maybe have a family history of type 2—but then [their blood tests] come back positive" for type 1, Kaufman says.

Diabetes has been undertreated and undermanaged. Now we have good tools to manage it.

Stuart Weiss, MD

Alternatively, other young patients, who have had type 1 since childhood, become obese in adolescence "and then begin to look like they have elements of type 2 diabetes," Kaufman explains. "They are becoming more and more insulin-resistant."

OBESITY DRIVES THE TREND

America's obesity epidemic is clearly driving the trend toward double diabetes, experts say. And while links between obesity and type 2 diabetes have long been clear, research is only just beginning to suggest that obesity can also trigger late-onset type 1 diabetes.

Dr. Stuart Weiss, a clinical assistant professor of medicine at the New York University School of Medicine, says he is diagnosing more and more people in their 20s and 30s with double diabetes. "Many are type 1s who have already been diabetic for years, and who are also eating a hypercaloric diet and require a lot more insulin," he says. "They become obese, and then become insulin-resistant."

COMPLEX TREATMENT

Kaufman says treatment for double diabetes may be more complex than what is needed for patients who have either type 1 or type 2 alone. "It may mean that someone needs insulin *and* pills," she says.

"Whether it's type 1 or type 2, we have to look at the cardiovascular risk factors, waist-to-hip ratios, blood triglycerides and cholesterol issues that are common to all diabetics," Weiss says. "That's where I think the focus should be—not just in managing glucose, but in managing the consequences."

And, he says, good treatments are available. "Diabetes is a real problem—it has always been there, but it has been undertreated and undermanaged," Weiss says. "Now we have good tools to manage it, so there's less of an excuse for physicians not to treat it well."

PREVENTION IS BEST

Of course, prevention remains the best way to fight the disease. For parents, that means trying to have your child maintain a healthy weight, be active and eat appropriate foods in appropriate quantities, Kaufman says.

"We're looking at a world now in which the rate of diabetes just continues to increase," she says. "We should all be aware of this disease and try to minimize it in every way we can."

■ ■ ■ ■

What Type Are You?

In type 1 diabetes, which affects 5% of all diabetics, the body's immune system turns against beta cells in the pancreas that produce the insulin needed to regulate blood sugar. Type 1 diabetics typically must take daily insulin via injection to remain healthy.

Type 2 diabetes is the most common form of the disease and is often linked to obesity. In type 2 diabetes, either the body doesn't produce enough insulin—a hormone needed for the body to convert blood sugar into energy for cells—or the cells ignore the insulin. If left untreated, complications that can result include heart disease, blindness, and nerve and kidney damage, according to the American Diabetes Association.

info For more information on diabetes, visit the American Diabetes Association Web site at *www.diabetes.org*.

How to Make Sure You Don't Get Diabetes

Robert Rizza, MD, professor of medicine, Mayo Clinic College of Medicine, Rochester, MN, and president, American Diabetes Association. *www.diabetes.org.*

The epidemic of type 2 diabetes is alarming—and more dangerous than many people ever imagine. The disease, which affects 20 million Americans, increases the risk for heart attack and stroke. Complications from the disease include blindness, kidney failure, impotence and poor wound healing that can lead to amputation.

Until recently, doctors diagnosed diabetes only when a patient had full-blown symptoms, which typically develop gradually over a period of years.

Now: You can stop diabetes in its tracks if you recognize and take action against "prediabetes," which affects more than 40 million people between the ages of 40 and 74. *Here's how...*

WHEN SUGAR ISN'T SWEET

Glucose, a simple sugar molecule that is metabolized from the food you eat, is basic fuel for your body. It is broken down in cells to produce energy that powers your muscles, lets you think and keeps your heart pumping and your lungs breathing.

The hormone *insulin*, which is produced by your pancreas, plays a key role in this process, escorting glucose from the bloodstream into the cells. When there isn't enough insulin to do the job or the insulin is not effective, sugar builds up in the blood. That's when the trouble begins.

To diagnose diabetes, doctors order blood tests that measure the amount of glucose in your bloodstream. One test, *fasting plasma glucose* (FPG), checks the glucose level first thing in the morning, before you have eaten anything. A normal glucose level is less than 100 milligrams per deciliter (mg/dL).

The *oral glucose tolerance test* (OGTT) is a bit more complicated—after fasting all night, you drink a sugary liquid, and your glucose level is tested two hours later. A normal result is less than 140 mg/dL.

If your FPG is 126 mg/dL or higher...*or* the two-hour OGTT is higher than 200 mg/dL, you likely have diabetes. Your pancreas no longer secretes enough insulin for proper glucose metabolism or your body has become more resistant to its effects. This means that your risk of developing complications, such as heart disease, kidney failure or vision loss, has more than doubled.

AN EARLIER DIAGNOSIS

There is also an intermediate condition—between normal and diabetes. Fasting blood sugar of 100 to 125 mg/dL is called *impaired fasting glucose*. If the two-hour OGTT is between 140 and 200 mg/dL, it is known as *impaired glucose tolerance*.

Today, these conditions are called *prediabetes*, meaning your insulin activity has already started to fall short of the amount your body needs. And if something isn't done, there's a good chance you'll go on to develop full-blown diabetes.

What are the odds? Fasting blood sugar between 100 and 110 mg/dL means you have a 20% chance of developing diabetes within five to 10 years. If it's higher than 110, you have a 40% chance of getting diabetes. If both the fasting blood sugar and two-hour glucose tolerance tests are elevated, the odds increase even more.

At the prediabetes level, excess blood sugar has already started to take its toll. For example, the risk of heart disease is 1.5 times higher for a prediabetic than for someone who has normal blood sugar.

DO YOU HAVE PREDIABETES?

To determine whether you have prediabetes, ask your doctor for a fasting glucose test—especially if you are at increased risk due to...

- **Excess body weight.**
- **Family history of diabetes** (parent, brother or sister).
- **Diabetes during pregnancy** (gestational diabetes).
- **Asian, African-American or Hispanic ethnicity.**

If any of these risk factors applies to you, have your blood sugar checked at your next physical. After age 45, you should have it checked at least every three years. Given the high rates of diabetes today, *everyone* older than 45 should consider getting tested.

TREATMENT FOR PREDIABETES

Slightly elevated blood sugar doesn't mean you're destined to get diabetes. Fairly moderate lifestyle changes can reduce that risk by more than 50%.

Obesity increases diabetes risk. If you are overweight, bring your weight down by 5% to 10%. Ideally, your weight should be brought down to the normal range, which means a body mass index (BMI), a ratio of weight to height, of 18.5 to 24.9. To find your BMI, use the free calculator at the National Heart, Lung and Blood Institute Web site at *http://nhlbisupport.com/bmi*. Or use the formula (weight in pounds × 703) ÷ height in inches squared.

Important finding: A Finnish study of 522 middle-aged, overweight people who had prediabetes found that diabetes risk was reduced by 58% among those who participated in diet *and* exercise programs for three years compared with those in a control group, who experienced no reduction.

How to stop prediabetes…

•**Diet wisely.** Consuming fewer calories than you burn is the key to weight loss. Some research also suggests that reducing saturated fat (most beef and some dairy products), and the resulting weight loss that can occur, helps reverse prediabetes, allowing your body to use insulin more efficiently. A diet that is rich in complex carbohydrates, such as fruits, vegetables and whole grains, will meet these goals—and is best for *everyone's* general health.

•**Exercise regularly.** Physical activity helps control your weight and improves your body's ability to use insulin. Aim for at least 30 minutes of exercise five or more days a week. The type of exercise doesn't seem to matter, as long as it requires modest exertion—brisk walking, swimming, riding a bike, etc.

•**Forgo medication.** Blood sugar in people who have prediabetes can be reduced using prescription diabetes medication such as *metformin* (Glucophage). However, research suggests that this drug is not as effective as diet and exercise in preventing diabetes.

Important finding: In a *New England Journal of Medicine* study, 3,234 men and women who had prediabetes were randomly assigned to a lifestyle program or to the drug metformin.

After three years, weight loss and exercise reduced diabetes incidence by 58%, while drug treatment reduced diabetes incidence by only 31%.

■■■■

Diabetes Improves After Weight-Loss Surgery

In a study, 84% of obese diabetics who underwent gastric bypass surgery had normal blood sugar (glucose) levels after surgery. Most of these patients were able to discontinue their diabetes medication shortly after surgery.

Theory: The weight-loss surgery, which allows food to bypass part of the small intestine, may alter the secretion of gastrointestinal hormones that increase insulin levels.

David E. Cummings, MD, associate professor of medicine, division of metabolism, endocrinology and nutrition, University of Washington, Seattle.

Beyond Glucose: Better Ways to Know Your Risk

Amir Tirosh, MD, internist and researcher, department of internal medicine, Sheba Medical Center, and former head of the research and project development section, Israeli Defense Forces Medical Corps., Tel-Hashomer, Israel. *The New England Journal of Medicine*.

Blood sugar levels at the high end of "normal," coupled with other risk factors for type 2 diabetes, may help identify apparently healthy men who are at an increased risk of the disease, a new Israeli study suggests.

THE STUDY

For the study, the researchers obtained fasting glucose levels for more than 13,000 men from the Israeli Defense Forces, all between the ages of 26 and 45. During the average 5.7 years of follow-up, 208 of the men were diagnosed with type 2 diabetes.

Men who had fasting blood sugar levels at the high end of normal—95 to 99 milligrams per deciliter (mg/dL) of blood—had approximately three times the risk of developing type 2 diabetes as men who had blood sugar levels that were less than 81 mg/dL.

Men who had other risk factors, such as obesity, as well as high-normal blood glucose readings were even more likely to develop type 2 diabetes. Obese men who had fasting glucose levels between 91 and 99 mg/dL had eight times the risk of developing the disease, compared with nonobese men who had blood glucose readings of less than 86 mg/dL, the study found.

> *A 'normal' glucose level may have to be defined in a more individualized manner.*
>
> Amir Tirosh, MD

High triglyceride levels and a family history of the disease also increased the risk of diabetes for those men who had high-normal blood sugar levels.

Study author Dr. Amir Tirosh, an internist and researcher at the department of internal medicine at Sheba Medical Center, says he believes the study's findings also apply to women.

ADDITIONAL RISK FACTORS

The National Institute for Diabetes and Digestive and Kidney Diseases considers normal fasting blood sugar to be below 99 mg/dL. Fasting blood sugar between 100 and 125 mg/dL is considered prediabetic, and above 125 mg/dL is diabetic. However, the study suggests that these current standard guidelines are not appropriate for everyone.

"The results suggest that a 'normal' glucose level [one that is not associated with increased diabetes risk] may have to be defined in a more individualized manner depending on a person's additional risk factors," says Tirosh.

"People and physicians should not look only at the current definition of normal and abnormal blood glucose levels when assessing an individual's risk to develop diabetes. A careful interpretation of the body mass index, the triglyceride level and the patient's family history of diabetes is [also] needed in order to better identify those at high risk," Tirosh adds.

"Identifying individuals at high risk for diabetes, particularly among young adults, will hopefully prove beneficial in reducing the epidemic proportions of the disease," says Tirosh, the former head of research and project development section of the Israeli Defense Forces Medical Corps.

The new study suggests that more people may be prediabetic even if their glucose levels are in the normal range. If these people are identified early, they can take steps to reduce potential health problems. Those steps can include exercise, improved diet and/or medication.

info For more information on how type 2 diabetes is diagnosed and how to prevent it, visit the National Diabetes Information Clearinghouse at *http://diabetes.niddk.nih.gov/dm/pubs/diagnosis.*

■ ■ ■ ■

61% of Diabetics Don't Know About this Critical Test

The *A1C* test shows average blood sugar levels over the past 120 days. The test is done by a lab or in your doctor's office in addition to home monitoring of blood sugar. The A1C test tells whether diabetes treatment is working effectively —but 61% of diabetics recently surveyed did not know what it was. The A1C test can help diabetics adjust diet, activity and medication to avoid possible complications from the disease. Ask your doctor how often you should have an A1C test.

Robert Rizza, MD, professor of medicine, Mayo Clinic College of Medicine, Rochester, MN, and president, American Diabetes Association. *www.diabetes.org.*

Blood Sugar: Why It's Important Even If You're Not Diabetic

Thomas M.S. Wolever, MD, PhD, professor of nutritional science, University of Toronto Faculty of Medicine, Ontario, Canada, and coauthor of *The Glucose Revolution: The Authoritative Guide to the Glycemic Index.* Marlowe & Co.

Although all carbohydrates share the same basic chemical composition, all carbohydrates are *not* equal. Eating the right type of "carbs" will help you control your weight...cut your risk for heart disease and diabetes...and minimize your risk for the low blood sugar condition known as *hypoglycemia*.

More good news: Cakes, cookies and other carbohydrate-rich foods that are often considered taboo can be part of a healthful diet—in moderation.

WHAT *ARE* CARBOHYDRATES?

People often describe bread, potatoes, pasta and certain other foods as carbohydrates. Actually, carbohydrates are a chemical constituent of many different foods. *They encompass...*

●**The simple sugars** *glucose* and *fructose.*

●**More complex sugars,** such as *sucrose* and *lactose*, which are made up of two simple sugars that are linked.

●**Starches,** even more complex molecules, which are made up of thousands of linked glucose molecules.

Bread contains carbohydrates, but it also contains protein, fat, vitamins, minerals and other nutrients.

Milk isn't generally thought of as a carbohydrate, but it contains significant amounts of lactose...as well as protein, fat, calcium and, of course, water.

CARBS AND YOUR BODY

The digestive process converts carbohydrates into glucose (blood sugar). That's the basic "fuel" used by every cell in the body.

As the amount of glucose that's circulating in the bloodstream rises, the pancreas boosts its production of insulin. That's the hormone needed to "burn" glucose for energy.

Foods that have roughly comparable carbohydrate content can have *very* different effects on blood sugar. Some carbs raise blood sugar levels sharply. Others have little effect.

To gauge a particular food's effect on blood sugar levels, scientists use what is known as the *glycemic index.* At the top of this 100-point scale is glucose. Consumption of glucose causes the sharpest rise in blood sugar. Other foods fall lower on the scale. The higher a food's glycemic index, the greater its effect on blood sugar levels.

The chief determinant of the glycemic index of a particular food is the *speed at which it is digested.* Carbs that break down into glucose quickly raise blood sugar sharply. Slow-digesting carbs keep blood sugar levels on an even keel.

What determines the speed of digestion? A food's particle size. The smaller the particles, the faster the food is digested and the higher its glycemic index.

Milling, baking, cooking in water and other forms of processing increase starch *gelatinization*, which increases the glycemic index. That's why processed foods have high glycemic indices.

Example: Canned pasta, which is cooked for a long time, has a higher glycemic index than pasta cooked *al dente.*

GLYCEMIC INDEX AND HEALTH

The body operates best when blood sugar stays at a constant level. *Increasing the proportion of low-glycemic index foods in your diet...*

●**Promotes weight loss.** Carbs are natural appetite suppressants. Low-glycemic index foods remain in the digestive tract longer and so provide a lasting feeling of satiety.

●**Lowers the risk of diabetes.** The risk of developing *adult-onset* (type 2) diabetes is determined largely by heredity. But diet may be what determines which at-risk people go on to develop diabetes.

Cells that are repeatedly subjected to surges of insulin eventually become less sensitive to its effects. Eventually, the pancreas can't produce enough insulin to overcome the cells' *insulin resistance*...and diabetes develops.

By preventing blood sugar surges, low-glycemic index foods help forestall insulin resistance. A Harvard study that involved more than 100,000 people found that a high-glycemic index, low-fiber diet more than *doubled* diabetes risk.

If you have diabetes, eating a low-glycemic index diet helps keep glucose levels—and therefore, insulin levels—in check. That helps prevent insulin resistance, allowing insulin or antidiabetes drugs to work more efficiently. This may help reduce the risk of complications, such as kidney disease.

●**Guards against heart disease.** Because low-glycemic index foods help prevent diabetes and obesity, they reduce the risk of developing heart disease.

Low-glycemic index eating also fights heart disease by raising the levels of HDL ("good") cholesterol, which carries fat away from the coronary arteries. And while a carbohydrate-rich diet can boost heart attack risk by raising triglyceride levels, this won't occur if most of the carbs have a low glycemic index.

Evidence: In the famed Harvard Nurses' Health Study, women who ate a low-glycemic index diet had *half* the heart attack risk as similar women who consumed many high-glycemic index foods.

•**Reduces the risk of hypoglycemia.** Some people experience weakness, drowsiness and/or anxiety after eating—because abnormally high insulin levels cause blood sugar to fall precipitously. Low-glycemic index eating helps dampen these swings.

LOW GLYCEMIC EATING

You needn't eliminate all high-glycemic index foods from your diet. Just include enough low-glycemic index foods to bring down the average glycemic index.

Breakfast: Choose oatmeal (glycemic index, 49)…muesli (56)…or cereals like Kellogg's Bran Buds with Psyllium (45).

Bread: Whole-grain pumpernickel (51)…sourdough (52)…and stone-ground whole wheat (52) have lower glycemic indices than whole-wheat or white bread (69 to 70).

Starches: Pasta (30 to 45) should be a mainstay of your diet. Pearled barley (25) and bulgur (48) have lower glycemic indices than white rice (72). Boiled potatoes (62) are better than baked potatoes (85) or instant mashed potatoes (86).

Legumes: Lentils (30), chickpeas (33), kidney beans (27) and other beans are low in fat and high in fiber.

Fruits and Vegetables: Fruits have glycemic indices ranging from 40 to 55. Vegetables are a bit higher, but their carbohydrate content is too low to affect blood sugar very much.

Snacks: Flavored, low-fat yogurt is a good snack—it has a glycemic index of 33. While pastries, candy and ice cream are too fatty and calorie-dense to be more than an occasional indulgence, their glycemic indices are the same as the glycemic index of bread.

You might expect table sugar and honey to have the highest glycemic indices. In fact, each has a glycemic index that is approximately the same as white or whole-wheat bread.

Explanation: Honey and table sugar break down into fructose as well as glucose. Fructose is converted into glucose very slowly.

Women Lower Diabetes Risk with Coffee

Mark A. Pereira, PhD, associate professor of epidemiology and community health, University of Minnesota, Minneapolis.
Rob van Dam, PhD, research scientist, Harvard School of Public Health, Boston.
Archives of Internal Medicine.

In an 11-year study, drinking coffee cut women's risk of developing diabetes. The greatest reduction in risk was seen in participants who drank decaffeinated coffee, according to researchers.

THE STUDY

In the study, researchers gathered data on nearly 29,000 older women who answered questions about their risk factors for diabetes, such as age, body mass index (BMI), physical activity and smoking. They also reported on their consumption of various foods and beverages, including regular and decaffeinated coffee.

Adjusting for these risk factors, the researchers found that women who drank more than six cups of any type of coffee daily were 22% less likely to develop type 2 diabetes compared with those who did not drink coffee.

Diabetes risk dropped even more—by 33%—for those who drank more than six cups of decaf per day, the study authors found.

THE ANTIOXIDANT EFFECT

"In our study, for whatever reason, it doesn't look like caffeine has anything to do with [the reduction in diabetes risk]," says lead researcher Mark A. Pereira, an associate professor of epidemiology and community health at the University of Minnesota, Minneapolis.

Pereira points out that coffee has many components, including powerful antioxidant chemicals similar to those found in berries and grapes. "When you get up to four or five or more cups per day, you might have very powerful antioxidant activity," he says.

Rob van Dam, who was part of a research team in the Netherlands that first reported the protective effect of coffee, was not surprised by the results of this study.

"People think that if coffee causes it, it must be the caffeine. But coffee is a very complex mixture," van Dam says.

One component of coffee, *chlorogenic acid*, seems to be able to slow the absorption of sugar by cells. Studies in rats found that this molecule lowered blood-sugar levels, he says.

In addition to coffee, chlorogenic acid is abundant in both red wine and chocolate. "People think that nutritionists are always recommending things they don't like, but that's not true," he says.

Still, van Dam and Pereira agree that it's much too early to single out any one component of coffee as beneficial. "Clearly, the next step is experimental studies in humans," van Dam says.

info Find out if you're at risk for type 2 diabetes at the American Diabetes Association Web site, *www.diabetes.org/risk-test/text-version.jsp.*

■■■■

Cheers! Moderate Drinking May Cut Diabetes Risk

People who consume one or two standard alcoholic drinks per day are approximately 30% less likely to develop type 2 diabetes than people who don't drink at all. The risk reduction is the same whether a person has one or two drinks.

Caution: Drinking more than three alcoholic beverages a day raises diabetes risk. Ask your doctor if daily alcohol is right for you.

Lando L.J. Koppes, PhD, researcher, VU University Medical Center, EMGO Institute, Amsterdam.

The Hormone that May Stop Type 1 Diabetes

Franck Mauvais-Jarvis, MD, PhD, assistant professor, department of medicine, division of diabetes, endocrinology & metabolism, and department of molecular and cellular biology, Baylor College of Medicine, Houston.
Robert Rizza, MD, professor of medicine, Mayo Clinic College of Medicine, Rochester, MN, and president, American Diabetes Association.
Proceedings of the National Academy of Sciences.

Animal research suggests that a naturally produced estrogen hormone known as *estradiol* might help protect against diabetes by preventing the death of pancreatic cells that are critical to the production of insulin.

The findings are based on research using mice and have not yet been tested in a human trial.

"This is the first study that shows that the female hormone estradiol is important to ensuring pancreatic beta-cell survival in both females and males," says study coauthor Dr. Franck Mauvais-Jarvis, an assistant professor in the department of medicine in the division of diabetes, endocrinology & metabolism at Baylor College of Medicine in Houston.

THE STUDY

Knowing that the death of insulin-producing pancreatic beta-cells causes type 1 diabetes, Mauvais-Jarvis and his colleagues attempted to isolate estradiol's impact on this beta-cell destruction.

The researchers looked at both male and female mice that were either unable to produce estradiol or had abnormal estradiol functioning.

All of the mice experienced severe beta-cell death as well as dramatically lower-than-normal levels of insulin production—leading to the onset of type 1 diabetes.

However, after the scientists administered targeted doses of estradiol to the mice, the pancreatic beta-cells were "rescued" from death, insulin production resumed and diabetes was averted.

The researchers conclude that—at least in mice—estradiol appears to protect against the chain of events that leads to type 1 diabetes.

CAUTIOUSLY OPTIMISTIC

Mauvais-Jarvis is cautiously optimistic that his study might one day benefit humans who are at risk for diabetes. "One has to be cautious, because this study has been performed in mice, and although the mouse is the best available model to study human diseases, mice are not humans," he says.

Still, Mauvais-Jarvis says the study indicates that estradiol may offer a new clinical route for the prevention of diabetes in women and men.

He stresses, however, that estrogen-replacement therapy isn't always an option, given the recent findings that such treatment appears to raise the risk of breast cancer, heart disease, stroke and blood clots. Rather, he suggests that, "the future goal is to try to dissect the good and the bad uses of estradiol," in an effort to develop medicines that could prevent beta-cell deaths and diabetes without causing harmful side effects.

Dr. Robert Rizza, a professor of medicine at the Mayo Clinic College of Medicine, and president of the American Diabetes Association, calls the findings of the study "intriguing."

"There have been various studies that have shown that estrogen may lower the risk for developing diabetes, and this study shows why this might be the case," he says.

"It may or may not be true for humans. But it will teach us more about how estrogen works. And if it turns out to be [true], it could be used for other novel therapies to prevent diabetes."

Breast-Feeding May Lower Moms' Risk of Diabetes

Alison Stuebe, MD, clinical fellow in maternal–fetal medicine, Brigham and Women's Hospital, and instructor, Harvard Medical School, both in Boston.

Loren Wissner Greene, MD, endocrinologist, New York University Medical Center, and clinical associate professor of medicine, New York University School of Medicine, New York City.

The Journal of the American Medical Association.

Breast-feeding can lower the risk of developing type 2 diabetes, according to recent research.

THE STUDY

Scientists have suspected that breast-feeding might affect the risk of developing type 2 diabetes because previous research has shown that it improves insulin sensitivity and glucose tolerance.

However, no long-term studies had examined the effect of breast-feeding on the mother's risk of diabetes.

Study author, Dr. Alison Stuebe, a clinical fellow in maternal–fetal medicine at Brigham and Women's Hospital, and an instructor at Harvard Medical School, and her colleagues used data from the Nurses' Health Study and the Nurses' Health Study II, which together included more than 150,000 women who had given birth during the study period. More than 6,000 of these women were diagnosed with type 2 diabetes.

After controlling for *body mass index* (BMI) (a high BMI is a known risk factor for type 2 diabetes) the researchers discovered that long-term breast-feeding reduced a woman's risk of developing diabetes. The risk was reduced by 15% for each year of breast-feeding for women in the Nurses' Health Study, and by 14% for each year of breast-feeding for those in the Nurses' Health Study II.

POSSIBLE EXPLANATIONS

Stuebe says the researchers were not able to determine how breast-feeding might offer some protection against diabetes, but they suspect that it may help keep blood sugar in balance.

Breast-feeding mothers burn almost 500 additional calories daily, according to the study. That's equivalent to running approximately four to five miles a day, Stuebe notes. "If done for a year, it's not surprising that it might have an effect on how the body takes care of insulin and glucose," she says.

Dr. Loren Wissner Greene, an endocrinologist at New York University Medical Center, says the explanation could be simple—"The small weight changes from lactation can make a significant impact on diabetes risk."

In fact, Wissner Greene says, the best advice for anyone to avoid type 2 diabetes is to achieve and maintain a healthy weight.

Another possible explanation is that women who breast-feed for a long time are more health-conscious than other women—they may have a healthier diet, they may exercise more and they may do other health-promoting activities that could reduce their diabetes risk.

Stuebe says the researchers tried to take these lifestyle factors into account and they still saw an association between breast-feeding and reduced diabetes risk.

The bottom line, concludes Stuebe, is that breast-feeding is "an intervention that doesn't cost anything, has no side effects and has other potential benefits."

■ ■ ■ ■

Breast-Feeding Benefits

Breast-feeding offers a host of health benefits for babies. Along with providing optimal nutrition, breast milk also provides compounds that boost babies' immune system and help protect them from bacteria, viruses and parasites, according to the US Food and Drug Administration (FDA). In addition, breast-fed children have lower rates of childhood illnesses and tend to be leaner than their formula-fed counterparts.

And research has shown that breast-feeding benefits mothers as well, by helping the body return to normal faster after pregnancy, according to the FDA. Some studies have also suggested that women who breast-feed for a long time may have lower rates of breast and ovarian cancer.

info You can find out more about the benefits of breast-feeding for both mom and baby from The National Women's Health Information Center at *www.4woman.gov/breastfeeding*. Click on "Benefits of Breastfeeding."

The 4 Biggest Mistakes Diabetics Make

Paul S. Jellinger, MD, professor of medicine, voluntary faculty, University of Miami School of Medicine; endocrinologist, Center for Diabetes and Endocrine Care, Hollywood, FL; immediate past president, American College of Endocrinology; and past president, American Association of Clinical Endocrinologists (AACE).

Only one-third of the 18 million Americans who have type 2 diabetes can successfully control their blood sugar, according to a discouraging report presented at an American Association of Clinical Endocrinologists (AACE) conference.

This means that approximately 12 million diabetics are at a dramatically increased risk for heart attack, stroke, blindness, kidney failure and other complications that can result when elevated blood sugar (glucose) permanently damages nerves and blood vessels.

Good news: Although increases in obesity rates and a sedentary lifestyle have made diabetes three times more common today than it was 40 years ago, the disease almost always can be controlled—or prevented—by avoiding mistakes in treatment and self-care…

Mistake 1: **Not knowing (or controlling) A1C levels.** Controlling glucose is the key to effective diabetes treatment. The best indicator of long-term glucose control is the *A1C blood test*, which shows the average glucose level during the preceding three months. A blood glucose test is less meaningful because it reveals the person's glucose level only at the time of testing.

A recent study of 157,000 diabetes patients showed that two-thirds had A1C scores that were higher than 6.5…and one-fifth to one-third had levels above 9. (A normal A1C level is less than 6.)

A survey found that 81% of people who have type 2 diabetes *think* they're doing a good job of managing blood sugar, even though most don't even know what the A1C test is.

It's critical for patients to maintain an optimal A1C level. For every one-point drop in elevated A1C, the risk for serious diabetes complications, such as kidney failure or blindness, drops by 25% to 40%.

Recommendation: If your A1C levels have remained normal for six months, get the test twice annually. If you have been recently diagnosed with diabetes or have trouble maintaining tight control of your glucose levels, get the test every three months.

Caution: If glucose control is poor and you have had substantial changes in medications and/or dosages, the test may need to be performed at six- to eight-week intervals.

Mistake 2: **Misusing home tests.** Home glucose testing provides valuable information about foods that cause excessive increases in glucose as well as the physical symptoms (headache, fatigue, etc.) that often accompany these glucose swings. But these tests work only when used properly. *Common errors...*

●Testing too infrequently. All type 2 diabetics should self-test blood glucose levels. Most should test once a day.

Even better: Many patients benefit from testing two or three times daily because it gives a more accurate assessment of glucose fluctuations.

●Testing only before meals. Experts have traditionally recommended premeal testing to obtain a fasting glucose level. It's just as important—perhaps more so—to test after meals, since most of the day is spent in the postmeal, or *postprandial*, state. (Three to five hours after each meal is considered postprandial, making a total of 9 to 15 hours daily.) Diabetics should know whether their glucose levels rise after meals because these increases appear to be linked to blood vessel damage.

Recommendation: Vary the times of testing.

Example: Always do a fasting test in the morning, then check before dinner one day, and before bedtime on another. Perform a test two hours after eating at least a few times a week.

Red flag: A glucose reading of 140 or higher two hours after the beginning of a meal...or 110 or higher before a meal. Talk to your doctor if you get these readings more than half the time.

Mistake 3: **Delaying drug treatment.** More than 40% of people who have prediabetes (a fasting glucose level of 100 to 125) eventually will develop full-fledged diabetes. Starting drug treatment during the prediabetes stage greatly reduces the risk for future diabetes-related complications.

Recommendation: In most cases, if you don't achieve normal glucose levels after trying lifestyle changes (improving your diet, losing weight, exercising, etc.) for three months, ask your doctor about starting medication. *Examples...*

●Metformin (Glucophage) is an oral drug that inhibits the release of glucose from the liver and reduces the body's need for insulin. In a six-year study, prediabetics who took metformin reduced their risk of diabetes by 31%.

Bonus: Metformin is less likely than other diabetes drugs to cause weight gain. Nausea and other gastrointestinal side effects are usually temporary.

●Sulfonybureas, such as *glipizide* (Glucotrol) and *glyburide* (Glynase), stimulate the pancreas to produce more insulin. Side effects include low blood sugar and weight gain. These drugs are frequently combined with metformin, resulting in an additional decrease in A1C.

●Thiazolidinediones, such as *pioglitazone* (Actos) and *rosiglitazonte* (Avandia), increase the body's sensitivity to insulin. They are often combined with metformin, insulin or other medications to further lower A1C levels. Side effects include fluid retention and weight gain.

●Insulin injections may be required when a patient is unable to achieve adequate glucose control after taking two or three oral drugs for three months. Injections are simple to administer and virtually painless.

Breakthrough: The US Food and Drug Administration (FDA) recently approved a new drug, *exenatide* (Byetta), for people who cannot adequately control glucose levels using other drugs. Taken by injection twice daily, it's called a "smart" drug because it stimulates the pancreas to produce insulin based on the level of blood sugar.

Exenatide mimics the effects of the intestinal hormone *incretin*, which is not produced adequately in diabetics. The drug slows stomach emptying...inhibits increases in postprandial glucose levels...and acts as an appetite suppressant. Nausea may occur but it's usually temporary.

Mistake 4: **Not eating and/or exercising properly.** These two factors are the cornerstones of diabetes prevention and management. If people who are at risk for diabetes eat nutritiously and lose as little as 5% to 10% of body weight, they are better able to use their natural insulin to remove glucose from the blood.

Exercise is equally important. Prediabetics who engage in 30 minutes of moderate-intensity aerobic exercise five days per week can reduce their risk of progressing to diabetes by 58%.

Recommendation: Substitute whole-grain products for refined grains, such as white bread ...limit fat consumption...and exercise for at least 30 minutes on most days of the week.

Elderly Diabetics Twice as Likely to Fall

Columbia University news release.

Diabetic nursing home residents are much more likely to have dangerous falls than those who do not have diabetes, researchers report.

THE RESEARCH

A study of 139 residents at the Hebrew Home at Riverdale in Riverdale, New York, found that 78% of those who had diabetes fell during the 299-day study period, compared with 30% of residents who were not diabetic.

"Our study clearly indicated that nursing homes, assisted-living facilities and others that care for the elderly should consider diabetes a significant risk factor for falling," says researcher Dr. Mathew S. Maurer, assistant professor of medicine at Columbia University Medical Center and director of the Clinical Cardiovascular Research Laboratory for the Elderly at New York-Presbyterian/The Allen Pavilion.

REDUCING THE RISK

"In an era of limited resources, knowing that diabetics are more likely to fall may facilitate identifying older individuals who are likely to benefit from interventions aimed at reducing falls and their consequences," Maurer says.

He says diabetics may be at an increased risk of falling due to problems with the peripheral nerves that affect sensation in the feet.

"We will now add diabetes to the list of risk factors for falling and expect this to become standard practice," says Dr. Robert Zorowitz, chief medical officer of the Hebrew Home at Riverdale. "By controlling diabetes, addressing the complications it causes and being vigilant about the other factors that contribute to falls, we may substantially reduce the risk."

Falling is the leading cause of accidental death among elderly people in the United States. Previous studies identified gait or balance disorders, vision impairment and medications as risk factors for falls among frail elderly nursing home residents. However, diabetes has not been recognized as an important risk factor.

info The National Institute on Aging can provide more information on how to prevent falls and fractures at *www.niapublications.org/agepages/falls.asp.*

■ ■ ■ ■

When 'Going Downhill' Is Good

A study has found that walking downhill increases glucose tolerance (a person's ability to use blood sugar) by 25%, compared with only a 9.4% increase when walking uphill. That's important for people who are obese or who have diabetes, heart failure or another condition that makes it difficult to perform vigorous exercise.

Theory: Eccentric muscle work (as in stepping down) helps the body make more efficient use of glucose.

Self-defense: Talk to your doctor about starting a downhill walking regimen or adding one to your current workout.

Heinz Drexel, MD, professor of medicine, Academic Teaching Hospital, Feldkirch, Austria.

6

Drug News

More 'Black-Box' Drugs Are Being Prescribed Incorrectly

In a recent sampling, nearly 42% of US patients were receiving prescriptions for drugs that had "black-box" warning labels. The labels—printed in a black frame in the package insert as well as on all promotional materials—advise people of the potential risks of using that medication and represent the US Food and Drug Administration's (FDA) highest warning.

"We need to think about communicating the risks of drugs more effectively," says study author Anita Wagner, an assistant professor of ambulatory care and prevention at Harvard Medical School in Boston.

THE STUDY

Although approximately 200 classes of drugs (including birth control pills) carry black-box warnings, there has been little information on how prescribers' actual practice conforms with the recommendations.

In what may be the first large study on the subject, Wagner and her colleagues looked at the medications that currently carry black-box warnings, and sought to determine how frequently these drugs are used and if they are prescribed in compliance with the stated recommendations for patient safety.

The study was a retrospective look at the records of people enrolled in 10 managed-care organizations.

RESULTS

"We found that drugs with black-box warnings are used very frequently, with more than 40% [of the people studied] receiving such drugs," Wagner says.

Guidelines suggesting that a lab test be performed before certain drugs were prescribed

Anita Wagner, PharmD, MPH, DrPH, assistant professor, department of ambulatory care and prevention, Harvard Medical School, Boston.

B. Jay Brooks, Jr., MD, chairman, hematology/oncology, Ochsner Clinic Foundation, Baton Rouge, LA.
Pharmacoepidemiology and Drug Safety.

were not followed in nearly half (49.6%) of the prescriptions.

The most common omission was the recommendation for a pregnancy test when a woman was given a new prescription.

In addition, almost 13% of the patients who were taking drugs that required them to be monitored by ongoing lab tests did not receive such monitoring, according to the study.

> *We need to think about communicating the risks of drugs more effectively.*
>
> Anita Wagner, PharmD, MPH, DrPH

Also, 9% of the prescriptions were written on the same day as a prescription for another drug that could be hazardous when combined with the first.

These prescriptions involved *methotrexate* (a cancer drug) that was prescribed along with *nonsteroidal anti-inflammatory drugs* (NSAIDs) or *ketorolac* (for pain relief) that was also prescribed along with other NSAIDs.

IMPROVEMENTS

More precise wording on the warning labels may help make people more aware of the potential risks, the researchers say.

The study authors also recommend that the FDA establish and maintain a list of current black-box warning medications, as well as illnesses and conditions that may be adversely affected by these drugs.

Another suggestion is for the pharmacist to give the patient the literature that is in the black-box warning before they take the medication, says Dr. B. Jay Brooks, Jr., chairman of hematology/oncology at the Ochsner Clinic Foundation in Baton Rouge, Louisiana. "That would force another level of safety to be added," he says.

info To find out more information on the medications that have black-box warnings, visit the US Food and Drug Administration's Office of Drug Safety at *www.fda.gov/cder/offices/ods.*

The Many Dangers of Over-the-Counter Drugs

Larry Sasich, PharmD, MPH, a licensed pharmacist, public policy expert and pharmaceutical research analyst for Public Citizen, a nonprofit consumer advocacy organization, Washington, DC. He teaches drug information and policy at the School of Pharmacy, Lake Erie College of Osteopathic Medicine, Erie, PA, and is coauthor of *Worst Pills, Best Pills: A Consumer's Guide to Avoiding Drug-Induced Death or Illness.* Pocket. *www.worstpills.org.*

Just because a medication is available without a doctor's prescription doesn't mean that it's risk-free. Over-the-counter (OTC) drugs can be dangerous.

Example: The leading cause of acute liver failure isn't alcohol or hepatitis but an overdose of *acetaminophen*, the active ingredient in Tylenol.

OTC drugs can be dangerous even when taken in the recommended dosages. *Here are common OTC medications and their dangers…*

NSAIDs

The class of medications called *nonsteroidal anti-inflammatory drugs* (NSAIDs) relieve pain, tenderness, inflammation and stiffness.

Popular brands: Ibuprofen is in Advil, Excedrin IB, Midol Cramp, Motrin and Nuprin… *naproxen* is in Aleve… *ketoprofen* is in OrudisKT.

Dangers: Gastrointestinal irritation as well as bleeding…peptic ulcers…kidney complications …reduced effectiveness of some blood pressure–lowering medications…rebound headaches (the pain reliever itself can cause headaches as the medication builds up in the body).

What to do: Before taking an NSAID, consult a doctor if you are older than age 60 and you are taking a prescription anticoagulant, steroid, diuretic or hypertension drug daily.

ASPIRIN

Aspirin is a type of NSAID that relieves mild to moderate pain…reduces fever and swelling… and reduces the risk of heart attack and stroke.

Popular brands: Alka-Seltzer Effervescent Pain Reliever and Antacid, Bayer Aspirin, Excedrin Extra Strength, St. Joseph Adult Chewable Aspirin.

Dangers: Stomach upset…vomiting…ulcers …inhibited blood clotting. Children younger than age 18 who have chicken pox or flu can develop a rare, life-threatening condition called Reye's syndrome.

What to do: Take aspirin with a full glass of water or milk, or try coated tablets to avoid stomach upset.

Consult your doctor if you are taking blood thinners, corticosteroids, such as *hydrocortisone* or *prednisone,* or medications for gout or hypertension—all can react negatively with aspirin.

ACETAMINOPHEN

Relieves pain and fever.

Popular brands: Tylenol, Excedrin Quick-Tabs. Many OTC products contain acetaminophen along with other active ingredients. These include Allerest, Sine-Off, St. Joseph Cold Tablets for Children, Sudafed Non-Drowsy Sinus Headache.

Dangers: Liver damage.

What to do: Avoid taking multisymptom OTC medicines that duplicate ingredients.

Important: If you regularly have more than three alcoholic drinks daily, consult your doctor.

CALCIUM CARBONATE

Relieves heartburn, acid indigestion and other stomach upset.

Popular brands: Alka-Mints, Caltrate 600, Rolaids Calcium Rich, Tums.

Dangers: May decrease the effectiveness of certain prescription medicines, including the heart drug *digoxin,* the anticonvulsant *phenytoin* and the antibiotic *tetracycline.*

What to do: Consult your doctor if you are taking any prescription drug. Do not take calcium carbonate within two hours of taking any other medication.

DIPHENHYDRAMINE

An antihistamine that relieves red, irritated, itchy, watery eyes…sneezing…and runny nose caused by hay fever, allergies and the common cold. It also may relieve the itching that is caused by insect bites, sunburn and poison ivy. It is used in sleep aids as well because it causes drowsiness.

Popular brands: Benadryl, Excedrin PM, Sominex, Tylenol PM, Unisom.

Dangers: Drowsiness, decreased mental alertness, memory loss.

What to do: Avoid exceeding the maximum dosage (generally 100 milligrams [mg] every four to six hours). This can easily happen if, for example, you're taking an antihistamine and a sleep aid that both contain diphenhydramine. Don't drive a car or operate machinery until you know how this drug affects you.

PSEUDOEPHEDRINE

A decongestant that relieves stuffy nose and clogged sinuses caused by colds, allergies and hay fever.

Popular brands: Sinutab, Sudafed. Some OTC products, such as Advil Cold and Sinus Caplets and Tylenol Sinus Daytime, contain pseudoephedrine along with other active ingredients.

Dangers: Increased blood pressure…rapid heart beat…insomnia.

What to do: Avoid caffeinated beverages because they can increase restlessness and insomnia. Do not use pseudoephedrine if you have taken an MAO inhibitor (a type of antidepressant) within the last two weeks—the combination can cause dangerously high blood pressure.

Consult a doctor if you have hypertension, an overactive thyroid gland or difficulty urinating due to an enlarged prostate gland—pseudoephedrine can aggravate these conditions.

DEXTROMETHORPHAN

An antitussive that relieves a dry (nonproductive) cough caused by a cold or flu.

Popular brands: Benylin Cough Suppressant, Robitussin DM Cough Syrup, Sucrets 8-Hour Cough Suppressant, Vicks 44 Cough Relief.

Dangers: Dizziness, even hallucinations and seizures, if taken in excessive doses (more than 10 times the recommended dosage of 30 mg daily).

What to do: Follow the dosage recommendation on the label. Use the measuring device that comes with the medication, not a household tablespoon or teaspoon. If you misplace the device, ask your pharmacist for an appropriate replacement.

info For more information, contact the Office of Nonprescription Products at the US Food and Drug Administration Web site, *www.fda.gov/cder/index.html.* Click on "Drug Information," then "Over-the-Counter Drug Information." Or call 301-827-2222. For a chart of drugs that contain acetaminophen or NSAIDs, go to *http://familydoctor.org/otc/knowmeds.html.*

■■■■

Don't Play Doctor with Over-the-Counter Drugs

It's Sunday night, and your child has a cough. Should you run to the pharmacy and grab a bottle of cough syrup?

The US Food and Drug Administration's (FDA) Center for Drug Evaluation and Research has some sound advice for parents who are trying to help ease their child's symptoms without making a trip to the doctor...

•**Don't estimate the dose based on your child's size.** Read the label and follow all directions carefully.

•**Follow any age limits** on the label.

•**Some over-the-counter (OTC) products come in different strengths.** Make sure you know what strength you are using.

•**Know the difference between TBSP (tablespoon) and TSP (teaspoon).** They are very different doses.

•**Be careful about following dose instructions.** If the label says two teaspoons, it's best to use a measuring spoon or a dosing cup marked in teaspoons, not a common kitchen spoon.

•**Don't play doctor.** When in doubt, call your physician.

Acetaminophen Overdose —A Growing Threat

Anne M. Larson, MD, assistant professor of medicine and director, Hepatology Clinic, University of Washington, Seattle.
Marc Siegel, MD, clinical associate professor of medicine, New York University School of Medicine, New York City, and author, *False Alarm: The Truth About the Epidemic of Fear.* Wiley.
Kathy Fallon, spokeswoman, McNeil Specialty & Consumer Pharmaceuticals, Fort Washington, PA.
Hepatology.

An overdose of *acetaminophen*, the active ingredient in Tylenol, is now the most common cause of acute liver failure in the United States, accounting for at least 42% of all cases that are seen at liver centers, researchers report. Approximately half of these cases are due to unintentional poisoning as opposed to attempted suicides, the researchers add.

Compared to the millions of acetaminophen tablets taken by Americans every day, the number of poisonings still remains low. But the researchers find it troubling that the percentage of acute liver failure cases linked to the drug have almost doubled since 1998.

THE STUDY

Lead researcher Dr. Anne Larson, director of the Hepatology Clinic at the University of Washington in Seattle, and her colleagues examined the records of 662 patients who were treated for acute liver failure at 22 liver centers in the United States over the six-year period from 1998 through 2003.

We make the assumption that over-the-counter drugs are somehow safer.

Marc Siegel, MD

In total, 275 patients (42%) had acetaminophen-related acute liver failure. Within this group, 48% were unintentional overdoses, 44% were suicide attempts and 8% were of unknown intent, the study found.

The median dose ingested was 24 grams (g) —the equivalent of 48 extra-strength tablets. Some patients, however, reported taking significantly less than that, suggesting that smaller doses may also be hazardous.

People who had unintentionally overdosed tended to be older, were taking several medications containing acetaminophen, and waited longer to seek help. Most of the people in the study were taking the medications for pain. Many were also depressed and were taking alcohol or narcotics.

More than one-third (38%) of those who unintentionally overdosed took at least two acetaminophen preparations simultaneously. Almost two-thirds (63%) used narcotic-containing compounds in addition to acetaminophen, according to the study.

One-third of the patients (35%) who had acute liver failure died, and 27% died without ever undergoing a transplant.

A SIGNIFICANT PROBLEM

"This is not a problem of epidemic proportions, [but] there is still a significant problem," says Larson.

Dr. Marc Siegel, a clinical associate professor of medicine at New York University School of Medicine, and author of *False Alarm: The Truth About the Epidemic of Fear*, adds, "This is already known. This study just increases our perception that Tylenol is potentially a dangerous drug."

Although best known by the brand name Tylenol, acetaminophen is found in more than 100 over-the-counter (OTC) products, including cold-and-cough remedies, such as Benadryl, Contac, Robitussin and Sinutab, as well as in medications for menstrual cramps, such as Midol and Pamprin. According to background information from the study, more than one-third (36%) of Americans take the drug in one form or another at least once a month.

In the past, some experts have suggested changing Tylenol's OTC status. "We make the assumption that over-the-counter drugs are somehow safer," Seigel says. "Just remember that Tylenol was approved to be over-the-counter before we even looked at these things, and I submit that maybe Tylenol, in some sense, shouldn't be over-the-counter."

The makers of Tylenol defend their products. "The results of this study update do not change what is known about the safety of acetaminophen," says Kathy Fallon, a spokeswoman for pharmaceutical company McNeil. "When taken in recommended doses, acetaminophen is a safe and effective pain reliever."

POSSIBLE SOLUTIONS

The study's authors believe that one way to reduce the number of acetaminophen overdoses is to restrict the package size of OTC acetaminophen and of prescriptions of narcotic–acetaminophen combinations.

They cite statistics from the United Kingdom, that show a 30% reduction in the number of patients admitted to specialty centers for severe acetaminophen-induced acute liver failure in the four years after OTC sales of acetaminophen were restricted to 16 g. More severe restrictions in France also resulted in improvements.

Education is also needed, the study authors state. "We think it's important to educate the public—and even physicians, when they give a patient a narcotic–acetaminophen combination," Larson says. "They need to make sure patients know there's acetaminophen in it and not to go and take Nyquil and other things on top of it."

"Tylenol used occasionally, or Tylenol used properly or Tylenol, like any other over-the-counter drug, used with a physician's awareness, is safe," Siegel adds. "It should not be used indiscriminately. And any drug used more than occasionally should be under a physician's guidance, including Tylenol."

info Get detailed information about acetaminophen from the US National Library of Medicine's MedlinePlus Web site at *www.med lineplus.gov.*

Poison Centers Resolve 80% Of Medication Mistakes

Marjory Abrams, publisher, newsletters, Boardroom Inc., 281 Tresser Blvd., Stamford, CT 06901.

My aunt recently confessed to me that she and my uncle occasionally have taken each other's medications by mistake. That scared me a bit because they don't share any of the same ailments, but she told me that they have never experienced any ill effects.

Jay Schauben, PharmD, director of the Florida Poison Information Center in Jacksonville, says that mistakes like this are not unusual—but they're not always risk-free.

People who think that they may have taken the wrong medicine—or too high a dose—should immediately call the free National Poison Hotline, 800-222-1222. Callers are connected to the nearest poison center. Dr. Schauben notes that poison centers can resolve more than 80% of callers' questions over the phone.

Even better than treatment, of course, is preventing the problem in the first place. *Among the common—and potentially dangerous—mistakes that people make with their medicines...*

●**Taking several over-the-counter (OTC) medications that have the same or similar active ingredients.**

Examples: Sudafed and Nyquil both have *pseudoephedrine*...Benadryl and Tylenol PM have *diphenhydramine*.

Always check the labels. When in doubt, consult a pharmacist.

•**Measuring liquid medications incorrectly.** Tableware is not for measuring medications. The most accurate measuring devices are oral dosage syringes, calibrated medicine droppers and similar products. Some pharmacies distribute them free.

•**Not shaking suspensions before each use.** Certain medicines are mixed with—but not dissolved in—liquids, so the medicine particles settle to the bottom. If the suspension is not shaken before each use, the initial doses will contain too little medicine—and the later doses, too much. When in doubt, shake.

•**Chewing or crushing tablets or capsules.** If the integrity of the tablet or capsule is destroyed, the medication may enter the bloodstream too quickly, potentially heightening its effect in the short term and decreasing its effect later on.

•**Taking medications twice.** It's easy to get confused about whether or not you have taken a pill. Checking it off on a list or calendar can be helpful—but Dr. Schauben suggests that people who take multiple medications use a plastic medicine box that has compartments labeled for various times of the day and different days of the week. They're sold at most drugstores.

•**Not clarifying which parent is responsible for medicating a child**—or which caregiver is responsible for medicating an adult. This can lead to double dosing or missed doses.

•**Taking medication in the dark**—or in a hurry. Read labels carefully.

Chances are that nothing terrible will happen from one wrong dose...but why take the risk?

■ ■ ■ ■

Deaths from Medication Errors Spike

Deaths from medication errors spike by 25% at the start of each month, according to a recent study.

Presumed reason: Government checks go out at the beginning of the month. As a result, pharmacies have a surge in their workloads, increasing the risk of mistakes.

Safety: Have your prescriptions filled when your pharmacy isn't busy.

David P. Phillips, PhD, professor, department of sociology, San Diego Center for Patient Safety, University of California, San Diego.

Children Poisoned by Medications Is a Common Cause of ER Visits

Dan Budnitz, MD, Division of Healthcare Quality Promotion, National Center for Infectious Diseases, Centers for Disease Control and Prevention.

David L. Katz, MD, MPH, associate professor of public health, and director, Prevention Research Center, Yale University School of Medicine, New Haven, CT.

Morbidity and Mortality Weekly.

Medications that are taken accidentally by young children account for an estimated 53,517 nonfatal emergency room visits each year in the United States, a federal study has found.

THE RESEARCH

Reviewing the data from 3,600 cases of medication mistakes in young children, researchers discovered that approximately 42% had ingested common over-the-counter (OTC) drugs, including vitamins, and 39.2% had accidentally taken prescription drugs. The remaining children had ingested a combination of drugs or an unknown medication.

Any medicine is a potential poison.

David L. Katz, MD, MPH

Children who were one and two years of age accounted for 72% of the cases. In addition, 75% of accidental ingestions occurred in the home. Of the children taken to emergency rooms, almost one in 10 were hospitalized or transferred to another facility for specialized care, according to the report.

"Medications are far and away the most common ingestions for which children are treated in the emergency department," says study co-author Dr. Dan Budnitz, from the Centers for Disease Control and Prevention's (CDC) Division of Healthcare Quality Promotion.

"We found that from 2001 to 2003 there were approximately 53,000 young children treated in the emergency department after swallowing medications that were not intended for them," Budnitz reports.

WHAT PARENTS CAN DO

Budnitz says that there are three things parents or caregivers can do to prevent medication accidents…

1. Keep medication out of the sight and reach of young children.

2. Don't assume that keeping medications in purses or pillboxes will prevent children from getting them.

3. Pay close attention when giving medication to children to ensure that they are getting the right drug and the correct dose.

"Young children continue to swallow medications or doses of medications that are not intended for them," Budnitz says. "Parents should be vigilant, whether it's storing their own medications or properly administering medications to children."

Dr. David L. Katz, director of the Prevention Research Center at Yale University School of Medicine, agrees that most of these cases can be avoided. "Parents must recognize that any medicine is a potential poison when taken in a high dose or by the wrong person. The precautions we take with dangerous chemicals should also be applied to seemingly innocuous items, such as Tylenol, cold remedies and even vitamins," Katz says. "Pill vials should be securely closed, hidden away and stored at a height young children can't reach."

info The Centers for Disease Control and Prevention has more suggestions on how you can prevent poisoning at *www.cdc.gov/ncipc/fact sheets/poisonprevention.htm*.

Drug Expiration Dates: Take Them Seriously

Cynthia LaCivita, PharmD, director of clinical standards and quality, American Society of Health-System Pharmacists.
Rachel Bongiorno, PharmD, director, University of Maryland Drug Information Service, Baltimore.

Should you use a prescription or over-the-counter (OTC) medication that has an expiration date that has long past?

To answer this question, some pharmaceutical experts point to a study conducted for the US Army that found that many drugs are still usable nearly five years after the expiration date. However, other experts say using expired drugs isn't worth the risk and you should throw them out.

THE ARMY STUDY

The Army study examined 96 different drugs and found that 84% of them remained stable 57 months beyond the expiration date.

The longer you go beyond the expiration date, the more question there is about the activity of the drug.

Cynthia LaCivita, PharmD

But in their report, the researchers add that the additional stability period is "highly variable," depending on the drug.

STUDY LIMITATIONS

Cynthia LaCivita, a pharmacist and director of clinical standards and quality for the American Society of Health-System Pharmacists in Bethesda, Maryland, notes that the Army study "looked at drugs in their original, unopened containers. That is not usually how an individual would store a drug."

In fact, most consumers do not store medications in optimal conditions, making it even more crucial to pay attention to the expiration date, according to Rachel Bongiorno, a pharmacist and director of the University of Maryland Drug Information Service.

RECOMMENDATIONS

"To be on the safe side, I would never recommend anyone take medication past the expiration date," Bongiorno advises.

"I would take expiration dates seriously," agrees LaCivita. "The longer you go beyond the expiration date, the more question there is about the activity of the drug," she adds. "There are studies that show that, over time, some of these drugs are degraded."

LaCivita points to a recent study that found that liquid antibiotics, often prescribed for children's ear infections and meant to be stored no more than 14 days under refrigeration, begin to lose some therapeutic value after 14 days.

POTENTIAL PROBLEMS

"The biggest problem is [the medication] won't be as effective," Bongiorno says. But there are other reasons not to take old medicine. "You may start a new medicine that may interact with the old one [or] you may have another disease that could require a dose reduction," she says.

LaCivita recommends people go through their medicine cabinet once a year and throw out expired drugs. If you use medicine before its expiration date, you can be sure you're getting the medicine's best benefit, both experts say.

info To learn more about medication safety, visit the University of Michigan Web site at *www.med.umich.edu/patientsafetytoolkit/medication.htm.*

Breakthrough! Men and Women Need Different Drugs

Marianne J. Legato, MD, founder, Partnership for Gender-Specific Medicine, and professor of clinical medicine, College of Physicians and Surgeons, both at Columbia University, New York City. She is author of *Eve's Rib: The New Science of Gender-Specific Medicine and How It Can Save Your Life*. Harmony.

Medical researchers have long known that men and women differ in their susceptibility to common diseases, including diabetes, heart disease and cancer.

Now: Researchers are discovering that men and women often respond differently to the same medication.

Example: The allergy drug *terfenadine* (Seldane) was removed from the market in 1998 when it was discovered that women taking it were at an increased risk for potentially deadly heartbeat irregularities (*arrhythmias*). Men taking the drug did not have the same risk.

THE GENDER FACTOR

Until quite recently, the pharmaceutical industry mainly tested new drugs on men. Women were not included in drug trials in an effort to protect them and any children if the women became pregnant during the testing. In addition, the hormone fluctuations experienced by women were thought to make them less desirable study subjects than men.

In 1993, after researchers discovered that men and women respond differently to drugs, the US Food and Drug Administration (FDA) began requiring that women be included in drug trials for medications that would be taken by them.

Among the most popular theories to explain gender-related differences in drugs are...

•**Hormones.** The enzymes that metabolize drugs are affected by hormones, which differ greatly in men and women. For example, the "female" hormone *progesterone*, which increases just prior to menstruation, accelerates the breakdown of the steroid prednisone in the body. This means that a woman who has asthma might require a higher dose of the drug just before her menstrual period in order to avoid an attack.

•**Fatty tissue.** Some drugs are stored in fatty tissue. Because women typically have a higher percentage of body fat than men, women might require a lower drug dose in some cases because the drug is stored in the fatty tissue and is available for a longer period of time after dosing.

Following are five common medications that have sex-specific differences...

ANALGESICS

Women may be biologically more sensitive to pain than men—and they are known to experience more inflammation from infection and injury. Therefore, women may require higher doses of analgesics that have an anti-inflammatory component.

Women often do better with *ibuprofen* (Advil) or another *nonsteroidal anti-inflammatory drug* (NSAID), such as *naproxen* (Aleve), than with pain relievers, such as *acetaminophen* (Tylenol), that do not treat inflammation.

Best advice: For severe pain—following surgery, for example—women should ask their doctors for a "kappa opioid," such as *butorphanol tartrate* (Stadol), a morphine-like painkiller. This class of drugs is much more effective for women than other analgesics. In men, kappa opioids are not as effective as other drugs.

ANESTHESIA

Women tend to wake up quicker than men following anesthesia—an average of six minutes faster—even when they're given the same dose relative to their body weight. Women also experience more side effects from anesthesia than men and are more likely to report some consciousness during surgical procedures.

Despite this, women tend to be given less pain-relieving medication in the recovery room following surgery.

Reason: A man's blood pressure rises when he's in pain. Doctors rely on this to indicate when to use drugs and how much to give. Women in pain frequently have a drop in blood pressure—and a more rapid heart rate as a result, which is a better indicator of how much distress they are feeling.

Best advice: Before an operation, women should request that their heart rate be monitored as a pain indicator along with blood pressure. If their heart rate increases, their doctors should consider providing more pain medication.

ANTI-ARRHYTHMICS

This class of drugs is used to treat heart arrhythmias. One popular anti-arrhythmic, *sotalol* (Betapace), is more dangerous for women than for men. Due to differences in the characteristics of the cardiac cell membranes in men and women, sotalol, which acts on these cell membranes, can increase a woman's risk of *ventricular tachycardia*, a potentially life-threatening arrhythmia.

Best advice: A woman who needs an anti-arrhythmic drug can sometimes be treated using another drug in the same class. If she requires sotalol, she should be advised to stay in a hospital or another type of facility that can provide continuous heart monitoring—and cardiac resuscitation, if necessary.

ANTIDEPRESSANTS

These days, most people who are diagnosed with depression are prescribed a *selective serotonin reuptake inhibitor* (SSRI) antidepressant, such as *paroxetine* (Paxil) or *fluoxetine* (Prozac). These drugs increase brain concentrations of *serotonin*, a neurotransmitter that regulates mood.

However, a new study shows that men don't appear to benefit from SSRIs as much as women—perhaps because men are known to have approximately 50% more brain serotonin than women. Therefore, increasing the levels of this neurotransmitter through drug therapy has relatively modest effects in men.

Best advice: Tricyclic antidepressants, such as *amitriptyline* (Elavil) or *nortriptyline* (Pamelor), are often better choices for men. These older drugs have a higher risk for side effects, such as weight gain and dry mouth, than the SSRIs, but are more likely to be effective in men.

ASPIRIN

Millions of healthy Americans take aspirin daily or every other day to "thin" the blood and reduce the risk of clots, which can contribute to heart attack and/or stroke. However, doctors must weigh the potential benefits of aspirin therapy against the potential risks. In both sexes, regular aspirin use has been shown to increase the risk of gastrointestinal bleeding.

New finding: In men, daily aspirin can lower heart attack risk by 32%, according to a recent analysis of aspirin therapy conducted by researchers at Duke University Medical Center in Durham, North Carolina. Aspirin does not have this effect in all women. However, women who take a daily or every-other-day aspirin were found to have a 17% reduction in the risk for stroke.

Best advice: For men who are at risk of heart attack (due to smoking, high blood pressure or family history), aspirin therapy can often be a good choice.

Women younger than 65 who are concerned about heart protection alone may want to forgo aspirin therapy and focus on other protective strategies, including weight control, not smoking, regular exercise, etc.

In women older than 65, the heart benefits of aspirin therapy may outweigh the risks for stomach problems.

Because women have strokes almost as often as men—and their risk of dying from stroke is even higher—they should consider aspirin therapy if they have stroke risk factors, such as smoking, high blood pressure, etc.

Important: Consult your doctor before starting or discontinuing aspirin therapy.

■ ■ ■ ■

Drug Alert for Women

Women respond differently than men to certain drugs and, therefore, should be aggressive in researching their medications.

Women have been underrepresented in clinical drug studies, which long assumed that they respond to drugs in the same way that men do. But, in fact, women experience more adverse drug events than men do.

Steps: Understand the need for a drug. Ask a doctor or pharmacist about side effects and potential interactions with other drugs and be sure to understand correct dosage amounts and the timing of doses.

Rosaly Correa-de-Araujo, MD, PhD, MSc, director, women's health and gender-based research, Agency for Healthcare Research and Quality (AHRQ). *www.ahrq.gov.*

Generic Drugs Boast Greater Adherence Rates Than Brand Names

Brigham and Women's Hospital news release.

Patients who are prescribed generic drugs are more likely to continue taking them than patients who take brand-name drugs, a new study has found.

THE STUDY

Dr. William Shrank, of Brigham and Women's Hospital and Harvard Medical School, both in Boston, analyzed how well 6,755 patients who were enrolled in a three-tier pharmacy benefit plan stuck to their drug regimens. Under this plan, the patients had the highest copayment for nonpreferred brand-name drugs (third tier), smaller copayments for preferred brand-name drugs (second tier) and the smallest or no copayment for generic drugs.

There were six classes of drugs included in the study: cholesterol-lowering statins, oral contraceptives, orally inhaled corticosteroids (used to treat asthma) and three types of antihypertensives (calcium-channel blockers, angiotensin receptor blockers as well as angiotensin converting enzyme inhibitors). The group received 7,532 new prescriptions during the study.

Participants who took generic drugs showed 12.6% greater therapy adherence than patients who took brand-name third-tier drugs, the study authors report. Patients who took second-tier drugs had 8% greater adherence than those who used third-tier drugs.

These findings are another reason why "generic drugs should be prescribed for patients beginning chronic therapy, as long as there are no specific clinical reasons why a branded drug may be more appropriate," says Shrank.

"Physicians commonly prescribe chronic medications for important medical problems. Both physicians and patients should be aware of how the medication choice directly influences the patient's ability to follow the prescribed treatment," he says.

info The Center for Drug Evaluation and Research has more information about generic drugs at *www.fda.gov/cder/consumerinfo/ generics_q&a.htm.*

■ ■ ■ ■

How to Save Big on Drugs

Americans spend an average of $885 annually on prescription and over-the-counter (OTC) medications. But when it comes to cost, you have more options than you might think.

Example: An average daily dose of the popular cholesterol-lowering statin Lipitor costs approximately $98 per month. *Lovastatin*, a generic of the statin Mevacor that is used in lower-risk patients, is available for $37 a month.

The next time your doctor writes you a prescription, be sure to ask the right questions to save money, advises Diane Nitzki-George, RPh, a clinical pharmacist in Evanston, Illinois, and the author of *Generic Alternatives to Prescription Drugs* (Basic Health)...

• **Is a generic available?** On average, generics, which have the same active ingredients as brand-name drugs, cost 52% less.

• **Is there a cheaper drug in the same class?** The newest—and most expensive—drugs sometimes represent a significant advance over older medications in the same chemical class. But many people do just as well on older, less expensive medications.

Doctors may prescribe expensive drugs because they are often more convenient for patients to take.

Example: The blood pressure drug Toprol-XL (approximately $65 per month) is taken only once a day, while the generic version, *metoprolol* ($10 per month), is taken twice a day.

Finally, ask your health insurer if a prescribed drug is listed in its *formulary*, the list of drugs that are covered by an insurance plan. Patients usually must pay full price for medications that don't appear on the formulary.

Rebecca Shannonhouse, editor, *BottomLine/Health*, 281 Tresser Blvd., Stamford, CT 06901.

70% of Bacteria Are Resistant to Antibiotics— How to Fight Them

Stuart Levy, MD, professor of medicine, molecular biology and microbiology, and director, Center for Adaptation Genetics and Drug Resistance, Tufts University School of Medicine, Boston. He is founder and president of the nonprofit Alliance for the Prudent Use of Antibiotics (*www. apua.org*) and author of *The Antibiotic Paradox*. Perseus.

By now, we've all heard about the growing threat of antibiotic-resistant bacteria. We know not to ask our doctors to prescribe an antibiotic unnecessarily, and we've been told that frequent handwashing cuts down on the transmission of bacterial infections.

With such strong warnings, you might assume that antibiotic resistance is going away. But the reality is that it isn't.

Increasingly, bacteria that are responsible for sinusitis, ear and urinary tract infections and many types of pneumonia are resistant to one or more antibiotics. This means that many infections that were once easily cured by taking an antibiotic for a few days can now linger much longer—and even become life-threatening.

How antibiotic-resistance develops: Bacteria can become resistant to antibiotics by mutating to become insensitive to the drug. The surviving resistant organisms then multiply and create new strains of bacteria that don't respond to antibiotics that were previously effective. The potential for resistance is enhanced when patients do not finish a full course of an antibiotic—or when antibiotics are overused or misused in general. *Latest developments…*

LAX HANDWASHING

What's new: Many people still aren't washing their hands. Although 91% of American adults claim to wash their hands after using the restroom, only 83% actually do so, according to the American Society for Microbiology.

What this means for you: Because many viruses and bacteria are spread from hands to the mucus membranes of the mouth, nose or eyes, dirty hands are a prime means of transmitting infection.

Self-defense: In addition to washing your hands after using the restroom and before eating or preparing food, it's also important to wash after handling garbage…playing with a pet…changing a diaper…blowing your nose, sneezing or coughing…and inserting or removing contact lenses.

What to do: Use soap and warm, running water, and rub your hands together for at least 10 seconds. Don't forget the wrists and backs of your hands. Dry with a clean cloth or paper towel. Pocket-sized bottles of hand-sanitizing gels and disposable towelettes that contain alcohol are convenient ways to wash when water is not available.

MORE DRUG-RESISTANT STRAINS

What's new: The number of drug-resistant and multidrug-resistant strains of bacteria is up sharply from just a few years ago. Approximately 70% of the bacteria that cause infections in hospitals are now resistant to at least one common antibiotic.

What this means for you: If you are hospitalized, you are now at an increased risk of contracting an infection that can be difficult to treat and that may even result in death. Recent studies show that 5% to 10% of hospital patients in the United States get an infection during their stay, and nearly 100,000 die annually as a result. This compares with approximately 13,000 deaths from hospital-acquired infections in 1992.

Self-defense: Keep hospital stays as short as possible. Visitors and hospital staff should wash their hands before and after contact with you. With some infectious diseases, such as tuberculosis, visitors and staff may need to wear a mask, gown and gloves to prevent the spread of the infection.

ANTIBIOTIC BAN FOR POULTRY

What's new: In July 2005, the US Food and Drug Administration (FDA) announced a ban on the use of the animal antibiotic *enrofloxacin* (Baytril) in poultry. Enrofloxacin is a *fluoroquinolone* antibiotic in the same class as *ciprofloxacin* (Cipro). The ban followed the finding that fluoroquinolone-resistant bacteria that infected poultry were becoming increasingly less responsive to Cipro in human infections caused by the same bacteria. This was the first time the FDA had banned an antibiotic used in animal health because of the potential harm posed to people by the emergence of drug-resistant bacteria.

What this means for you: Greater attention is being given to antibiotic use in agriculture, animals and people. Europe has instituted a ban on the use of all growth-promoting antibiotics. In the US, antibiotics are still given to poultry to increase growth. The FDA is currently reviewing the issue, and many experts believe the US should also ban growth-promoting antibiotics.

Self-defense: To find poultry that is totally free of antibiotics, check with your local butcher or at a natural-food store.

CIPRO RESISTANCE

What's new: Ciprofloxacin, one of the first-line antibiotics that is used to treat anthrax (a leading bioterror weapon), is becoming increasingly ineffective against other infections.

What this means for you: For now, other antibiotics can fill the gap for ear, sinus and urinary tract infections. Experts do not believe that

Cipro's effectiveness against anthrax has been compromised—but this could change in the future if the antibiotic is overused.

Self-defense: Some of the experts believe that doctors are too quick to prescribe Cipro when another antibiotic would be sufficient. If your doctor prescribes Cipro, ask if another antibiotic could be used.

NEW STAPH INFECTIONS

What's new: A drug-resistant strain of *staphylococcus* bacterium—*community-acquired methicillin-resistant Staphylococcus aureus* (CA-MRSA) —formerly found only in hospitals, is now increasingly being detected within communities.

What this means for you: This particular staph bacterium appears to be more virulent than others and spreads from person-to-person, particularly through skin-to-skin contact sports, such as football and wrestling.

Self-defense: To prevent infection, wash well with soap and water immediately after any contact sports, being especially careful to clean any cuts. Never share towels or washcloths in a gym.

LATEST ANTIBIOTICS

What's new: *Tigecycline* (Tygacil), the first in a new class of antibiotics called *glycylcyclines*, was introduced in June 2005. It was approved by the FDA as a first-line treatment for hospital-based skin and soft tissue infections caused by bacteria that are resistant to other antibiotics. A new class of antibiotics called *diarylquinolones*, which treats drug-resistant tuberculosis, is now in clinical trials.

What this means for you: Despite these new drugs, antibiotic research is getting short shrift. That's because many major pharmaceutical companies have found that it is more profitable to fund research and development for new drugs that treat chronic illnesses, such as diabetes, arthritis and high cholesterol.

Self-defense: Write to your representatives in Congress and tell them that you support efforts to boost incentives (via tax credits and other means) for pharmaceutical companies to develop new antibiotics.

To write to your congressional representatives online, go to *www.firstgov.gov*. This Web site also gives mailing addresses and phone numbers for your congressional representatives.

45 Million Antibiotics Prescribed, but May Not Be Necessary

Philip Tierno, PhD, director, clinical microbiology and immunology, New York University Medical Center, New York City, and author of *The Secret Life of Germs.* Atria.

Jeffrey Linder, MD, MPH, associate physician, Brigham and Women's Hospital, and instructor in medicine, Harvard University Medical School, both in Boston.

The Journal of the American Medical Association.

Despite widespread concern about the growing problem of antibiotic resistance, too many people are still receiving prescriptions for antibiotics that they don't need, according to two recent studies.

"In the United States approximately 150 million prescriptions are written each year, and 60% of those are for antibiotics," says Philip Tierno, director of clinical microbiology and immunology at New York University Medical Center. "So, approximately 90 million antibiotic prescriptions are written and approximately half of those are either unnecessary or inappropriate, which is the leading cause of antibiotic resistance in this country. These studies represent a beginning effort in trying to break the cycle of inappropriate antibiotic use," he says.

THE FIRST STUDY

The first study looked at the rate of antibiotic prescriptions and included 4,158 American children between the ages of three and 17 who were examined in a physician's office, hospital outpatient department or emergency room for a sore throat.

According to the study, most sore throats are not caused by bacteria, but by viruses. Only 15% to 36% of all sore throats are caused by the *streptococcus* (strep) bacteria.

For those infections that are caused by strep, the antibiotics penicillin or amoxicillin are the recommended first-line treatments. For patients who are allergic to penicillin, erythromycin and some cephalosporin medications are recommended, the study authors say.

Overall, 53% of the children seen were tested for strep. Of those who received an antibiotic prescription, 51% received the strep test.

"Almost 100% of these kids should have had the strep test," says study author Dr. Jeffrey Linder, an associate physician at Brigham and Women's Hospital and an instructor in medicine at Harvard University Medical School, both in Boston. "That was surprising. This is an example where there's a good test available and what you should do is pretty clear," he says.

At most, 35% of the children would be expected to have strep, but more than 50% were given antibiotics, according to the study. The good news is that that number is 12% lower than it was in 1995. The bad news is that almost one in five of these prescriptions is probably unnecessary, the researchers say.

Linder says that in addition to concern about antibiotic resistance, parents should be cautious about giving children unnecessary medications because all drugs, including antibiotics, have certain risks.

"Exposing kids to medicine they don't need may not help them, and it exposes them to all the risks of the drug," he says.

THE SECOND STUDY

The second study included 334 primary-care doctors from 12 rural areas in Idaho and Utah. Half of the communities received community intervention, which included press releases, educational materials and a direct mailing to parents who had children younger than age six about the appropriate use of antibiotics.

The other half of the communities received the same community intervention. The doctors were also given a *clinical decision support system* (CDSS), which is a step-by-step guide for the appropriate diagnosis and treatment of acute respiratory infections.

The antibiotic prescription rate dropped by nearly 10% in the CDSS group and went up slightly in the community intervention-only group. Antibiotic prescriptions deemed "never indicated" by study guidelines dropped 32% in the CDSS group, but only fell 5% in the community intervention-only group.

The results of these studies indicate that the use of a clinical decision-making tool for physicians and the consistent use of strep testing might help reduce the number of inappropriate antibiotic prescriptions.

info For advice on when antibiotic use is appropriate, visit the American Academy of Family Physicians Web site at *http://familydoctor. org/680.xml.*

Are Your Medications Making You Sick?

John Abramson, MD, clinical instructor in primary care, Harvard Medical School, Boston, and author of *Overdosed America: The Broken Promise of American Medicine.* HarperCollins.

With our national pharmacy bill now topping $200 billion each year, and recent disclosures about harmful and ineffective drugs, more people are asking, *Are all those pills really necessary?*

To learn more, we talked with John Abramson, MD, a clinical instructor at Harvard Medical School who is widely recognized for his in-depth research of the drug industry…

•**Are most Americans overmedicated?** They sure are. Americans take many drugs unnecessarily, and when drugs *are* needed, people often take the wrong ones. For example, before *rofecoxib* (Vioxx) was withdrawn from the market because it was found to cause heart attacks and strokes (and did not provide better relief of arthritis symptoms than older, much less expensive anti-inflammatory drugs), approximately 80% of the Vioxx that was prescribed worldwide was used in the US.

•**Are doctors to blame?** The vast majority of physicians prescribe medication because they think it's in their patients' best interest. But there have been radical changes in the way that our medical knowledge is provided. Prior to 1980, most clinical research was publicly funded, but now most is funded directly by the drug industry and other medical industries, whose primary mission is to maximize the return on investments for investors.

Now, 90% of clinical trials are commercially funded—as well as 75% of published clinical research. When a pharmaceutical company sponsors a study, the odds are five times greater that the findings will favor its product.

Drug and medical industries fund 70% of continuing education lectures and seminars, which are among the activities that doctors are required to attend to maintain their licenses to practice. Wherever doctors turn for sources of information, drug companies dominate.

•**Who should be monitoring doctors' relationships with drug companies?** The real failure is on the part of government agencies, such as the US Food and Drug Administration (FDA) and the Agency for Healthcare Research and Quality. Medical journals and academic researchers have become dependent on drug company money and/or are vulnerable to drug company lobbying. Doctors and the public still trust these institutions to independently oversee the integrity of the knowledge that informs our medical care, when they simply are not able to do this anymore.

•**We all know that cholesterol-lowering statins are widely prescribed. Are they unnecessary?** Despite being on the market for 18 years and becoming the best-selling class of drugs, statins have never been shown in randomized, controlled trials to provide a significant health benefit when used by women of any age and men older than 65 who do not have heart disease or diabetes. Even so, millions of people in both groups are now taking a statin drug.

•**Is it ever advisable to take a statin?** Yes, there is good evidence that statins are beneficial for people who already have heart disease and for at least some people who have diabetes. A good case can also be made for men who are at very high risk of heart disease (LDL, or "bad," cholesterol approaching 200 in addition to other risk factors).

•**What other drugs do you think are being prescribed because of drug company influence?** Antihypertensives—drugs used to treat high blood pressure—are good examples. Newer medications, such as calcium channel blockers and angiotensin converting enzyme (ACE) inhibitors, are among the most popular. One of them, *amlodipine* (Norvasc), was the second most commonly prescribed drug for older adults in 2003. But a study funded by the National Heart, Lung, and Blood Institute (NHLBI) found that diuretics, which have been around for decades, are as good as or better than Norvasc in protecting against the complications of hypertension, such as heart attack and stroke. A diuretic might cost $29 per year, compared with $549 to $749 for Norvasc, depending on the dose. The patents for diuretics expired decades ago, so drug companies do not make much profit from them.

●**Should everyone who has high blood pressure just take a diuretic?** High blood pressure is a complex problem. Some people respond to one drug, some to another, and some need more than one. It would make sense, though, to start by taking a diuretic, and use expensive drugs such as Norvasc only when other alternatives haven't worked.

●**Are natural therapies a better alternative to some drugs?** If you look at all of the data rather than listen to the drug ads, you will see that natural alternatives, such as improved diet and routine exercise, are often far more effective than drugs at achieving real health improvements, such as reducing heart disease and extending life.

Probably the most important test of a healthy diet's effect on heart disease is the Lyon Diet Heart Study conducted in Lyon, France. Heart attack patients were randomly counseled to eat a Mediterranean diet (high in unprocessed grains, fruits, vegetables and olive oil...very low in red meat, dairy fat and cholesterol) or a "prudent" post-heart attack diet (no more than 30% of calories from total fat and no more than 10% from saturated fat).

During the next four years, the people who were counseled to eat the Mediterranean diet developed 72% less heart disease than those in the prudent-diet group. There were 56% fewer deaths in the group that was counseled to eat the Mediterranean diet—that's two to three times the benefit achieved by statin drugs.

The same holds true for exercise. A study conducted at the Cooper Institute for Aerobics Research in Dallas looked at 25,000 men who had undergone physical exams. During the next 10 years, the men whose exercise endurance (as measured on a treadmill) was in the lowest 20% of the group were at a much higher risk of dying than those who had high total cholesterol levels (above 240)—confirming that exercise is even more important than cholesterol control.

●**But many patients prefer pills because they're easier.** There is no question that many of us would rather take a pill than change our lifestyle. If the pills worked, it would simply be a question of how we want to spend our money. The problem is that the pills are often closer to folk medicine—empowered by our cultural beliefs but without a genuine scientific basis. Approximately two-thirds of our health is determined by the way we live our lives, and—for better or worse—no pills can change that.

●**What's the solution?** Most doctors do not invest much time or energy helping patients to make healthy changes in diet and exercise or teaching stress reduction. If you are willing to consider these approaches before trying drug treatment, tell your doctor.

When medication is necessary, ask your doctor if a generic drug is just as effective as the expensive brand-name product. Remember, drug ads that tell you to "ask your doctor" about a particular drug have a single purpose—to sell more drugs, not to improve your health.

Prescription drug ads have become a normal part of our cultural landscape, but the US and New Zealand (that has a population of less than 4 million) are the only two industrialized countries that allow them. The remaining industrialized countries feel that assessment of the scientific information about prescription drug treatment should be left to doctors, who should work in partnership with each patient to determine optimal medical care based on his/her individual situation.

Are Cholesterol-Lowering Drugs Right for You?

Jay S. Cohen, MD, adjunct associate professor of family and preventive medicine and of psychiatry, University of California, San Diego. He is author of *What You Must Know About Statin Drugs & Their Natural Alternatives.* Square One. *www.medicationsense.com.*

In the fight against heart disease, statin drugs are heavy artillery. Their cholesterol-lowering power has the potential to reduce heart disease, stroke and cardiac death by 25%.

Yet these medications are not for everyone. In two recent surveys, both published in *The Journal of the American Medical Association*, 60% to 75% of 100,000 people who started taking statins said they discontinued them within an average of eight months.

What goes wrong? If a patient has no insurance, cost is a factor—a month's supply of some statins exceeds $300. More often, people discontinue this medication because of side effects, which are largely avoidable—if the drugs are prescribed properly.

STATIN SIDE EFFECTS

To reduce cholesterol levels, statins alter liver metabolism. Cholesterol is manufactured in the liver, and statins inhibit an enzyme that is needed for cholesterol production. These drugs also prevent the inflammation that lodges cholesterol deposits inside arteries.

Although statins have fewer side effects than other cholesterol-lowering drugs, an estimated 15% to 30% of the people taking them experience abdominal discomfort, muscle or joint pain, muscle weakness and/or memory problems.

More serious side effects occur in 1% to 2% of statin users, whose liver enzymes rise—a warning of possible liver damage if uncorrected. *Rhabdomyolysis*, a breakdown of muscle tissue, is an extremely rare side effect but can be fatal. Approximately one in 2,000 long-term (more than five years) statin users develops a painful nerve condition known as *peripheral neuropathy.*

These adverse effects—both uncomfortable and dangerous—are dosage-related. The more powerful the statin and the greater the dosage, the greater the risk.

Side effects can be minimized, if not avoided altogether, by taking the lowest effective dosage.

MORE ISN'T BETTER

Many people are getting excessive doses of statins because of the way the FDA assesses new drugs for approval. To gain FDA approval, a drug manufacturer must show that its medication works for the majority of people who take it. Therefore, manufacturers design clinical trials using dosages that are high enough to meet that benchmark.

However, people respond very differently to medication. Women may need less of a particular drug than men, and people who weigh less often don't need as much as those who weigh more. Older people often respond to lower dosages. And some people need less—or more—just because everyone's biochemistry is different.

Result: Many people could do well on far less than the "recommended" dosage that was proven to be most effective in clinical trials.

What's more, not everyone needs the same amount of cholesterol reduction.

PRECISION PRESCRIBING

The key question when your doctor prescribes a statin is, how much cholesterol reduction do you need? Depending on your risk for heart disease, aggressive treatment using statins may—or may not—be a good idea.

To determine your optimum cholesterol level, check with your doctor. National Institutes of Health guidelines advise LDL ("bad") cholesterol levels of 100 to 160, depending on cardiovascular risk factors, such as family history of heart disease, age, if your HDL ("good") cholesterol is higher than 40 mg/dL, etc.

Regardless of your LDL level, it makes sense to incorporate lifestyle changes. A diet that is low in saturated fats (10% or less of total calories) and high in fruits and vegetables (at least nine daily servings) and whole grains can often lower cholesterol as much as a moderately powerful statin. Regular exercise also helps. Walking 45 minutes per day reduces cardiac mortality by 50%. And if you do go on medication, a healthy diet and regular exercise will enable you to use a lower dosage.

To ensure that you're being prescribed the appropriate amount of medication, ask your doctor what percentage of LDL cholesterol reduction you need. Then you and your doctor can determine what statin dosage is best for you.

Example: Your LDL cholesterol is 165, and your target is 130 (a 21% reduction). A daily 10-milligram (mg) dose of *lovastatin* (Mevacor) or *pravastatin* (Pravachol) is a good place to start.

After one month, have your cholesterol tested again. If it hasn't dropped enough, you may need to increase the dosage. Or, if it has dropped to desired levels, particularly if you also have made dietary changes, you may be able to decrease the dosage.

This approach can identify your lowest effective dosage and minimize side effects.

WHICH STATIN?

All statins work the same way, so the key difference among them is potency. LDL reductions of 50% to 60% are possible using *atorvastatin* (Lipitor) and *simvastatin* (Zocor), compared with an average reduction of approximately 40% using older statins, such as lovastatin, pravastatin and *fluvastatin* (Lescol).

Rosuvastatin (Crestor) is the newest, strongest and riskiest statin. There have been reports of rhabdomyolysis, kidney damage and kidney failure in some patients taking this drug. I recommend it only if no other drug lowers cholesterol adequately.

If you need a significant reduction in cholesterol, particularly if you already have heart disease or risk factors, one of the high-potency statins makes sense.

For a more modest reduction, you may consider an older, less powerful drug. Lovastatin is a particularly attractive choice if cost is a factor—it is the only statin available in generic form and costs up to four times less than the other statins.

Aggressive Statin Therapy May Reverse Hardening Of the Arteries

Steven E. Nissen, MD, interim chairman, department of cardiovascular medicine, The Cleveland Clinic, and president, American College of Cardiology (ACC).

Peter Lurie, MD, deputy director, Health Research Group, Public Citizen, Washington, DC.

Sidney Smith, MD, professor of medicine, University of North Carolina at Chapel Hill, former president, American Heart Association (AHA), and cochairman, ACC/AHA Task Force on Practice Guidelines.

American College of Cardiology annual meeting, Atlanta. *The Journal of the American Medical Association.*

In a study, intensive cholesterol-lowering therapy using *rosuvastatin* (Crestor)—a powerful (and controversial) member of the statin family of drugs—not only reduced low-density lipoprotein (LDL, or "bad") cholesterol levels but actually reversed *atherosclerosis*, also known as hardening of the arteries.

THE STUDY

For the trial, 507 patients at 53 health-care centers in the United States, Canada, Europe and Australia were given 40 milligrams (mg) of Crestor daily.

Plaque build-up was measured at the beginning of the study and two years later using *intravascular ultrasound* (IVUS). The researchers were able to report information on 349 of the participants.

In total, 64% of the patients showed a regression of atherosclerosis. The average LDL level fell from 130.4 mg/dL (milligrams per deciliter of blood) to 60.8 mg/dL, a reduction of 53.2%. High-density lipoprotein (HDL, or "good") cholesterol levels rose from an average of 43.1 to 49 mg/dL, a 14.7% increase.

With very, very low levels of LDL, we can remove some of the plaque from the coronary artery, and that's a pretty good thing.

Steven E. Nissen, MD

"That's the lowest LDL ever that's been achieved in a clinical trial of this kind," says lead author of the study, Dr. Steven E. Nissen, interim chairman of the department of cardiovascular medicine at The Cleveland Clinic and president of the American College of Cardiology (ACC). "The 14.7% increase in HDL is also unprecedented. With that combination, we saw a large-scale regression" of artherosclerosis.

IMPLICATIONS

The introduction of statins in 1987 brought with it the hope that atherosclerosis could one day be reversed. That hope, however, has been elusive.

LDLs were reduced to 79 in previous studies. "We thought that was fantastic," Nissen says. "But all we got was no [disease] progression. Now, we can say that if you can get your patients to these very low levels of LDL with an intense statin regimen, particularly if it's accompanied by a major increase in HDL, then you are capable of partially reversing the disease," he says. "We think it's good news for patients because it means that with very, very low levels of LDL, we can get to the point where we're removing some of the plaque from the coronary artery, and that's a pretty good thing."

Several questions still remain unanswered. One is whether the same benefits could be achieved using other statins instead of Crestor because of concerns about its safety.

The consumer advocacy group Public Citizen has petitioned the US Food and Drug Administration (FDA) to take Crestor off the market. But the agency concluded that the available evidence about Crestor's safety does not warrant its withdrawal from the market. Public Citizen isn't likely to change its stance, despite this new research.

"The study is a bit less impressive than perhaps is put forth," says Dr. Peter Lurie, deputy director of Public Citizen's Health Research Group. "Many patients were lost to follow-up. And there is no comparison group, so we have no way of knowing if some other drug might not have accomplished exactly the same thing," he says. "It leaves many questions unanswered. I don't see a fundamental shift here in our position."

Even those who support the study acknowledge that medical practice will not be altered by this one study.

"Usually a single study doesn't change everybody's practice," Nissen says. "It changes the momentum and, with that momentum, you'll see more interest in people lowering LDL levels."

Another question is whether reducing plaque build-up in the coronary artery actually correlates with fewer cardiac events.

Although the findings are "potentially very helpful and an important addition to our understanding, in terms of broad treatment recommendations, we really need to see how these findings correlate with outcomes," says Dr. Sidney Smith, professor of medicine at the University of North Carolina at Chapel Hill, former president of the American Heart Association (AHA) and cochairman of the ACC/AHA Task Force on Practice Guidelines.

In addition, the study only looked at people who had already experienced one coronary event, such as a heart attack. It is unclear whether statins would reverse artherosclerosis in people who had not yet experienced such an event.

ER Doctors Overprescribe Powerful Heart Drugs

Karen Alexander, MD, associate professor of medicine, Duke University, Durham, NC.
The Journal of the American Medical Association.

Emergency room doctors treating heart attack patients often fail to administer powerful clot-preventing drugs in the proper doses, according to a recent study.

One common error is overprescribing—giving a dose large enough to cause potentially dangerous bleeding, the researchers say.

THE STUDY

The researchers analyzed data from an ongoing study that is tracking adherence to treatment guidelines at more than 400 US hospitals. The researchers identified more than 30,000 patients who had been rushed to hospitals with heart attack symptoms during a nine-month period.

Within the first 24 hours of symptoms, these patients often get anticlotting drugs, most notably *heparin*, to help open arteries or keep them open. The analysis showed that 42% of the patients got doses outside the recommended range.

Patients who got too-large doses were more likely to have bleeding episodes. They were also more likely to need extended stays in the hospital or to die.

ONE-SIZE-FITS-ALL APPROACH DOESN'T WORK

The problem is that the doctors tend to follow the rules *too* closely, says study author Dr. Karen Alexander, an associate professor of medicine at Duke University.

"In many cases, doctors resort to standard dosing, which is appropriate for middle-aged men of normal body size and normal renal [kidney] function," she says. "But one size doesn't fit all."

For many patients—the elderly, women, thin people, those who have kidney problems—"certain calculations are required to make sure the doses are in the clinical range," Alexander says. She believes that too often those calculations are not being made.

Alexander stresses that anticlotting drugs are unquestionably helpful in the treatment of heart attacks and are safe when dosed correctly. "There are a lot of data encouraging physicians to use these medications because they are beneficial," she says. "There haven't been much data looking at how they are given."

IMPLICATIONS

Although the study was funded by four drug companies, "the message in this paper is not a particularly good one for drug companies—the idea that these drugs might be harmful," Alexander notes.

"Hopefully, this will begin to get providers to be aware that it is important to consider dosing adjustments, particularly among high-risk populations, such as women, the elderly and those who are small," she says.

info For more information on heparin, visit the US National Library of Medicine's MedlinePlus Web site at *www.medlineplus.gov.* Click on "Drugs & Supplements."

Self-Monitoring Blood Drug Saves Lives

Carl Heneghan, MD, clinical research fellow, Oxford University, England.
Gary Liska, director, disease management group, Quality Assured Services, Melbourne, FL.
The Lancet.

People who take the anticlotting medication *warfarin* (Coumadin) get substantial benefits if they monitor their own blood levels rather than have a laboratory do it for them, British researchers report.

THE STUDY

An analysis of 14 controlled trials found that patients' self-monitoring of warfarin led to a 55% reduction in harmful clotting events, a 39% lower death rate from all causes and a 35% reduction in major bleeding crises, compared with laboratory monitoring.

The study was initially intended simply to show that self-monitoring in warfarin patients was safe, says study author Dr. Carl Heneghan, a clinical research fellow at Oxford University. Finding that it actually provided a substantial benefit came as something of a surprise.

"Each of the trials alone was not statistically significant, but combining them showed that you get a benefit in terms of mortality," he says.

ADVANTAGES

Warfarin is a notoriously difficult drug to manage, requiring patients who are taking it to have frequent blood tests to make sure that their blood-clotting ability is within the normal range. They often need to be tested every few weeks—or even every week—for many years. Self-monitoring "offers a sense of freedom, not being tied to a clinic," Heneghan says.

EQUIPMENT

The method that patients use to self-monitor warfarin is basically the same as what diabetics do when they check their blood sugar levels—a drop of blood from a fingerstick is placed on a monitoring device. If the reading is outside the range set by the doctor, the patient can call him/her for instructions about changing the dose.

> *Self-monitoring offers a sense of freedom, not being tied to a clinic.*
>
> Carl Heneghan, MD

Self-monitoring equipment has been approved for use by the US Food and Drug Administration (FDA), but fewer than 1% of physicians allow their patients to use it, notes Gary Liska, director of the disease management group at Quality Assured Services, a company that markets this type of monitor.

One reason these devices are not used more is that Medicare pays for them only for people who have artificial heart valves, Liska says. However, warfarin can be taken for a number of other reasons, such as to control the abnormal heartbeat, called *atrial fibrillation.*

In addition, doctors worry that patients will not be able to adequately control their blood levels, Liska says. "We feel that, in reality, the opposite is true—that patients have better control than ever before."

Another issue is the fear of malpractice suits should something go wrong when patients are self-monitoring. Many people who take warfarin are elderly and are also taking a number of other medications that could interact with warfarin.

Finally, intensive patient training is required to use the equipment and the test strips are expensive.

info You can find out more information about warfarin from Drug Digest at *www.drug digest.org*. Click on "Drugs & Vitamins" in the pull-down menu under "Drug Library."

Anticlotting Drug Only Half as Effective as In Clinical Trials

Brian F. Gage, MD, associate professor of medicine, Washington University, St. Louis.
Stroke.

Two recent studies examined the difficulties of using the drug *warfarin*, a clot-preventing drug that is often prescribed for people who have *atrial fibrillation*, an abnormal heartbeat. Common among older individuals, atrial fibrillation increases the risk that a clot will form in the heart and travel to the brain, causing a stroke.

Warfarin is a difficult drug to manage—for both the doctors who prescribe it and the people who take it. Frequent blood tests are necessary to make sure that the dosage prescribed creates just the right amount of clot-preventing activity. Too much warfarin can cause dangerous bleeding episodes.

THE FIRST STUDY:
WHY IT'S NOT PRESCRIBED

One study at Boston University followed the treatment of 405 people, age 65 and older, who had atrial fibrillation. According to the researchers, only 51% of the patients were taking warfarin when they left the hospital. Doctors gave several reasons for not prescribing the drug.

In one-third of the cases, doctors cited current or chronic bleeding episodes as the reason for not prescribing warfarin. In another one-third, the physicians cited falls by patients that had caused a head injury or a broken bone. And the reason given in 14% of the cases was the patient's refusal to take the drug or a history of not taking prescribed drugs.

"We need to better understand the underlying mechanism of clotting to find novel drugs that lessen the risk of hemorrhage," says study author Dr. Elaine M. Hylek, an associate professor of medicine at Boston University.

THE SECOND STUDY:
REAL-LIFE EXPERIENCES

The second study looked at the real-life experiences of more than 17,000 Medicare beneficiaries who were taking warfarin for atrial fibrillation.

> *What we need
> are easier drugs to handle.
> In a few years, we should have
> alternatives to warfarin.*
>
> Brian F. Gage, MD

"It was pretty disappointing," says lead researcher, Dr. Brian F. Gage, an associate professor of medicine at Washington University in St. Louis. "Warfarin was only half as effective in these Medicare beneficiaries as in clinical trials."

Even when warfarin use was clearly indicated—in people who had no reason for not taking the drug and had other risk factors for stroke—it was used in only 65% of the cases, the study found.

One major reason for the underuse of warfarin was the need for constant monitoring through a blood test every few weeks, Gage says. "Monitoring for many patients was infrequent," he says. "Tests were done every three months or sometimes at longer intervals."

Gage thinks the infrequent monitoring could be due to some Medicare policies. For example, most people get their blood test results by phone, but Medicare doesn't reimburse patients unless the assessment is made in a doctor's office, he says. "It's a hassle for patients, physicians and staff," Gage explains. "This kind of reimbursement is a disincentive for monitoring."

But, "In the long term, what we need are easier drugs to handle. In a few years, we should have alternatives to warfarin," Gage predicts.

Don't Lose Sleep Over Ambien Reports

Donna Arand, PhD, clinical director, Kettering Sleep Disorders Center, Dayton, OH, and spokeswoman, American Academy of Sleep Medicine.

Michael H. Silber, MB, ChB, professor of neurology, Mayo Clinic College of Medicine, codirector, Mayo Sleep Disorders Center, Rochester, MN, and president, American Academy of Sleep Medicine.

Michael Thorpy, MD, director, Sleep–Wake Disorders Center, Montefiore Medical Center, and associate professor of neurology, Albert Einstein College of Medicine, both in Bronx, NY.

American Academy of Sleep Medicine.

Reports in the media of bizarre behaviors —including eating, driving and even shoplifting—that occurred during Ambien-induced sleep have raised concerns among the millions of Americans who take the popular prescription sleep aid. But according to most experts, there is no need to panic.

THE NUMBERS

"It may seem like there's an explosion of these cases, but when you've got 26 million prescriptions written and just 48 cases reported to the US Food and Drug Administration [FDA]—most of which involved inappropriate use of the medication—the numbers are extremely small," says Donna Arand, clinical director of the Kettering Sleep Disorders Center in Dayton, Ohio, and a spokeswoman for the American Academy of Sleep Medicine (AASM).

These figures are from the FDA's adverse events reporting database, which has tracked patient reports of medication-associated sleepwalking since 1997. Based on those numbers, Arand says she believes, "Overall, the medications that are available are safe for almost everyone."

Michael H. Silber, codirector of the Mayo Clinic's Sleep Disorders Center, and president of the AASM, who has studied the phenomenon of Ambien-linked binge sleep-eating, says, "There's little doubt in my mind or those of my colleagues that Ambien can do this. I don't think it's common; I think it's a very small minority of patients who use Ambien who do this."

In sleep-eating, individuals gain weight after repeated bingeing at night, with no recollection of it when they awake. "We've had patients who, as soon as they started using Ambien, started sleep-eating," Silber says. "Then they stopped Ambien, and the sleep-eating went away. We first published on this a few years ago, and in the five years since, we have not seen it with other sleep medications."

EXPLANATION

According to Dr. Michael Thorpy, director of the Sleep–Wake Disorders Center at Montefiore Medical Center in New York City, specialists have long known that the risk of sleepwalking and other *parasomnias* rise when people take a sleeping pill.

> *There's little doubt in my mind that Ambien can cause parasomnias. I don't think it's common; I think it's a very small minority of patients.*
>
> *Michael H. Silber, MB, ChB*

Sleepwalking occurs when the brain doesn't catch up with the body as it emerges into wakefulness. "These parasomnias are related to the amount of time people have been in fairly deep, slow-wave sleep," Thorpy says. "So, if a sleep agent makes you sleep more consistently, with less arousals, you're more likely to have more of these behaviors."

Sanofi-Aventis, the French company that manufactures Ambien, says that it is aware that parasomnias are associated with this medication. In fact, Ambien's package insert states that parasomnias are a rare but potential side effect, as is temporary memory loss.

According to Arand and Thorpy, there's no hard evidence that Ambien users are more likely to experience parasomnias than people who use other sleep aids. Ambien, approved in 1993—and its two newer rivals in the billion-dollar sleep-aid market, Sonata (approved in 2002) and Lunesta (approved in 2005)—all work in much the same way.

"Maybe there is something specific that makes Ambien more likely to produce this type of behavior than other hypnotics, but that's hard to say at this point, because it's, by far, the largest medication used out there," Thorpy says.

Experts speculate that the reason these parasomnias are seen in Ambien users is related to the drug's *half-life*, or the amount of time the drug stays active in the brain. "It lingers [for] a shorter time than Lunesta and a longer time than Sonata," Silber says. "So, it may have something to do with that half-life—the fact that it stays around for three to five hours may be just the length that's needed to do what it does. But we're not entirely sure."

TAKE AS DIRECTED

One thing that experts are sure of is that Ambien, like all drugs, must be taken as directed. In many of the reported cases, users had combined Ambien with alcohol or other drugs, or had taken it too soon before a hazardous activity, such as driving. "People may also be exceeding the [recommended] dose," Thorpy says. "The usual dose is 5 or 10 milligrams [mg], but sometimes people will take 20 mg. That could be a factor."

The AASM recommends that consumers read the fine print on the package inserts that come with all prescription sleep medications, to familiarize themselves with the proper usage and any potential side effects.

Silber says he still routinely prescribes Ambien to his patients, but added there's a real need for awareness—not panic—about the drug. "I'm hoping people will learn that if they are prescribed Ambien, [they should] be aware that there are potential side effects—as there are with any drug. And [they should] be prepared to stop using it if these side effects develop."

According to Sanofi-Aventis, the most common side effects of Ambien include daytime drowsiness, dizziness and coordination difficulties. Many of these side effects can be avoided by taking the proper dose and avoiding alcohol.

info To get a good night's sleep, visit the American Academy of Sleep Medicine Web site at *www.aasmnet.org/pdf/insomnia.pdf.*

Medications to Help You Get a Good Night's Sleep

Michael Thorpy, MD, director, Sleep–Wake Disorders Center, Montefiore Medical Center, and associate professor of neurology, Albert Einstein College of Medicine, both in Bronx, NY. He is coauthor of *Sleeping Well: The Sourcebook for Sleep and Sleep Disorders.* Checkmark.

More and more Americans are taking medications to help them fall asleep. Spending on drugs to treat insomnia

and related disorders surged by 20% last year, according to Medco Health Solutions.

Insomnia is defined as trouble falling asleep or staying asleep for three or more nights per week for one month or longer, accompanied by daytime fatigue.

Don't let insomnia go on for days, weeks or months. The sooner you get episodes of insomnia under control, the less likely you will be to develop chronic insomnia.

Sleeping pills can provide relief from occasional insomnia and can help prevent chronic insomnia. *Here's what you need to know about today's sleep medications...*

NONBENZODIAZEPINES

This class of sleeping pills was introduced in the US in 1992 with the drug *zolpidem* (Ambien). These drugs target receptors in the brain that trigger the release of *gamma-amino butyric acid* (GABA), a chemical that reduces brain activity and induces sleep.

Compared with previous classes of sleeping pills, *nonbenzodiazepines* are more effective and cause fewer side effects, such as daytime drowsiness. Also, unlike the older class of *benzodiazepines*, they are not addictive. (If you are addicted to medication, you get an adverse reaction when you stop taking it, such as an increase in anxiety, irritability or heart rate.) Nonbenzodiazepines can be taken safely long-term.

Some people worry that if they take a sleeping pill, they won't be able to wake up if there is an emergency—but in the usual doses, that should not be a problem.

You should not take these medications with alcohol. However, if you have a glass or two of wine with dinner several hours before bedtime, there should be no adverse effects.

•**Zolpidem** (Ambien) is the most widely prescribed sleeping pill in the US. It works quickly and induces sleepiness for approximately six hours. It has a low rate of very mild side effects, such as headache and nausea. (See the preceding article on page 107 for information on the recent controversy about Ambien.)

Best if you: Have difficulty falling asleep and/or tend to wake up in the middle of the night and are not able to fall back asleep. Take at bedtime.

•**Zaleplon** (Sonata) also works quickly, but only lasts for two to four hours.

Best if you: Wake up in the middle of the night and don't intend to get up for at least four hours. For example, take it at 4 am if your rising time is 8 am. It's also good if you just have trouble falling asleep but don't have trouble sleeping through the night.

• **Eszopiclone** (Lunesta) was approved by the US Food and Drug Administration (FDA) in 2004. Research indicates that Lunesta may be the most effective nonbenzodiazepine for preventing nighttime waking. It lasts eight hours—two hours longer than Ambien—but it's still too soon to tell if daytime drowsiness is a commonly experienced side effect.

Best if you: Need help increasing the amount of time you sleep to a full seven or eight hours.

BENZODIAZEPINES

This class of drugs includes *temazepam* (Restoril), *estazolam* (ProSom), *triazolam* (Halcion) and *flurazepam* (Dalmane). They relax muscles and reduce anxiety—but can have serious side effects, including daytime drowsiness. They are potentially addictive, causing *rebound insomnia*, a worsening of sleeplessness when you stop taking them, as well as anxiety and nightmares.

Restoril is the most widely used benzodiazepine, but most doctors prefer to prescribe nonbenzodiazepines.

ANTIDEPRESSANTS

The so-called sedating antidepressants—*nefazodone* (Serzone), *trazodone* (Desyrel) and *amitriptyline* (Elavil)—are prescribed for people who are depressed and also have insomnia. Taken at night, they induce sleep and relieve depression during the day.

Downside: Serious side effects, such as cardiac irregularity, low blood pressure in the elderly and/or impotence.

Best if you: Have mild depression along with sleeping problems.

Another option: Use a newer, safer antidepressant during the day, such as *sertraline* (Zoloft), and a nonbenzodiazepine, such as Ambien, at night. Studies show that this combination is safe and effective.

NONPRESCRIPTION SLEEPING AIDS

• **Antihistamines,** including *diphenhydramine* (Benadryl, Nytol, Sleep-eze, Sominex, Tylenol PM) and *doxylamine* (Unisom) have drowsiness as a side effect. Unfortunately, it can last into the day. Also, antihistamines are not as effective as nonbenzodiazepines.

Best if you: Experience occasional insomnia.

Caution: If you start to experience insomnia regularly, discontinue antihistamines. See your doctor for a prescription medication that treats insomnia effectively and quickly.

• **Melatonin** is a hormone that affects the body's sleep–wake cycle. A recent review by the National Institutes of Health (NIH) showed that it is not an effective sleeping pill but is useful in changing the timing of sleep.

Best if you: Have trouble getting to sleep before 3 am or 4 am and then sleep until noon. This is most common among the elderly, adolescents who have insomnia and travelers who have jet lag. Melatonin can help bring bedtime back toward 11 pm. Take melatonin—following the dosage recommendation on the label—around 6 pm or 7 pm.

• **Valerian.** The research on this herb is mixed. Some studies indicate that valerian can reduce stress and help more quickly...others have shown no benefit. It is unlikely to cause side effects at the doses recommended on labels. Higher doses have been linked to blurred vision and changes in heart rhythm.

Best if you: Want to try an herbal remedy for occasional insomnia.

• **Herbal tea/warm milk.** Teas believed to be calming include chamomile, lemon balm and lavender. The active ingredients in these and other teas don't appear to have significant effects on insomnia. The same is true for milk. However, the nighttime ritual of a cup of tea or a glass of warm milk may reduce stress and help some people fall asleep more easily.

EVEN BETTER SLEEP

Insomnia medications are even more effective if you...

• **Don't stay in bed too long.** People who don't get enough sleep tend to go to bed earlier and get up later, trying to catch up. Over time, the sleep period spreads out over a larger portion of the day, which disturbs the normal sleep pattern. Never stay in bed longer than eight hours, no matter how you have slept.

•**Go to bed and get up at the same time every day.** This will help restore normal sleeping patterns.

•**Take medication at the right time.** The medication has to work in conjunction with a sleep–wake cycle, at a time when there is a physiological drive to sleep. If you had a good night's sleep and took the pill at 10 am, you would not sleep for the next eight hours.

■ ■ ■ ■

Where Do People Sleep Best?

Based on the number of days residents reported not getting enough sleep and certain other criteria, Minneapolis was named the "Best City for Sleep." It was followed by Anaheim, San Diego, Raleigh-Durham and Washington, DC.

Worst places to sleep: Detroit, Cleveland, Nashville, Cincinnati and New Orleans.

Bert Sperling, author of "Best Places" studies and founder of the research firm Sperling's Best Places, Portland, OR.

The Lowdown on the New Antidepressants

David L. Ginsberg, MD, clinical associate professor of psychiatry, New York University, and director, outpatient psychiatry, Tisch Hospital, New York University Medical Center, both in New York City.

Antidepressants have been getting negative reviews lately. Pharmaceutical companies have been called to task for the credibility of their research, and fears have emerged that the drugs may increase suicide risk—especially among teenagers.*

In the face of such controversy, why would anyone want to take an antidepressant?

Problem: Up to 19 million Americans experience depression. And self-help strategies, such as exercise, diet and natural remedies, don't help

*Antidepressants now carry a warning label because research shows increased suicidal thoughts (not actual suicides) in children and adolescents who are taking these drugs. When taking an antidepressant, call your doctor if you experience agitation, physical restlessness or have suicidal thoughts.

everyone. For many people who are depressed, medication offers the best hope for relief.

New: Drugs that relieve depression but do not cause intolerable side effects are now available.

DO YOU NEED AN ANTIDEPRESSANT?

Depression affects both the mind and the body. Emotionally, you feel sad or "numb" much of the time. You may no longer enjoy things that once pleased you (including hobbies, seeing friends and shopping)…you feel unmotivated…find it difficult to concentrate…experience decreased libido…feel guilty or worthless. You may be more prone to abuse alcohol or drugs and might even think of suicide.

Physically, you may experience fatigue, too little (or too much) sleep, changes in appetite and/or a sense of slowing down. In some people, depression manifests as headaches and/or backaches.

If you have several of these symptoms, see your doctor or a mental health professional to determine whether depression is to blame. This is especially true if your symptoms have caused trouble in your relationships and/or at work.

When depression is relatively mild—especially if it seems linked to a situation (a bad job or troubled marriage, for example) or traumatic event (such as a death in the family)—it may be worthwhile to try psychotherapy first. But if depression interferes seriously with your life—particularly if you or family members have had depression and/or anxiety before—medication combined with psychotherapy may be a better choice.

A GROWING ARSENAL

For nearly 50 years, doctors have prescribed *tricyclic antidepressants*, such as *amitriptyline* (Elavil) and *imipramine* (Tofranil)…and *monoamine oxidase inhibitors* (MAOIs), such as *tranylcypromine* (Parnate). They are not widely used today, largely because of side effects, such as weight gain, sedation and dietary restrictions.

In the last 18 years, antidepressants known as *selective serotonin reuptake inhibitors* (SSRIs) have received significant attention. They work by increasing the activity of *serotonin*, a brain chemical that is linked to depression. SSRIs include *fluoxetine* (Prozac), *sertraline* (Zoloft), *paroxetine* (Paxil) and *citalopram* (Celexa). In 2002, *escitalopram* (Lexapro) joined this group.

Drugs that work on other brain chemicals instead of, or in addition to, serotonin include *bupropion* (Wellbutrin), *venlafaxine* (Effexor), *mirtazapine* (Remeron) and the newest, *duloxetine* (Cymbalta), which was introduced in 2004.

FINDING THE RIGHT MEDICATION

Individuals respond differently to antidepressants. You may do better on Drug A while another person does better on Drug B. This is largely due to differences in individual biology. Any antidepressant will substantially relieve symptoms in approximately two-thirds of the people who take it.

Regardless of the drug being used, you may begin to feel better in a week or two, but it takes four to six weeks for symptoms to substantially improve. If you are still depressed after six to eight weeks, your doctor may suggest increasing the dosage or trying a different antidepressant.

SIDE EFFECTS

All medication, including antidepressants, may affect the body in undesired ways.

Example: SSRIs cause sexual problems (reduced desire, difficulty with arousal or orgasm) in many people. These problems are least likely with bupropion or mirtazapine.

Many people fear that antidepressants will change their personalities or blunt their emotions. With the right medication, however, this should not occur.

If side effects are troublesome, it may be necessary to reduce the dosage of the antidepressant or switch to another. *If the drug is otherwise working well, talk to your doctor about trying the following strategies to reduce side effects...*

•**Nausea.** Split the dose or take the medication at bedtime. Or take the pill with food.

•**Daytime sleepiness or fatigue.** If nighttime sleep is adequate, consider taking the antidepressant at night. Your doctor also may consider lowering the dosage, adding a low-dose stimulant, such as *modafinil* (Provigil), or switching to another drug.

•**Weight gain.** Diet and exercise are essential—but an antidepressant may lower metabolism, leading to weight gain. Consider one of the antidepressants that's least likely to affect weight, such as bupropion.

THE LONG HAUL

Once an antidepressant has eased depression symptoms, most people want to stop taking it.

But stopping too soon increases the risk of a recurrence.

•**If this is your first episode of depression,** talk to your doctor about staying on the medication for at least one year after you begin to feel better.

•**If this is your second bout, or if depression runs in your family,** consider continuing the medication for two years or longer.

•**If you've had three or more episodes of depression,** the risk of a recurrence is more than 90%. Many doctors advocate medication indefinitely—the way a diabetic takes insulin.

Important: If you stop taking an antidepressant, do so gradually—and under a doctor's supervision.

Popular IBS Drug Falls Short of Expectations

Mark A. Stengler, ND, naturopathic physician, La Jolla Whole Health Clinic, La Jolla, CA, and associate clinical professor, the National College of Naturopathic Medicine, Portland, OR. He is author of numerous books on natural healing, including *The Natural Physician's Healing Therapies.* Bottom Line. *www.bottomlinesecrets.com.*

The chronic condition known as *irritable bowel syndrome* (IBS) affects up to 20% of the US population. Symptoms include diarrhea and/or constipation, abdominal pain, cramping, gas and nausea.

In 2002, *tegaserod* (Zelnorm) was approved by the US Food and Drug Administration (FDA) for the short-term treatment of IBS in women who experienced constipation. Since then, it has been prescribed for 68% of IBS cases in the US, according to the drug's manufacturer, Novartis.

Is Zelnorm the drug that women who have IBS have been waiting for?

First, it's important to understand that Zelnorm was approved only for the short-term treatment of female IBS patients whose main symptom is constipation (hard stools or difficulty passing stools). Women who have diarrhea should not use Zelnorm because it can worsen this condition.

Zelnorm has never been shown to be effective for men who have IBS, but it is used for chronic *idiopathic* (from an unknown cause) constipation in men and women younger than age 65. Also, it is not recommended for people who have a history of bowel obstruction and/or gallbladder disease because it can worsen both conditions.

Zelnorm is one of a new class of drugs called *serotonin-4 receptor agonists*, which activate receptors for *serotonin*, a relaxing neurotransmitter, in the digestive tract. This action is thought to normalize digestive tract movement.

Studies involving Zelnorm show a mild benefit, such as improved bowel movements and reduced abdominal pain, discomfort and bloating, but the drug's long-term safety and effectiveness have not been established. The most common side effects include headache, abdominal pain, diarrhea, nausea and dizziness.

In April 2004, the FDA warned people to stop taking Zelnorm immediately if they developed rectal bleeding, bloody diarrhea or new or worsening abdominal pain. These are symptoms of *intestinal ischemia*, a potentially fatal condition in which the supply of blood and oxygen to the intestines is compromised. The FDA's caution was based on information from clinical trials and "postmarketing reports." This means that, essentially, people who had taken Zelnorm—just as those who take other new drugs—had unwittingly served as guinea pigs to determine the drug's side effects.

A BETTER OPTION

In summary, Zelnorm has undergone no long-term studies, has the potential for some very serious side effects and has not been shown to be effective in men or in patients who have diarrhea-associated IBS. I believe most people can find better relief with nontoxic natural therapies.

IBS is a disease of modern times, which are marked by fast food, high stress and the overuse of drugs. (Antibiotics and steroids, in particular, destroy "friendly" bacteria that help digest food.)

I have found that natural therapies for IBS have a very high success rate in both men and women. I'm confident that the benefits of a holistic approach using a healthful (high-fiber, low-sugar) diet, nutritional supplements that aid digestion (probiotics, enzymes and digestive herbal tonics) and stress-reduction techniques (exercise, prayer and counseling) far exceed the mild benefits of Zelnorm. And, of course, the drug's serious side effects would not be an issue using a natural approach.

In my opinion, Zelnorm is a waste of time and money and not worth the risk. Save the $170 you would spend on Zelnorm each month and invest it instead in healthful food and supplements that aid digestion.

■ ■ ■ ■

Identifying IBS

Contrary to popular belief, *diverticulosis*—the existence of noninfected pockets in the colon—rarely causes symptoms. But how then do you explain why one in every three people who has diverticulosis also reports having abdominal discomfort?

These symptoms are usually caused by *irritable bowel syndrome* (IBS), a separate (and very common) condition marked by pain, bloating, constipation and/or diarrhea.

If you're experiencing any of these symptoms, see your doctor, who will give you a physical exam and perhaps run some tests to rule out other possible conditions.

IBS can have a wide variety of causes, including muscle spasms in the colon as well as emotional stress.

Helpful: IBS treatment typically includes stress reduction, a shift to a high-fiber diet and possibly medication.

Important MS Drug Back on the Market

Steven K. Galson, MD, MPH, director, Center for Drug Evaluation and Research, US Food and Drug Administration.

Patricia O'Looney, MD, director, biomedical research, National Multiple Sclerosis Society.

Russell Katz, MD, Office of Drug Evaluation 1, Division of Neurology Products, Center for Drug Evaluation and Research, US Food and Drug Administration.

Setting strict guidelines, the US Food and Drug Administration (FDA) has allowed the return of the multiple sclerosis (MS) drug *natalizumab* (Tysabri).

BACKGROUND

Tysabri had received FDA approval in November 2004, only to be pulled from the market three months later after several patients in clinical trials developed a rare but deadly viral infection of the brain called *progressive multifocal leukoencephalopathy* (PML).

The FDA put the clinical trials on hold in February 2005, but allowed them to resume one year later, in February 2006, with no additional cases of PML reported.

"This is one of the very rare cases in which a drug withdrawn from the market for safety reasons has been returned back to the market after appropriate steps have been taken," says Dr. Steven K. Galson, director of the FDA's Center for Drug Evaluation and Research.

"In this case, we made the assessment that the benefits of this drug outweigh the risks," Galson adds. "We are certain that patients are willing to take this risk because of the potential benefits of the drug."

BENEFITS

Studies have found that treatment using Tysabri reduced the rate of relapse in MS patients by as much as two-thirds after two years, and reduced the number of patients whose symptoms worsened.

"We are very pleased with the review and the outcome from the FDA," says Dr. Patricia O'Looney, director of biomedical research at the National Multiple Sclerosis Society. "It's good news for people with MS. It's good news because it provides an option for treatment.

"The important thing is to have the drug back on the market, so that patients and doctors can discuss whether or not to use the drug for a particular patient," O'Looney says.

RISKS

Still there are risks. "Currently, the best estimate we have of the rate of occurrence of PML is about one in 1,000 patients treated," says Dr. Russell Katz, of the FDA's Division of Neurology Products. "We know little about what the risk would be in a larger population or what the risk would be if treatment continues beyond two years," he says.

With the drug's return to the market, there will undoubtedly be other cases of PML and additional deaths, Katz adds. But, he says, "This is balanced against the significant benefit that the drug confers."

THE NEW GUIDELINES

Tysabri will only be available through a risk-management plan, called the TOUCH Prescribing Program. To receive Tysabri, patients must confer with their doctor, understand the risks and benefits of the drug and agree to all of the guidelines of the program. *Some of those guidelines include...*

•**Only those registered with the program and who agree to comply with it** will be able to prescribe the drug.

•**Only infusion centers registered and authorized** will be able to administer Tysabri intravenously.

•**Only pharmacies registered with the program** will be able to dispense Tysabri to authorized infusion centers.

•**Only patients enrolled in the program and who agree to comply with it** will be able to receive the drug.

•**All program prescribers, pharmacies, infusion centers and patients will be educated** about the program as well as the risks of Tysabri.

O'Looney says the FDA restrictions are warranted. "We don't know enough about the drug. The results from the two-year study were remarkable in terms of its impact on disease activity and progression, but there is a concern about PML. So all of these restrictions are justified," she says. "It's all for the protection of the patient."

In addition, safety surveillance—including regular *magnetic resonance imaging* (MRI), monitoring and reporting of PML and other serious infections and deaths, and systematic tracking of patients and drug disposition—will be carried out, according to the FDA.

■ ■ ■ ■

What Is Multiple Sclerosis?

Multiple sclerosis (MS), which affects approximately 350,000 Americans, is an unpredictable disease of the central nervous system. Most MS patients experience muscle weakness in their extremities and difficulty with coordination and balance. Symptoms may be severe enough to impair walking or even standing. Its cause is not known and there is no cure, according to the National Institutes of Health (NIH).

info The National Multiple Sclerosis Society can tell you more about multiple sclerosis at *www.nationalmssociety.org.*

New Drug Helps Smokers Quit for Good

Serena Tonstad, MD, attending physician, department of preventive cardiology, Ulleval University Hospital, Oslo, Norway.
The Journal of the American Medical Association.

The drug *varenicline* (Chantix) quadrupled the success rate of people trying to quit smoking, according to three recent studies. Approved by the US Food and Drug Administration (FDA), Chantix was also found to be twice as effective as *bupropion* (Zyban), another smoking-cessation drug.

The research—all of which was funded by the drug's maker, Pfizer Inc.—is encouraging, experts say, because smokers do not have many medications that are useful in helping them quit.

Unlike Zyban and nicotine-replacement methods (patches and gums), Chantix works by stimulating the release of the brain chemical *dopamine*, to reduce cravings, while simultaneously blocking the brain cell receptors that help sustain addiction.

TWO STUDIES

In one study, researchers led by David Gonzales at the Oregon Health & Science University in Portland, compared the effectiveness of Chantix, Zyban and a placebo in helping 1,025 adult smokers quit over the course of one year.

After 12 weeks, 44% of the people taking Chantix had been smoke-free for at least one month, compared with 29.5% of those taking Zyban and just under 18% of those in the placebo group, the researchers report.

Long-term quit rates were lower, however. The rate of "continuous abstinence" from week nine to the one-year mark was just under 22% for Chantix, approximately 16% for Zyban, and 8.4% for the placebo.

A second, similar trial led by Douglas Jorenby of the University of Wisconsin found almost identical results.

THE THIRD STUDY

A third trial of more than 1,900 smokers living in seven countries looked specifically at relapse rates after quitting.

All of the smokers first underwent 12 weeks of Chantix therapy. Approximately two-thirds (1,236) were deemed to have kicked the habit by the end of the three-month period.

The researchers then gave these "quitters" either Chantix or a placebo daily for the next 12 weeks.

By the end of the 24-week study period, 70.5% of the people who continued on Chantix remained nonsmokers, compared with 49.6% of those taking a placebo for the second 12 weeks.

"An additional 12 weeks of treatment was more beneficial than placebo," says lead researcher of the study, Dr. Serena Tonstad, an attending physician in the department of preventive cardiology at Ulleval University Hospital in Oslo, Norway.

'NOT A PANACEA'

Robert Klesges and his colleagues at the University of Tennessee Health Science Center in Memphis say that when a new smoking-cessation aid gets FDA approval, "there is often unbridled enthusiasm regarding the potential to solve the problems associated with smoking." However, because of high rates of both side effects and treatment failure, Chantix "definitely is not a panacea for smoking cessation."

While on Chantix, almost 30% of the trial participants reported nausea, and many others experienced "abnormal dreams."

Dropout rates were also high, although that is consistent with what is usually seen in smoking-cessation trials.

In the Norwegian trial, only those smokers who had quit by 12 weeks were allowed to enter the second, relapse-focused phase of the trial. "The authors have eliminated [from their analysis] approximately one-third of individuals for whom this drug does not appear to be effective," the Tennessee experts note.

Finally, they say, all of these Pfizer-funded trials took place under the very best conditions—at academic research centers where smokers were closely monitored and instructed on the proper use of the drugs. That's quite different than a "real world" situation where the average smoker is given a prescription and then left more or less on his/her own.

So, while the results of these trials are promising, nicotine addiction remains a tough challenge. In fact, "the majority of participants in these three studies did not quit smoking—even with varenicline," the experts point out.

 For help on quitting smoking, visit the Web site, *www.smokefree.gov.*

▪▪▪▪

Easing Withdrawal Symptoms

A recent study found that *selegiline* (Deprenyl) reduces withdrawal symptoms of smokers who are trying to quit. Another study to confirm those results is under way and will be finished in 2008. Selegiline helps users maintain higher levels of *dopamine*, a brain chemical associated with pleasure. People trying to quit smoking produce less dopamine, which can cause them to be irritable and nervous. The drug is currently used for Parkinson's disease patients.

Tony P. George, MD, associate professor of psychiatry, Yale University, New Haven, CT.

▪▪▪▪

Even Casual Smoking Can Be Deadly

People who smoke only one to four cigarettes a day are 50% more likely to die prematurely than nonsmokers. Their risk of death from heart disease is three times higher than the risk for nonsmokers.

Bottom line: There is no level at which smoking is safe.

Kjell Bjartveit, MD, PhD, National Health Screening Service, and Aage Tverdal, PhD, Norwegian Institute of Public Health, both in Oslo.

▪▪▪▪

Quitting Reaps Rapid Health Benefits

Even people who have already had a heart attack quickly benefit from stopping smoking, according to a new study.

The study looked at 1,000 patients who had recently experienced an *acute coronary syndrome* event, such as a heart attack or unstable angina. The people who quit smoking saw a 30% reduction in their risk of having a second event during the following year, compared with those who didn't quit.

Dorothee Twardella, PhD, research fellow, department of epidemiology, German Centre for Research on Ageing, Heidelberg.

Ricin Vaccine Is Safe and Effective

Ellen Vitetta, PhD, director, Cancer Immunobiology Center, University of Texas Southwestern Medical Center, Dallas.

Christopher P. Holstege, MD, associate professor of emergency medicine and pediatrics, and director, Blue Ridge Poison Center, division of medical toxicology, University of Virginia, Charlottesville.

Proceedings of the National Academy of Sciences online.

The first human tests of a vaccine to prevent *ricin* poisoning show that it is safe and effective, researchers at the University of Texas Southwestern Medical Center report.

> *Ricin is a bioterrorism agent that is very potent. This is something that is a risk to the general public.*
>
> *Christopher P. Holstege, MD*

Ricin is a lethal poison made from the remains of processing castor beans. With more than 50,000 tons of castor bean extract available globally, public health officials warn that ricin could easily be obtained and used by terrorists.

THE NEW RESEARCH

In the pilot study, 15 participants were divided into three groups of five. Each group received a different dose of the vaccine, called RiVax, in a series of three injections. The group that received the highest dose produced ricin-neutralizing antibodies in their blood, indicating that their immune systems had responded, the researchers found.

"A vaccine that we developed against ricin is safe and it elicited antibodies in human volunteers," says lead researcher Ellen Vitetta, director of the Cancer Immunobiology Center.

To determine whether the antibodies would prevent ricin poisoning, Vitetta's team tested the human antibodies in mice that had been injected with active ricin. The mice survived.

DEVELOPMENT WILL TAKE TIME

While this small study is encouraging, the actual development of the vaccine may take some time, Vitetta says. First, the researchers need to establish a large stockpile of the vaccine to test on many people, and they must find the best way to store the vaccine to keep it stable. In addition, the researchers need to test its effectiveness against the various ways that ricin can be delivered. "We need to determine whether the vaccine will protect against ricin aerosol, ricin given orally or in water or food," Vitetta says.

Dr. Christopher P. Holstege, director of the Blue Ridge Poison Center in the division of medical toxicology at the University of Virginia, thinks that developing a successful vaccine against ricin is important to thwart a potential bioterror attack. There is a pressing need for an effective vaccine for ricin poisoning, Holstege says. "Ricin is a bioterrorism agent that is very potent," he says. "This is something that is a risk to the general public and to the military."

■ ■ ■ ■

What Is Ricin?

Ricin is a lethal poison that is considered a potential bioterror threat. It is made from castor bean extract, a byproduct of castor oil production, and can come in the form of a powder, mist or pellet or be dissolved in water or weak acid.

Depending on how the ricin is given, victims develop fever, nausea and abdominal pain or lung damage, and die within a few days of exposure. There is no antidote after the first few hours of exposure, and because symptoms do not appear until later and can mimic other illnesses, people often do not know they have been exposed until it is too late for treatment.

In recent years, there have been several incidents involving ricin in the United States and Europe. In 2004, three US Senate office buildings were closed after ricin was found in the mailroom of Senate Majority Leader Bill Frist's office. There were no injuries reported.

The Centers for Disease Control and Prevention (CDC) classifies ricin as a Category B biological agent, meaning it is "relatively easy to disseminate."

info The Centers for Disease Control and Prevention has more information about ricin at *www.bt.cdc.gov/agent/ricin/facts.asp.*

Injectable Osteoporosis Drug Shows Promise

Nieca Goldberg, MD, former chief, women's cardiac care, Lenox Hill Hospital, New York City, spokeswoman, American Heart Association, and author of *The Women's Healthy Heart Program*. Ballantine.
The New England Journal of Medicine.

A recent study has found that a new, injectable drug to treat osteoporosis—*denosumab*—boosts bone mineral density and decreases the rate of bone loss in postmenopausal women.

THE STUDY

This study looked at 412 postmenopausal women who had low bone mineral density. Participants were randomly assigned to one of four groups—one group received denosumab every three months; the second group got denosumab every six months; another group took open-label oral *alendronate* (Fosamax) once a week; and the final group received a placebo.

At the end of 12 months, the women who were taking denosumab had an increase in bone mineral density at the lumbar spine (lower back) of 3% to 6.7%, compared with a 4.6% increase in bone mineral density for those taking Fosamax, and a loss of 0.8% bone mineral density for those taking a placebo.

At the hip, women taking denosumab experienced a gain of 1.9% to 3.6% bone mineral density, versus a 2.1% increase for those who were taking Fosamax and a loss of 0.6% for those taking a placebo.

At the wrist, women taking denosumab experienced an increase of 0.4% to 1.3% in bone mineral density, versus declines of 0.5% and 2% for those on Fosamax and for those on a placebo, respectively.

Three days after denosumab was administered, researchers say there were reductions in blood levels of *C-telopeptide*, indicating less bone destruction.

CONCLUSIONS

In conclusion, the researchers report that denosumab, given at three- or six-month intervals, resulted in an increase in bone mineral density, similar to that achieved using Fosamax, and a decrease in the rate of bone destruction.

Denosumab, which only needs to be administered a few times a year, is injected under the skin, most likely eliminating any gastrointestinal upset, a side effect of the currently prescribed osteoporosis medications known as *bisphosphonates*, says Dr. Nieca Goldberg, former chief of women's cardiac care at Lenox Hill Hospital in New York City and author of *The Women's Healthy Heart Program*.

IMPLICATIONS

According to the study authors, one of the problems with the current treatments for osteoporosis is a lack of adherence. For whatever reason, many patients stop taking medications that are designed to add calcium and other strengthening substances to their bones. One group of researchers reported that fewer than 25% of women consistently took their medication during the course of one year.

■ ■ ■ ■

What Is Osteoporosis?

An estimated 10 million Americans currently have osteoporosis, and another 34 million are considered to be at risk for the disease. Women are four times more likely than men to develop the condition.

People who have osteoporosis experience low bone mass and a weakening of the bone structure. This can eventually result in debilitating fractures, particularly of the hip, spine and wrist.

info Visit the National Osteoporosis Foundation Web site for more information on this condition at *www.nof.org*.

■ ■ ■ ■

Milk Not Enough to Build Strong Bones

Drinking milk is not enough to build strong bones, according to a recent study.

Recent finding: Women who drank one or more glasses of milk per day were just as likely to fracture a hip or wrist as those who drank less than one glass of milk per week.

Reason: Most women don't get enough vitamin D, which is necessary for calcium absorption.

Best way to get adequate vitamin D: Sit in the sun for 15 minutes a day, without sunscreen. Sunlight is necessary for the skin to manufacture the body's own supply of vitamin D. Vitamin D also can be found in fortified orange juice, certain fortified cereals and fatty fish, such as salmon and sardines. The recommended daily intake of vitamin D is 400 international units (IU), but many researchers now believe that much higher daily intakes are necessary.

Diane Feskanich, ScD, assistant professor, Channing Laboratory, department of medicine, Brigham and Women's Hospital and Harvard Medical School, both in Boston.

7

Emotional Well-Being

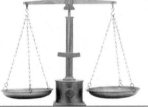

Antidepressants *Do* Raise Kids' Suicide Risk: Study

There is new evidence that the use of common antidepressants increases the risk of suicide in children and adolescents. Though much of the previous research had focused on users' suicidal thoughts and actions, this study "focused on things that are at the far more severe end of the spectrum—kids coming into the emergency room following suicide attempts and those who actually die," says Dr. Mark Olfson, lead author of the study and a professor of clinical psychiatry at the New York State Psychiatric Institute at Columbia University Medical Center in New York City. "These are things that are many, many times less common, thankfully, than the sorts of things that have been studied."

THE STUDY

The researchers looked at nearly 5,500 Medicaid beneficiaries across the country who had received inpatient treatment for depression. They divided the people into two groups—those who had received antidepressants and those who had not.

They found that children between the ages of six and 18 who were taking antidepressants were 1.5 times more likely to attempt suicide and 15 times more likely to die in that attempt than individuals not treated with an antidepressant. This trend was not seen among adults who used the drugs.

However, the authors caution, the statistics on the suicide deaths were based on only eight individuals, and these eight may have been among the sickest, which may have skewed the results.

In particular, children and adolescents who used antidepressants seemed to be at heightened risk of suicide in the period immediately

Mark Olfson, MD, MP, professor of clinical psychiatry, New York State Psychiatric Institute, Columbia University Medical Center, New York City.

Alec Miller, PsyD, chief, child and adolescent psychology, Montefiore Medical Center, and associate professor of psychiatry and behavioral sciences, Albert Einstein College of Medicine, both New York City.

Archives of General Psychiatry

after a hospitalization, especially if they were just starting on the medication, Olfson notes. The risk appeared to be linked to only certain types of antidepressants.

Children using *venlafaxine* (Effexor)—a *serotonin–norepinephrine* reuptake inhibitor (SNRI)—had a 2.3 times greater risk of suicide attempts compared with no drug treatment at all. Tricyclic antidepressants were also significantly linked with suicide attempts.

With the exception of (sertraline) Zoloft, selective serotonin reuptake inhibitors (SSRIs), were not significantly associated with suicide attempts, the study authors report.

IMPLICATIONS

It is likely that the differences in suicidal thoughts and behaviors among children were, in fact, due to the drugs they were taking, Olfson surmises.

"In order to be due to the depression, there would have to be differences in depression between groups," Olfson explains. "I can't completely exclude that possibility—and those that are more severely ill get more medications—but I think if depression were responsible, we would expect to find the same kind of relationships in adults. The fact that we see it with kids should raise our concern about this risk."

"This reinforces what the [US] Food and Drug Administration [FDA] has been warning about for the last couple of years," says Olfson.

"Parents and teachers and health-care professionals should pay close attention to changes in mood and actions of depressed children and take them seriously if they report that they feel more anxious or restless or develop thoughts of wanting to harm themselves," he adds.

"It appears that there are still reasons to be concerned about the antidepressant treatment of child and adolescent depression," says Alec Miller, chief of child and adolescent psychology at Montefiore Medical Center in New York City.

THE FUTURE

Miller, who is also an associate professor of psychiatry and behavioral sciences at Albert Einstein College of Medicine in New York City, says that children who are battling depression need more and better treatment options.

The Columbia study "makes the argument for really establishing more effective psychosocial interventions so that we don't need to rely on medication treatment," he says.

BACKGROUND

Pediatric use of antidepressant medications—especially SSRIs—has been the subject of extended controversy.

In October 2004, the FDA directed manufacturers of SSRIs, which include (*citalopram*) Celexa, (*paroxetine*) Paxil, (*fluoxetine*) Prozac and Zoloft, to put a special "black-box" warning on the drugs' labels to alert health-care providers of an increased risk of suicidal thoughts and behaviors in children and teens who are using the medications.

In July 2005, the FDA issued a public health advisory saying that this same risk may also apply to adults taking SSRIs, after several studies pointed to that possibility.

info For more information on depression, visit the Web site of the US National Alliance on Mental Illness at *www.nami.org*. Click on "About Mental Illness" under "Inform Yourself."

■ ■ ■ ■

Depression May Be Genetic

Recent research indicates that there is a genetic variation that could predispose some people to depression. This may explain why some individuals who experience depression are not helped by certain drugs. These findings may also allow scientists to formulate a genetic test for depression and pinpoint the most effective treatment.

Marc G. Caron, PhD, department of medicine, Duke University Medical Center, Durham, NC.

Depression: The #1 Hidden Health Threat

Peter D. Kramer, MD, clinical professor of psychiatry and human behavior, Brown University, Providence, RI, and author of *Listening to Prozac* (Penguin) and *Against Depression* (Viking).

Depression is one of the most misunderstood health problems. Some people still stigmatize it as a "character flaw."

Others romanticize it, claiming that it lends creativity, sensitivity—even wisdom.

However: Few people are aware that depression actually fuels the development of other serious medical conditions.

Unfortunately, the 19 million Americans who experience depression—and their families—are paying the price for the misconceptions. Only one in eight depressed Americans gets treatment.

To learn more, we spoke with Dr. Peter Kramer, a renowned psychiatrist…

●**As a health problem, how serious is depression?** In a very real sense, depression is the most devastating disease known to humankind—both in the developing world and industrialized nations. It is extremely widespread; it often strikes first in young adulthood or middle age and it frequently returns or becomes chronic. It robs more people of more years of active life than AIDS, heart disease or cancer. The disability that accompanies episodes of major depression is exceeded only in conditions such as dementia and quadriplegia.

And all this doesn't even take into account the effect that depression has on other diseases. Over the last 10 years, it's been firmly established that depression significantly raises the risk for heart attack and stroke, as well as accelerating bone loss and perhaps impairing immune function. Even if depression didn't cause terrible emotional suffering, it would be important to treat it for these medical reasons.

There's also evidence that certain physical conditions and medical treatments can cause depression. In older adults, for example, tiny strokes that cause changes to the *prefrontal cortex*—a part of the brain that seems to be involved in depression—can lead to depression symptoms, such as altered sleep and appetite and impaired self-image. Some doctors call this "vascular depression."

Thyroid disorders that affect hormone levels can be a direct cause of depression, while painful ailments, such as rheumatoid arthritis, can be an indirect cause. Fortunately, these types of depression are quite treatable with medication and other therapies. Drugs, such as the cancer medication *interferon*, steroids and some antihypertensives, can induce very severe depression.

●**Isn't depression a type of mental illness?** Research in the last decade has found that depression is associated with physical changes in the brain, similar to those that might occur with any neurological disease, such as epilepsy, Parkinson's or Alzheimer's. Depression causes *atrophy*—that is, brain cells die—and a loss of connections between brain cells. The longer the depression persists—or goes untreated—the greater the damage.

One study conducted by researchers at Washington University in St. Louis found that the *hippocampus*—a brain region linked to memory—was smaller in women who had a history of depression. The longer they had the disease without treatment, the greater the shrinkage. Their loss of memory was proportional to the time they had spent depressed.

●**Can treating depression reduce the risk for heart attack, stroke and other related illnesses?** The evidence isn't as strong as we'd like, but some research does suggest that this is true. A recent study of 1,834 patients who had had a heart attack and were depressed found that the risk of death or a second heart attack was approximately 40% lower in the patients who were prescribed an antidepressant.

Among stroke patients, one study conducted in Denmark showed that those who did not take an antidepressant were two to three times more likely to have another stroke within the next year.

●**How effective are the current treatments for depression?** The prescription antidepressants we have today are far from perfect, but they work pretty well. Approximately 80% of patients who are treated properly get substantially better. But all researchers agree that depression is underdiagnosed and undertreated. Most people still don't get the treatment they deserve.

●**Aren't many people wary of antidepressants because of side effects?** Yes. However, while side effects do occur, they are usually well tolerated compared with the side effects of many other medications. For someone who has major depression, minor side effects are tolerable. Although rare, antidepressants have been known to induce suicidal thoughts. (For more information on the link between antidepressants and suicide, see page 118.) When you start taking a new antidepressant, you should follow up with your doctor consistently.

•How depressed do you need to be for treatment to make sense—and how do you gauge this? Many more people should be evaluated for depression than currently are. Minor, or low-level, depression is just like major depression but with less intensity. There are many advantages to being assessed by a mental health professional to determine if you need treatment.

•Does depression ever mimic other illnesses? Yes. Some people may have a type of depression, often called *pseudodementia*, that has the pattern of a dementia illness. It resembles late-stage Parkinson's disease, resulting in problems in motivation, memory, concentration and word finding. Patients don't feel sad, but they do respond well to antidepressants.

•What should a person who has depression do to get help? If you think that you—or someone close to you—might be depressed, act as you would for any serious disease and get professional help from a doctor or mental health professional. If you're under treatment for depression, expect to see some sign that it's working. If you are using antidepressants and/or psychotherapy, you should start feeling at least somewhat better after four to six weeks. Don't settle for halfway—once you begin to improve, stay with the treatment until you and your doctor agree that you have achieved optimal results.

■ ■ ■ ■

Symptoms of Depression

In addition to feeling sad, hopeless and/or sluggish, people who are depressed may gain or lose weight, sleep too much or too little, feel irritable, anxious or emotionally numb, and/or lose interest in pleasurable activities, including sex.

If you experience two or more of these symptoms for more than two consecutive weeks, seek professional help immediately.

Some symptoms of depression that are commonly overlooked include chronic aches and pains, as well as problems with memory and concentration.

Switching Meds Can Help Beat Depression

A. John Rush, MD, professor of psychiatry, University of Texas Southwestern Medical Center, Dallas.

Thomas Insel, MD, director, National Institute of Mental Health.

Madhukar H. Trivedi, MD, professor of psychiatry, University of Texas Southwestern Medical Center, Dallas.

Eva Ritvo, associate professor of psychiatry, Miller School of Medicine, University of Miami, and chairwoman, department of psychiatry, Mount Sinai Medical Center, Miami Beach.

Maurizio Fava, director, Depression Clinical and Research Program, Massachusetts General Hospital, Boston.
The New England Journal of Medicine.

Approximately half of the people battling depression can achieve complete remission by either adding one more drug to their regimen or by switching to a new medication, according to researchers.

Selective serotonin reuptake inhibitors (SSRIs) —which include *citalopram* (Celexa), *paroxetine* (Paxil), *fluoxetine* (Prozac) and *sertraline* (Zoloft)—are considered effective medications to treat depression. However, doctors have not had good evidence on the best course of action if a patient fails to respond to a particular SSRI.

THE TRIAL—PART 1

The Sequenced Treatment Alternatives to Relieve Depression (STAR*D) trial, the largest effectiveness study ever done on depression, examined the benefits of antidepressants in "real world" settings.

The trial looked at rates of *remission* (full recovery)—as opposed to *response* (partial relief of symptoms)—in people who had nonpsychotic major-depressive disorder. Unlike many other clinical trials, most of the STAR*D participants also had coexisting psychiatric and/or medical conditions, or were unemployed or lacked health insurance.

For the first part of the study, more than 700 adults who had not responded to Celexa or who could not tolerate this drug were randomly assigned to receive instead either sustained-release *bupropion* (Wellbutrin, not an SSRI), Zoloft or *venlafaxine* (Effexor, not an SSRI) for up to 14 weeks.

Approximately 25% of the participants in the trial achieved total remission, regardless of the drug used.

"Three different 'switch' medications were tested," says Dr. A. John Rush, principal investigator of the study and professor of psychiatry at the University of Texas (UT) Southwestern Medical Center in Dallas. "No one was clearly better than another, even though these treatments do differ in how they work in the brain. Which treatment may be less important than the drugs being used diligently."

The study also indicated that four weeks of drug therapy, the amount of time doctors believe is necessary before improvements are noticed, is often not long enough to see a benefit, Rush says.

THE TRIAL—PART 2

The second part of the study looked at the value of adding Celexa to the drug regimens of 565 adult outpatients who were taking either Wellbutrin or Buspar (*buspirone*) for depression.

---

*Two steps produced full recovery
in over 50% of patients.*

Madhukar H. Trivedi, MD

"One in three patients went into remission with the addition of another medication," Rush says. "Again, despite differences in how the drugs work, both worked with approximately the same degree of efficacy and tolerability, and therefore, both are reasonable choices for patients who have not gotten fully well with the first treatment step."

Patients who did not respond to a second-tier treatment are being followed-up to see if other treatments are effective.

IMPLICATIONS

"Remission can be achieved in 50% of those who receive two treatment steps," Rush concludes. "Thus, for patients, it's important to not give up if the first treatment doesn't work fully or if it causes side effects."

"Treatment does work for most people if it's delivered in an adequate dose and over an appropriate period of time, meaning 12 weeks," adds Dr. Thomas Insel, director of the National Institute of Mental Health, which funded the trial. "For someone who's not well at 12 weeks, another medication can bring remission. That's an extremely important and hopeful message. One size doesn't fit all."

"In this kind of real-world, chronic medical illness, two steps produced full recovery in over 50% of patients," says Dr. Madhukar H. Trivedi, coprincipal investigator of the trial and professor of psychiatry at UT Southwestern Medical Center, Dallas. "When you compare that to most major medical illnesses, these are very encouraging results."

Dr. Eva Ritvo, an associate professor of psychiatry at the Miller School of Medicine at the University of Miami, agrees. "It's real-world data with big numbers, which are so hard to get. There's tremendous value in the study," she notes.

"This is by no means the end game," explains Dr. Maurizio Fava, director of the Massachusetts General Hospital's Depression Clinical and Research Program in Boston. "In the near future, we may be able to predict who is going to respond to what."

Depression is a chronic, disabling condition affecting approximately 15 million Americans —almost 7% of the adult population in the United States, Insel says. Approximately 4% of the people who have depression will end their own lives, resulting in 30,000 suicides each year. "That's almost twice the number of homicides," Insel points out. "It's a very real public health challenge."

In addition, approximately half of the people who experience depression don't receive treatment, and of those who do get treatment, only approximately 40% receive the best, "evidence-based" treatment.

info For more information about depression, visit the National Institute of Mental Health Web site at *www.nimh.nih.gov.* Click on "Health Information," and then scroll down to "Depression."

■ ■ ■ ■

High-Tech Depression Fighter

People who experience depression but are resistant to medication may find relief from *vagus nerve stimulation* (VNS) therapy. The stimulator is a pacemaker-like device implanted in the chest and attached to the vagus nerve on the left side of the neck. It sends a regular pulse of electricity to stimulate mood-regulating regions of the brain. VNS therapy is currently approved for treating epilepsy.

Mark George, MD, director, brain stimulation laboratory, Medical University of South Carolina, Charleston.

Stigma Still Shadows Psychiatric Care

Charles Goodstein, MD, clinical professor of psychiatry, New York University School of Medicine, New York City, and president, Psychoanalytic Association of New York.

Bernice A. Pescosolido, PhD, director, Indiana Consortium for Mental Health Services Research, Indiana University, Bloomington.

A recent analysis has found that Americans are conflicted about psychiatric drugs. Although the majority say they believe these medications are effective, they still would not use them.

Although people are becoming more understanding of mental illness, there is still a stigma associated with taking antidepressants and other psychiatric drugs, according to a report from researchers at the Indiana Consortium for Mental Health Services Research at Indiana University, Bloomington. The report was funded, in part, by the National Institute of Mental Health.

THE STUDY

In the study, the research team reviewed data from the 1998 General Social Survey of 1,400 Americans. *They found that...*

●**Approximately two-thirds said psychiatric drugs do help people** who have mental health problems deal with day-to-day anxiety, control their symptoms and improve family relationships.

●**If they were to start experiencing panic attacks,** only 56% said they would be willing to take medication.

●**If they were diagnosed with depression,** 41% said they would take medication.

● **For personal troubles or stress** only approximately one-third would be willing to take medication.

●**47% said they believed that once symptoms go away** psychiatric medications should be discontinued even though many doctors recommend that drug therapy be continued for several months or longer after symptoms abate.

POSSIBLE EXPLANATIONS

"Even though people say that they are accepting of psychological disorders of all kinds, there is this residual feeling that a psychological disorder is a character flaw," explains Dr. Charles Goodstein, a psychoanalyst and clinical professor of psychiatry at New York University School of Medicine. So, for many, "not using a psychiatric drug means they never had such a flaw at all," he says.

People may not want to take these medications because they think they will face harsh judgment from others, says sociologist Bernice A. Pescosolido, director of the Consortium. She recounts the story of a friend who, following her divorce, took her fifth grader to see a therapist. After the doctor prescribed an antidepressant, the boy said, "That's it! I can't run for president."

> *There is a real link in the public mind between mental illness and 'dangerousness,' and that is what is fueling the stigma.*
>
> *Bernice A. Pescosolido, PhD*

Although many people are reluctant to take psychiatric drugs, most would have little qualms about taking a drug to ease a physical problem.

"I think they are afraid of what is going to happen to them," says Pescosolido. "They've been primed by the media about what might happen in the first two weeks, when some people have a risk for suicide.

"There is a real link in the public mind between mental illness and 'dangerousness,' and that is what is fueling the stigma," says Pescosolido.

There is reason for concern, adds Goodstein. "Sometimes the drugs are prescribed excessively or for some type of performance enhancement, and they do have side effects," he says.

Pescosolido notes that people taking psychiatric medications should be closely monitored by a doctor who has experience prescribing these drugs.

"Americans have become more sophisticated and knowledgeable about mental illness, and everybody assumed the stigma was going away," Pescosolido says. However, this analysis seems to show that assumption is not true.

Now You Can Relieve Stress, Anxiety and Depression... Without Drugs

David Servan-Schreiber MD, PhD, clinical professor of psychiatry, University of Pittsburgh, and author of *The Instinct to Heal: Curing Stress, Anxiety, and Depression Without Drugs and Without Talk Therapy*. Rodale. *www.instincttoheal.org*.

When we are faced with emotional difficulties, doctors often recommend drugs or psychotherapy—but drugs have side effects, and some people are not comfortable with psychotherapy.

But there is another way. If you experience anxiety, depression or the effects of stress, you can try to regain balance by applying methods that have been proven to trigger the mind's own healing powers.

CALM THE HEART

As the nervous system adapts to changing conditions inside and outside the body, the heart rate adjusts, speeding up and slowing down. Under stressful conditions, it becomes chaotic, like the driving of someone who incessantly shifts between the brake and the accelerator. You can train your heart to run smoothly, and researchers have found that smoothing out the heart's rhythm calms the brain.

Example: In a Stanford University study of people who had heart failure, stress declined by 22% and depression by 34% after six weeks of *cardiac coherence training* (CCT). CCT involves using biofeedback to control the moment-to-moment changes in heart rate.

Exercise to calm your heart: Take slow, deep breaths, and center your attention on your heart. Imagine that you are breathing in and out through your heart...imagine how each inhalation brings in oxygen to nourish your body and each exhalation dispels waste.

Visualize your heart floating in a lukewarm bath. Be aware of a warm feeling in your chest. Focus on it and encourage it by taking slow and deep breaths.

Even when you're not under stress, practice this exercise so that you can easily do it whenever you need to. I find that 10 minutes before bed works well.

SYNCHRONIZE BODY RHYTHMS

Our ancestors followed the rhythms of nature, rising with the sun and resting when it got dark. Electric lights changed all that. Now our busy lives often follow "unnatural" schedules.

The brain thrives on regularity. Try to go to bed and get up at the same time each day. It's important to awaken naturally. Being startled out of sleep, perhaps in the midst of a dream, sends you into the world off balance. Keep your shades open and rise with the sun.

If that's not practical, use a dawn simulator, a timer that gradually turns on your bedroom light. Set it to begin 30 to 45 minutes before you need to get up, to ease the transition from sleep to wakefulness. These devices cost $100 to $150. Companies that distribute them include Natural Emporium (866-286-3227, *www.naturalemporium.com*) and Light Therapy Products (800-486-6723, *www.lighttherapyproducts.com*).

MAXIMIZE OMEGA-3s

Essential fatty acids (EFAs), which come from the foods we eat, make up 20% of the brain—primarily the cell membranes and the fibers that carry nerve impulses. Of particular importance are two types of fatty acids—omega-3s, which are found in fish and certain leafy vegetables...and omega-6s, a principal component of many vegetable oils. When the brain developed, the human diet had equal amounts of both. Today, the average American diet has at least 10 times as much omega-6s as omega-3s. This imbalance plays a role in heart disease, arthritis, even Alzheimer's disease. It also raises the risk of depression.

A study in *The Lancet* found that people who ate fish more than twice a week were less likely to be depressed than those who ate fish less frequently. Other research has shown that supplements rich in omega-3s reduce depression, moodiness and other emotional ills. *To get more omega-3s in your diet...*

• **Eat ocean fish,** such as mackerel, herring, tuna and salmon, two to three times a week.

• **Eat dark-green, leafy vegetables,** particularly spinach and watercress.

• **Substitute oils that are rich in omega-3s,** such as flaxseed and walnut oil, for those that are high in omega-6s, such as soy, corn and sunflower oils.

• **Take a fish oil supplement daily.** It should contain 1 gram (g) of omega-3s. Be sure to check with your doctor—especially if you're taking aspirin or a blood thinner.

INCREASE ACTIVITY

Exercise is as important for the mind as it is for the body. Studies have shown that it promotes relaxation, reduces anxiety and increases energy. Active people cope with stressful situations better than people who are sedentary.

Example: In a Duke University Medical Center study, middle-aged people who were depressed gained as much benefit from 30 minutes of walking three times a week as a comparison group who took an antidepressant.

Exertion spurs the release of *endorphins,* natural opiate-like brain chemicals that evoke feelings of pleasure. It interrupts the cascade of negative thoughts that perpetuate anxiety and depression. Regular exercise may also raise levels of brain chemicals that promote the growth of new brain cells.

Exercise intensity matters less than regularity. Aim to walk briskly, run, cycle or swim for at least 30 minutes a day, three times a week.

Wayne Dyer's Simple Plan For a Stress-Free Life

Wayne W. Dyer, PhD, renowned thinker and speaker in the field of self-development. He is author of *The Power of Intention: Learning to Co-Create Your World Your Way* and *Getting in the Gap: Making Conscious Contact with God Through Meditation,* both from Hay House. *www. drwaynedyer.com.*

Stress has become so ingrained in modern life that many people assume that the tension and anxiety they experience are normal and unavoidable. Not true.

There is nothing natural about living a life filled with stress and anxiety. Our bodies react by elevating blood pressure, increasing heart rate, causing indigestion, ulcers, headaches, breathing difficulties and other negative responses.

Believe it or not, our natural state is joy. *Here's how to return to that state and live a more tranquil life...*

• **Understand that you are the source of your stress.** Stress and anxiety are choices that we make to process unpleasant events rather than entities that are waiting to invade our lives. If you blame outside forces for making your life stressful, you'll only make stress more difficult to beat.

When you admit that your own mind is the source, stress becomes manageable. You always have a choice—do I stay with the thoughts that produce stress within me or do I work to activate thoughts that make stress impossible?

Example: I had to drop off a prescription at the drugstore, and the customer ahead of me was asking the pharmacist a series of, what seemed to me, inane questions. I started thinking, *There's always someone just ahead of me in line who asks silly questions or fumbles with money or can't find what's needed.*

I knew that was a signal to change my inner dialogue. I reminded myself of my intention to live a stress-free life. I stopped judging and actually saw the virtue in having to take a moment and slow down. My emotion shifted from discomfort to ease, making stress impossible at that moment.

• **Expel stressful thoughts.** Stress can feed upon itself when left unchecked. Break the cycle of anxiety by banishing a stressful thought from your mind. Take a deep breath, and visualize yourself stamping "Next" or "Cancel" across the thought and pushing it out of your way.

If you're in a bad mood, repeat, *I want to feel good* until you believe it. Then say, *I intend to feel good* until you feel better. These new responses eventually will become habitual and replace your old habit of responding in stress-producing ways.

Sometimes, particularly worrisome thoughts run through your head. *Here is the thought and what you could say to yourself instead...*

●**I have so many things to do that I can never get caught up.** Instead, say, *I'll only think about the one thing I'm doing right now and will have peaceful thoughts.*

●**I can never get ahead in this job.** *If I choose to appreciate what I'm doing, I'll attract even greater opportunities.*

●**I worry about my health problems.** *I live in a universe that attracts healing, and I refuse to focus on sickness.*

●**I can't be happy when the person I love has abandoned me.** *I choose to focus on what I have rather than on what I'm missing. I trust that love will return to my life.*

●**I feel uneasy about the economy. I have lost so much money already.** *I choose to think about what I have, and I will be fine. The universe will provide.*

●**My family members are making me feel anxious and fearful.** *I choose thoughts that make me feel good, and this will help me uplift those family members in need.*

●**I don't deserve to feel good when so many people are suffering.** *I didn't come into a world in which everyone is going to have the same experiences. I'll choose to feel good, and by being uplifted, I will help eradicate some of the suffering.*

Here are some other things you can do to banish stress…

●**Return to your happiest moment.** Visualize a scene from your past that brings you joy. For me, it's a dock on a Michigan lake where I spent time with my family as a child. For others, it might be the greatest moment of a high school athletic career…the face of a loved one…a tree-lined road…even making love.

When you feel overwhelmed by stress, picture this happy image for several moments. Your mind will naturally return to the joyous mental state that you experienced originally.

●**Stop taking yourself so seriously.** Next time you're anxious about something trivial, take a step back and laugh at yourself for thinking that the problem is worth getting worked up over.

Example: Feel the anxiety building inside you because you're stuck in traffic? Ask yourself what you were going to do in those five minutes that was so important.

The world operates on its own time, not yours. If you plant tomatoes in your garden, they'll ripen when they ripen—wanting a tomato any sooner won't change anything. Yet in many phases of our lives, we expect the world to operate on our timetable and we become stressed when it doesn't.

●**Realize you will never get it all done.** There will always be something else to do or accomplish. Your desires, goals and dreams will never be finished—ever. As soon as you realize one dream, another will pop up. The secret is to live more fully in the moment.

●**Live in a state of gratitude.** It's impossible to be stressed and appreciative at the same time. Consider all the things that you have achieved in your life—your family, career success, anything that makes you proud and happy—and be grateful for them. Then search for a way to appreciate whatever is currently causing you stress. Perhaps the person in front of you who is driving too slowly is saving you from a speeding ticket or a traffic accident.

●**Meditate.** Nothing relieves stress, anxiety and depression like silence and meditation. The stillness of meditation relaxes the mind and gives us strength. Take time every day for moments of relaxation and quiet contemplation.

■ ■ ■ ■

Essential Traits for a Happy Life

There are a few personality traits that happy people have in common. *They are…*

●**Love of learning**—an interest in acquiring new skills.

●**Creativity**—trying new things just for fun and producing something surprising.

●**Humility**—recognizing your own abilities and appreciating those of others.

●**Humor**—being able to find something amusing even in difficult times and helping others do so, too.

●**Persistence**—working through to a goal despite obstacles.

•**Gratitude**—being thankful for all you have.

•**Forgiveness**—being able to let go of hurt and anger.

•**Appreciation of beauty.**

•**Spirituality.**

•**Vitality**—a feeling of being energized.

Martin E.P. Seligman, PhD, department of psychology, University of Pennsylvania, Philadelphia.

Don't Get Burned! Tanning May Be Addictive

Wake Forest University Baptist Medical Center, news release.

The effects of tanning may be more than just skin deep. According to a study, people who use tanning beds frequently experience effects similar to those of some addictive drugs.

Researchers at Wake Forest University Baptist Medical Center say that the ultraviolet (UV) light in tanning beds appears to trigger the production of *endorphins*, brain chemicals that are linked to pain relief and euphoric feelings.

THE STUDY

The study compared eight people who used tanning beds often (eight to 15 times per month) with eight people who used them infrequently (no more than 12 times per year).

All of the participants were given either a placebo or the drug *naltrexone*, which blocks the feel-good effects of endorphins and other opioids. The participants then used both UV and non-UV tanning beds.

At higher doses of naltrexone (15 milligrams), frequent tanners showed a preference for UV tanning, and four of the eight frequent tanners reported nausea or jitteriness. None of the infrequent tanners who took the drug reported these symptoms.

"The finding was unexpected and is consistent with the hypothesis that frequent tanning may be driven, in part, by a mild dependence

on opioids, most likely endorphins. The nausea and jitteriness induced by the medication are consistent with symptoms of mild opiate withdrawal," according to senior researcher Dr. Steven Feldman, a professor of dermatology.

"We had previously shown that ultraviolet light has an effect on mood that [people who use tanning beds] value," says Dr. Mandeep Kaur, lead author of the study. "Now, in this small study, we've shown that some tanners actually experience withdrawal symptoms when the 'feel-good' chemicals are blocked."

info The US Food and Drug Administration can provide more information about the dangers of tanning at *www.fda.gov/cdrh/fdaandyou/issue07.html*.

Real Reason Bipolar Teens Struggle Socially

National Institute of Mental Health news release.

A recent study has discovered that children who have bipolar disorder misinterpret facial expressions—believing these expressions to be hostile—more often than their healthy counterparts. This might explain why bipolar children often tend to be more aggressive and irritable and have poorer social skills than healthy children.

THE STUDY

Researchers at the US National Institute of Mental Health (NIMH) measured the brain activity in 22 bipolar children and 21 healthy children using *magnetic resonance imaging* (MRI).

When the children were asked to rate the hostility of a neutral facial expression, the area of the brain that registers fear showed more activity in the bipolar children than in the healthy children.

When the children considered a face to be hostile, other areas of the brain that are related to emotions also showed higher activity levels in the bipolar patients than in the healthy children. Activity was no different between the bipolar and the healthy children when they rated nonemotional features, indicating that the differences between the groups of children are specifically related to emotional processes.

IMPLICATIONS

"Our results suggest that children with bipolar disorder see emotion where other people don't. Our results also suggest that bipolar disorder likely stems from the impaired development of specific brain circuits," explains Dr. Ellen Leibenluft of the NIMH Mood and Anxiety Disorders Program.

"This line of research might help us refine our definition of pediatric bipolar disorder," says NIMH director Dr. Thomas Insel. "The researchers are following up with more imaging studies of children with bipolar spectrum disorders and healthy children who are at genetic risk for developing the disorder to see if they also have the same overactivation" of this particular area of the brain.

Studying children who have bipolar disorder may provide valuable insights into the development and treatment of adult bipolar disorder, according to Leibenluft. "Since children seem to have a more severe form of the disorder, they may provide a clearer window into the underlying illness process than adult onset cases," she says.

info For more information on bipolar disorder, visit the US National Library of Medicine's MedlinePlus Web site at *www.nlm.nih.gov/ medlineplus/bipolardisorder.html.*

■ ■ ■ ■

What Is Bipolar Disorder?

Symptoms of bipolar disorder differ in people of different ages. Bipolar children and adolescents have symptoms more continuously than adults. Children's symptoms are more varied and may include emotional difficulties or disruptive behaviors that are frequent or severe enough to interfere with academic or social activities.

Examples: Irritability, depression, anxiety, aggression, impulsive behavior.

Bipolar adults exhibit less obvious manifestations of impulsive behavior, such as excessive spending or traveling.

Helpful for diagnosis: If a parent has bipolar disorder and a child displays symptoms or has been diagnosed with a disruptive behavioral disorder such as *attention deficit hyperactivity disorder* (ADHD), the child may be bipolar.

Important: Mood and anxiety disorders and substance abuse often occur together.

Terence A. Ketter, MD, chief, Bipolar Disorders Clinic, Stanford University School of Medicine, Stanford, CA.

Don't Blame TV for ADHD Symptoms

Tara Stevens, EdD, assistant professor of educational psychology and leadership, Texas Tech University, Lubbock.
Jess Shatkin, MD, MPH, director, education and training, and child and adolescent psychiatrist, New York University Child Study Center, New York City.
Pediatrics.

Although previous studies have linked television exposure at an early age to attention problems, a recent study has not found a connection between *attention deficit hyperactivity disorder* (ADHD) and children's TV viewing habits.

> *I think these findings take a little bit of the pressure off parents.*
>
> *Tara Stevens, EdD*

"TV is designed to capture our attention and move us quickly from one subject to the next. The question is, does the young brain become different because of this?" wondered study co-author Tara Stevens, an assistant professor of educational psychology and leadership at Texas Tech University.

THE STUDY

Researchers randomly selected two groups of 2,500 children each from the Early Childhood Longitudinal Study–Kindergarten. That study includes information collected from parents and teachers on 22,000 youngsters who started kindergarten during the 1998–1999 school year. The researchers looked at the children's behavior in kindergarten and then again near the end of first grade. They included information on television exposure, limits that were placed on TV viewing, parental involvement, socioeconomic status and ADHD symptoms.

The study found no association between television exposure and symptoms of ADHD. It also found that parental involvement—such as the amount of time the parents spent participating in children's activities that did not involve TV—was not linked to ADHD symptoms.

Stevens says it's important to note that the children in the study who showed ADHD symptoms had not been diagnosed with the disorder.

POSSIBLE EXPLANATIONS

Stevens offers a number of explanations for why her study came up with different results than others.

One previous study that found an association between TV viewing and ADHD only looked at children younger than three years. It's possible that the age of the children affects the results, she speculates. The brain is much more "plastic," or malleable, at a younger age, she says. So, TV viewing at age two or three may have more of an effect than TV viewing at five or six.

Another possibility is that parents of hyperactive children may use the TV as a babysitter more often than other parents simply because they need a break or they need to capture their child's attention while they make dinner or take a shower.

Stevens is quick to point out that she and coauthor Miriam Mulsow are not advocating TV viewing in children. However, she says, "I think these findings take a little bit of the pressure off parents. It's very likely that you did not do something wrong to make your child develop ADHD."

MODERATION

Dr. Jess Shatkin, director of education and training at the New York University Child Study Center, says he isn't prepared to fully accept the new findings. "This is a thoughtful and interesting study, but there's not enough data to support the idea that we shouldn't be cautious about kids' exposure to all media. This doesn't change anything I would tell parents."

The bottom line, Shatkin says, is "all things in moderation."

info To learn more about attention deficit hyperactivity disorder, visit the Centers for Disease Control and Prevention at *www.cdc.gov/ncbddd/adhd*.

Violent Video Games Spur Aggression in Kids

Kevin Kieffer, PhD, assistant professor of psychology, Saint Leo University, Saint Leo, FL.

Kimberly Thompson, ScD, associate professor of risk analysis and decision science, and founder of the Kids Risk Project, Harvard School of Public Health, and cofounder/director of the Center on Media and Child Health, Children's Hospital, Boston.

Douglas Lowenstein, president, Entertainment Software Association, Washington, DC.

American Psychological Association annual meeting, Washington, DC.

Violent video games that involve protagonists who hunt, maim and kill are linked to short-term aggressive behavior in children, according to the first large-scale review of previous studies on the subject.

Although the long-term effects of these very realistic games remain unclear, their impact on kids' attitudes toward violence is worrisome, researchers say.

"Children and adolescents are becoming desensitized to this very violent content, so it doesn't surprise them. They expect to see blood squirting out of someone when they are shot," says coresearcher Kevin Kieffer, an assistant professor of psychology at Saint Leo University in Saint Leo, Florida.

THE RESEARCH

Kieffer and coresearcher Jessica Nicoll, also of Saint Leo, describe their review as an attempt to find recurrent "themes" in previous literature on the link between violent video games and aggression.

After looking at 16 studies of children younger than 18 years of age, all published between 1985 and 2004, Kieffer notes that three distinct trends emerged.

"First, we noticed in these studies that individuals who are subjected to violent media and video games tend to act more violent in the short-term," he says.

For example, one study of more than 600 eighth- and ninth-graders, published in 2004, found that kids who spent a lot of time playing video games also had "a greater number of arguments with authority figures such as teachers and were also more likely to be involved in physical altercations with other students," the researchers note.

In another study, children who were given either violent or nonviolent video games to play were subsequently presented with a "retaliation" activity where they could punish opponents by "blasting" them with a loud noisemaker.

"Participants who had played the violent game displayed more aggression against their opponents in the retaliation portion of the study than participants who played the nonviolent game," the authors of this latest study note.

Another study found that children who indulged in violent video game-playing were less "helpful" to other children during play.

Kieffer says strong gender differences also emerged in the research.

"Boys tend to play these games much more often than girls," Kieffer says. He and Nicoll suggest two theories as to why this might be so. First, it may simply be more socially acceptable for boys to play video games. Another explanation is linked to the "subordinate role women [characters] often take in these video games," not giving girls much to identify with as they play, he says.

STUDY LIMITATIONS

While these findings support links between violent video game use and short-term aggression, Kieffer says it is too soon to know whether this aggression will continue over the long term. "What's lacking is longitudinal data to suggest that [children] become more violent over time," he says.

Kimberly Thompson, a Harvard University researcher specializing in these types of issues, says that data isn't likely to arrive any time soon. "What's really amazing is that we aren't doing those [long-term] studies," she says. "We don't have the funds to do them."

There's also the chicken-and-egg problem of whether kids who might naturally be more aggressive are drawn to these types of games, or whether it's the game itself that is encouraging aggression.

"We have seen a lot of studies documenting that individuals with what we call 'low self-concept' and people that are going through difficult times, can act out their aggressive fantasies

through these games," Kieffer says. "I think there's a lot more research that needs to be done examining this."

According to Thompson, who founded the Kids Risk Project at Harvard, video games differ from more passive mediums, such as comic books. "They are interactive," she says. "When you play a video game, you get feedback, you're rewarded." In fact, her investigation into a wide range of popular, teen-rated games found that "players were being rewarded for committing acts of violence. So, basically, violence becomes just a part of how you move on in the game."

THE INDUSTRY SPEAKS

Douglas Lowenstein, president of the Entertainment Software Association, which represents the video gaming industry, calls the new review "little more than a rehash of old papers repackaged as 'new findings.'"

We do know that when it comes to kids and games, learning happens. So you really have to ask, just what is it they are learning?

Kimberly Thompson, ScD

"In truth," he adds, "it is neither new nor comprehensive. It is simply a highly selective review of previous research, much of which has been challenged as either weak, unpersuasive or flawed by independent sources." Lowenstein believes the reviewers ignored the studies that contradicted their "preconceived views."

WHAT PARENTS CAN DO

Parents who are concerned that their child is spending too much time staring into a video screen do have options, Kieffer says.

"Parents need to go out of their way to involve youth in other activities," says Kieffer, who is also a counseling psychologist. Too often, parents use gaming as a way to keep kids occupied. "It's easy to say, 'I'm going to plug you into your Gameboy or video game player—go have a good time for a couple of hours so I can do what I need to do.'"

He hopes parents learn to "be more in touch [with kids] and spend quality time getting their children involved in other activities."

Kieffer calls recent legislative efforts to rate video games according to their violent content "a step in the right direction," but adds that, ultimately, "kids are always going to get their hands on these games" if they want them.

"We do know that when it comes to kids and games, learning happens," Thompson says. "So you really have to ask, just what is it they are learning?"

info For more on the research into video games and their effects on kids, visit the American Psychological Association Web site at *www.apa.org/science/psa/sb-anderson.html.*

Don't Get Mad— Get Happy! Anger Can Harm Your Health

Daniel C. Vinson, MD, MSPH, professor of family medicine, University of Missouri–Columbia.
Hunter Champion, MD, PhD, assistant professor of medicine, Heart Institute, Johns Hopkins University School of Medicine, Baltimore.
Annals of Family Medicine.

Anger has been associated with everything from high blood pressure to road rage. Now, a new study links anger in men to injuries.

Researchers who interviewed emergency room patients found that men were likely to report being angry at the time of their injuries.

Although the findings may seem obvious, previous research into anger has found contradictory results, says study coauthor Dr. Daniel C. Vinson, a professor of family medicine at the University of Missouri–Columbia.

THE STUDY

Vinson and a colleague surveyed 2,517 emergency room patients in Missouri about their states of mind before they were injured. The researchers also randomly surveyed 1,856 uninjured Missouri residents about their anger levels during a regular day.

Nearly 33% of the injured people surveyed said they were irritable just before being injured; 18% said they were angry, and 13.2% described themselves as hostile.

Some of these numbers were similar to the anger assessments made by the uninjured people. However, the injured people—especially men and those who were injured by another person—were more likely to express greater anger, the study authors report.

"The association between anger and [self-]injury was much stronger in men than in women," according to Vinson. "Men may get more angry, may act on their anger or they may get distracted by their anger."

Surprisingly, the researchers did not find a link between anger and car accidents.

IMPLICATIONS

Although it's impossible to know how many of the injuries in this study were directly caused by anger, one anger specialist says the findings are important.

"They add significantly to our growing body of work that emotional stress—whether it be anger or grief or fear—has a profound effect on the body," says Dr. Hunter Champion, an assistant professor of medicine at Johns Hopkins University School of Medicine and its Heart Institute.

"When one begins to feel angry in some sort of situation, whether in interpersonal relationships or just because of what's going on in your own mind, it's wise to take a step back and move out of the situation that's escalating," Vinson advises. "Slow down and back off so you might be able to avoid injury."

Rage Disorder More Common than Thought

Ronald Kessler, PhD, professor of health-care policy, Harvard Medical School, Boston.
Rene Olvera, MD, MPH, assistant professor of psychiatry, University of Texas Medical School at San Antonio.
Archives of General Psychiatry.

A little-studied mental illness, marked by episodes of angry, potentially violent outbursts like those seen in road rage or spousal abuse, is more common than previously thought, researchers report. In fact, the illness, known as *intermittent explosive disorder* (IED), may affect 8.6 million Americans, the researchers found.

IED may also predispose people to other mental illnesses, such as depression and anxiety, as well as substance abuse problems.

THE RESEARCH

Researchers based their findings on an analysis of data on 9,282 adults who participated in the National Comorbidity Survey Replication conducted from 2001 to 2003. They found that 82% of the people who had IED also had depression, anxiety and alcohol or drug abuse disorders, although it was the IED symptoms that usually surfaced first.

"We found that IED is strongly related to depression and anxiety and other mental health problems," says the study's lead author Ronald Kessler, a professor of health-care policy at Harvard Medical School.

"An awful lot of people in America have IED," says Kessler. "IED is characterized by explosive anger attacks that they can't control and are out of proportion to what is going on in their lives and that lead to physical assault or breaking things," he says.

DEFINING THE DISORDER

According to the Diagnostic and Statistical Manual of Mental Disorders, Fourth Edition (DSM-IV), people who have IED overreact to certain situations with uncontrollable rage, experience a sense of relief during the angry outburst, and then feel remorse about their actions.

Because IED can first appear in childhood, Kessler wonders, "What would be the implications in the school years of finding these kids and getting them into treatment? Would it prevent later divorce, job loss, drug or alcohol addiction or legal problems?"

"Aggression is often a symptom that brings people for psychiatric attention," says Dr. Rene Olvera, an assistant professor of psychiatry at the University of Texas Health Science Center at San Antonio. IED appears to be a combination of a mood disorder and poor impulse control, he adds.

For adults, one hope is that they start seeing the problem in themselves, Olvera says. "These folks have a very narrow field of response in terms of their coping strategies—they have very few coping strategies that they use," he says.

TREATMENTS

Not many people who have IED are treated, Kessler says. "They usually don't think they have a problem. They think somebody else has a problem," he says.

However, there are effective treatments for IED, Kessler says, including cognitive-behavioral therapy, the antidepressants known as *selective serotonin reuptake inhibitors* (SSRIs) and/or mood stabilizers.

One expert thinks that early diagnosis and combination treatment—talk therapy and medication—is the best approach to treating IED.

info The American Psychological Association can tell you more about anger management at *www.apa.org/topics/controlanger.html.*

Irritable Male Syndrome: What It Is and How to Control It

Jed Diamond, founder and director, MenAlive, a therapy, information and education center, Willits, CA. *www.menalive.com.* He is author of *The Irritable Male Syndrome* (Rodale) and *Male Menopause* (Sourcebooks).

Many American men share an underdiagnosed condition known as *irritable male syndrome* (IMS). The term was first coined by a Scottish researcher, Dr. Gerald Lincoln. He found that when the testosterone levels dropped in the animals he was studying, they became more irritable and lethargic.

IMS is not the same as depression, although that often is one component. Rather, men who have IMS experience a constellation of symptoms, including episodes of hypersensitivity, anxiety, frustration, moodiness and anger. In addition to declines in testosterone, one of the main causes of IMS is stress—about money, relationships, sexual performance, etc. Nearly half of men surveyed reported feeling stressed much of the time.

Standard depression treatments, including antidepressants, can help to some extent, but they will not necessarily address all of the symptoms that may accompany IMS.

In addition to having a thorough health check-up, including a blood test for testosterone, most men who have IMS will gain relief by following this four-step plan…

Step 1: Acknowledge the problem. *Men who have IMS progress through the four stages of denial before they can begin to get better…*

- Failing to notice the initial symptoms.
- Downplaying the importance of the symptoms once they notice them.
- Recognizing that something is wrong but casting blame outward. They might say things like, *My wife has really been on my case lately* or *I can't believe the idiots I have to work with.*
- Understanding that other people are not to blame for the problem. Men can't begin to escape from the cycle of negativity until they reach this final stage.

Helpful: Keep a diary, and write down every incident that you consider "negative," such as snapping at your partner or having arguments with coworkers. Men need to see hard facts before they take action.

Step 2: Strengthen your body. We can't always control the amount of stress in our lives, but we can help dispel it. One way to do that is through daily exercise. Every man should set aside at least 30 minutes daily for strenuous exercise, such as fast walking, lifting weights, playing tennis, etc.

Bonus: Regular exercise increases brain levels of *serotonin*, the same neurotransmitter that is elevated by prescription antidepressants.

Step 3: Expand your mind. Men who have IMS tend to view the world through "irritable lenses," putting a negative spin on many situations and actions.

Example: One morning, my wife seemed unresponsive when I hugged her. My automatic thought was that she was angry with me. When I thought more about it, I reminded myself that she is never outgoing in the morning and that we had been very close the night before. Her behavior very likely had nothing to do with me.

Helpful: Fill out a "thought record" when you are feeling negative. Write down details of the situation…what automatic thoughts go through your mind…evidence that supports or disproves those thoughts…and an alternative, more positive way of looking at the situation.

Step 4: Deepen the spirit. There are times in our lives when we know we need to make changes but are held back by fear—and the feeling of being stuck increases our sense of powerlessness and anger.

Listen to your inner voice. Maybe you have always wanted to spend more time enjoying nature. Take up painting or photography, or volunteer for a community group. Make time for it. It will give you the energy and passion that you need to deal with the inevitable frustrations of day-to-day living.

DO YOU HAVE IMS?

If you check six or more of the following symptoms, you may have IMS. *I often feel…*

- Grumpy
- Angry
- Gloomy
- Impatient
- Lonely
- Hostile
- Annoyed
- Touchy
- Overworked
- Unloved
- Jealous
- Stressed

info You can take the full IMS questionnaire and have it scored for free at *www.theirritablemale.com.*

How Not to Worry Yourself Sick

Marc Siegel, MD, associate professor of medicine, New York University School of Medicine, New York City, and author of *False Alarm: The Truth About the Epidemic of Fear* and *Bird Flu: Everything You Need to Know About the Next Pandemic,* both from Wiley.

Being offered a regular flu shot doesn't seem to reassure my patients. Bird flu is what worries them.

Bird flu is indeed a threat—it has shown itself to be a ruthless killer of birds, and it has prompted humans to slaughter millions of birds that could be infected. But for people, the risk so far is close to zero for anyone except bird handlers in Southeast Asia. The virus has not

133

killed many people worldwide, and it will not spread widely among humans unless there are several more mutations of its genetic material.

Most of my patients understand all this. What scares them is the possibility of a pandemic. It's remote, but it's real—the hardest kind of risk to put in perspective. Yet focusing on a worst-case scenario can have grave consequences. Worst-case news reports, including comparisons to the terrifying flu pandemic of 1918, have scared my patients out of all proportion. The odds remain overwhelmingly on their side—in 1918 there were no vaccines for flu, no antiviral drugs, no antibiotics or steroids to treat flu patients who had pneumonia or asthma and no worldwide public-health network.

The current fear is reminiscent of the way many people blew out of proportion the risk for contracting anthrax, West Nile virus, SARS and mad cow disease.

I warn my patients that too much worry can lead to overeating, cigarette smoking and drinking too much alcohol. It also can increase levels of circulating stress hormones in the blood, which places more demand on the heart and appears to contribute to heart disease and stroke. But these very real diseases seem abstract when compared to the scary-looking chickens we regularly see on TV.

Our own brains make us easy prey to such distortions. Elizabeth Phelps, PhD, a psychologist and neuroscientist at New York University in New York City, has examined how the brain responds to envisioned threats. Using *magnetic resonance imaging* (MRI) scans, she discovered that the brain's fear center, known as the *amygdala*, can be activated in response to dangers that a person merely observes. "When you are watching it and you are told that it is going to happen to you, it causes the same robust response by the amygdala as if you actually experience it yourself," Dr. Phelps explains. She has also studied the safety signals that our brains use to turn off fear, and it seems that the brain's wiring heavily favors the "on" switch. In other words, it's easier to become frightened than to have that fear turned off.

Fear is meant to warn us against looming peril, not to provoke a generalized response to sensational videos of foreign lands. But since our fear radar doesn't discriminate, we release stress hormones unnecessarily, readying for a crisis that doesn't come. Heart rates and blood pressure increase, and we breathe harder. Like a car that revs constantly at high speed, we are more likely to break down.

Because the amygdala also processes positive emotions, I tell my patients to try to replace nervous negativity as much as possible with laughter, adventure and, above all, courage. I also recommend replacing obsessive voyeurism with more healthful regular routines, such as exercise, family meals and seven to eight hours of sleep each night. Worry also feeds on excessive exposure to news. Try to limit the amount of time you spend watching the news on TV.

Unfortunately, my treatments for unnecessary fear are not entirely successful. People continue to worry and obsess about things that don't directly threaten them. What bothers me most is that I see my patients being harmed by this, and there's not enough I can do to stop it.

■ ■ ■ ■

Up to 85% Feel Better After a Good Cry

Studies of hundreds of volunteers have discovered that 85% of women and 73% of men feel less sad and less angry after crying. Women cry four times as often as men—on average 5.3 times a month, while men cry only 1.4 times a month. Crying episodes in the majority of women involve tears running down their cheeks, but most male crying episodes only result in watery eyes. Research shows that emotional tears are chemically different from other types of tears, such as those shed when cutting onions. Emotional tears have a higher protein content.

William H. Frey II, PhD, neuroscientist, Regions Hospital, St. Paul.

■ ■ ■ ■

Dealing with Grief

Grieving is a journey, and it is normal to have a hard time when you reach certain milestones, such as an anniversary, birthday or holiday. Acknowledge these occasions in some special way—not necessarily at the cemetery. Come up with something meaningful to you.

Examples: Make a contribution or do some volunteer work on these days. Help someone in need, or plant a flower or a tree.

Accept your feelings—and don't try to hold them in.

Helpful: On difficult days reach out to empathetic friends, and spend some time with them—by phone if you cannot see them in person.

Rev. Z. Ann Schmidt, director, pastoral care, Stamford Hospital, Stamford, CT.

Sleep Inertia—What Happens to Your Brain When You Wake Up

Kenneth P. Wright, Jr., PhD, assistant professor, department of integrative physiology, and director, Sleep & Chronobiology Lab, University of Colorado at Boulder.
Robert Vorona, MD, assistant professor of sleep medicine, Eastern Virginia Medical School, Norfolk.
The Journal of the American Medical Association.

A small study has found that, on awakening, people are more mentally addled than when they are kept awake for 26 hours.

THE STUDY

To better understand this so-called "sleep inertia," study coauthor Kenneth Wright, Jr., director of the Sleep & Chronobiology Lab at the University of Colorado at Boulder, and his colleagues gave mathematical tests to nine men and one woman several times in the hours after waking from sleep. The participants took the same tests after being kept awake for 26 hours.

The researchers found that the subjects scored lower on the tests that were given just after waking from a normal night's sleep than they did on the tests that were given after 26 hours of no sleep. "We thought that [their performance] would be just as bad as sleep deprivation. But we were a little surprised that it was worse," Wright says. "The serious effects are probably gone within the first 10 minutes, but we still can detect impairments for up to two hours."

"It takes some time until we're able to be efficient in our ability to make decisions and think clearly," says Wright.

In most cases, the type of post-sleep "brain fog" noted in the study would not seriously affect a person's ability to perform. However, people do need to think fast and clearly in emergencies, and Wright says the research could be especially relevant for firefighters, doctors and other individuals who need to function at their best soon after awakening.

THE NEXT STEP

Unsure of why sleep inertia occurs, researchers would like to figure out how long it takes for people to think and function clearly after waking, Wright says. "We're also interested [in finding out] if someone is [experiencing] a very intense emergency, does that affect how long it takes for the brain to wake up?"

That could be a vital question for doctors, who are often woken up in the middle of the night to make important decisions, and for firefighters who must suddenly run out to fight a fire immediately after waking up, says Dr. Robert Vorona, an assistant professor of sleep medicine at Eastern Virginia Medical School.

It takes some time until we're able to be efficient in our ability to make decisions and think clearly.

Kenneth P. Wright, Jr., PhD

Ultimately, emergency workers may need to take the research into account when they figure out who makes the major decisions in a crisis, Wright says. "It may be more important for someone else to make those decisions until someone [who has just woken up] has gotten past that initial impairment."

The researchers didn't examine the brain-stimulating effects of coffee, but Wright says researchers have discovered that consuming caffeine before a nap actually helps people be more alert upon waking. The key, he says, is not to consume too much so that you can't sleep in the first place.

info Learn more about sleep inertia from the University of Denver Web site at *www.du.edu/~psherry/fatigue/sleep.html.*

Harvard Doctor Reveals What Your Dreams Really Mean

David Kahn, PhD, researcher and instructor, department of psychiatry, Harvard University Medical School, Boston. He is chair of the International Association for the Study of Dreams. *www.asdreams.org.*

We dream five dreams a night, on average. Sometimes dreams are exciting, sometimes troubling or confusing—and most of the time they're forgotten when we wake up.

Despite the considerable amount of time we all spend dreaming during our lives, dreams are not well-understood. *Here, David Kahn, PhD, a dream researcher at Harvard Medical School, answers some of the most common questions about dreams...*

•**Why do we dream?** This is still under debate. At one extreme, there are researchers who will argue that dreaming is simply an *epiphenomenon*, or a side effect, of chemical changes that occur in the brain during sleep. At the other extreme, some believe that dreaming is a mechanism that allows us to reconsider what's going on in our lives without the constraints that we impose on our thoughts when we are awake.

A theory known as the *threat simulation hypothesis* proposes that the purpose of dreams is to make us respond to artificial threats so we're better able to cope with the threats that come up in real life. Another theory suggests that our dreams help us interpret what other people are thinking, a useful skill for social beings.

I can only speculate on the purpose of dreaming. I think that dreams provide us with new ways to see ourselves and our relationships with people and the world—to think outside the box.

•**What does it mean if I don't dream?** You almost certainly do dream, but you don't remember that you do. The part of the brain that remembers what we've just said or done is essentially off-line when we sleep, so the vast majority of dreams are forgotten.

If you keep a pad or a tape recorder by your bed and jot down or dictate your dreams before they disappear, you are more likely to remember them.

There's also evidence that we can *will* ourselves to retain more dreams. Before you go to sleep and after you wake up, tell yourself you want to remember.

The only people who might not dream are those who have stroke damage or who have lesions on specific parts of the brain. Even in these extreme cases, it isn't clear whether these people don't dream or whether they are just incapable of remembering their dreams.

•**Is there any way to control our dreams or trigger good dreams?** The only way to control dreams is through something called *lucid dreaming.* During a lucid dream, the dreamer is aware that he/she is dreaming. Once armed with this awareness, it might be possible to take control of the dream—for example, by changing a frightening dream into something more pleasant. Perhaps the knife in a pursuer's hand becomes a piece of cake.

Lucid dreaming isn't easy, but it seems anyone can accomplish it with effort. If you'd like to try, think about the situations that are common in your dreams but impossible or unlikely in real life, such as flying without a plane or being chased by killers. Every night before you go to sleep, remind yourself, *If I'm flying, I must be dreaming.* It could take weeks or months, but eventually you may achieve a lucid dream. Some people who have mastered lucid dreaming say it becomes easier once you get the hang of it.

•**Can we use our dreams to improve our lives?** The things that appear in our dreams often carry an emotional tug for us during our waking lives. Since the dreaming mind is unconstrained, we might think of these things in different ways when we're asleep than we do when we're awake, potentially helping us gain some insight into ourselves.

For example, a woman dreamed that she missed her highway exit while driving to meet her boyfriend. In the dream, she was so concerned about being late that she put her car in reverse and backed up to the exit despite the dangers. When she was asked what this dream meant to her, the woman said that she didn't want to disappoint her boyfriend by being late. She hadn't previously realized how concerned she was about her boyfriend's opinion of her.

We should *not* let others tell us what our dreams represent. Such interpretations tend to be projections of the person doing the analysis, not the dreamer.

●**Are nightmares normal? Should I wake someone who is having a bad dream?** Nightmares are very normal. They usually don't suggest any mental or physical problem, though occasionally they might be related to stress.

Science really has no answer as to whether it's better to wake someone who is having a nightmare or let him/her sleep. My personal feeling is that it's best to let the person sleep because when we're dreaming, we're in the *rapid eye movement* (REM) stage. You don't want to deprive people of REM sleep, which is an important stage in our sleep cycle. If you're a parent and just can't stand to see your child upset during a nightmare, it's okay to wake him gently.

●**Why do some dreams recur? Is there any way to stop a recurring dream?** The content of recurring dreams frequently seems to be related to issues in our lives that lack closure or resolution. If you address the underlying issue, the dream is likely to go away.

Example: If you feel that you are not in control of your life, you might have recurring dreams about driving a car without brakes or rowing a boat that's being swept toward a waterfall. (The dream's details are likely to vary from night to night.) If you start to feel more in control of your life, you will probably have these dreams less often.

●**What is sleep paralysis?** Sleep paralysis while dreaming is perfectly normal. In fact, we would be at risk if we didn't experience it. Our bodies become paralyzed during the dream stages of sleep to prevent us from physically acting out whatever we're doing in our dreams. Without sleep paralysis, we might sleepwalk out a window or punch our spouse as we fight off a dream attacker. Medications are available for those who don't always experience sleep paralysis naturally.

Occasionally, sleep paralysis will continue momentarily after we wake up. This can be scary, but it generally lasts only a few seconds.

●**Why do dreams blend realistic and nonsensical images?** When we sleep, some areas of our brain become more active, while other areas become inactive. Thus, we're able to access certain realistic memories and images, but we can't always make the logical associations that go along with them. The nonsensical images in our dreams are our brain's attempts to fill in these missing pieces.

Interestingly, a dreaming brain is not all that different from a brain on hallucinogenic drugs. There are even similarities between dreaming brains and psychotic brains. The parallels are compelling enough to inspire some scientists to begin researching dreaming brains to better understand psychotic brains.

●**Why does it sometimes feel like the person you're dreaming about is actually present?** We don't really know why. Our best explanation is that the dreaming brain lacks the ability to say, *This doesn't make much sense.* If the person appears to be there in a dream, your brain simply might assume that he really is there.

●**Why do certain common themes occur in most people's dreams?** There do seem to be some universal dream themes. Among the most common are not being prepared, such as for a test…being chased or attacked…and not being in control. The details of these dreams differ from culture to culture—the out-of-control car in your dream might be a runaway horse in a part of the world without cars—but the themes appear everywhere.

Perhaps these dreams reflect something basic about the human condition. We all worry about being unprepared, being attacked and not being in control.

Decode Your Dreams to Improve Your Health

Gillian Holloway, PhD, a psychologist and instructor, Marylhurst University, Marylhurst, OR. She is author of *The Complete Dream Book: Discover What Your Dreams Tell About You and Your Life.* Sourcebooks. *www.lifetreks.com.*

D
ream interpretation has long been used to help people resolve troubling psychological issues.

But few people realize that dreams can also foretell health problems weeks to months before symptoms develop.

Landmark study: Vasily Kasatkin, a psychiatrist at the Leningrad Neurosurgical Institute, analyzed 10,240 dreams from 1,200 patients over a 40-year period. He concluded that illnesses, ranging from tooth infections to brain tumors, often caused distressing dreams that preceded the first symptoms.

Dreams related to health issues are typically recurring—and may include an intense physical sensation in the dream and/or pain or discomfort that lingers after awakening.

Here are some of the most common health-related dreams and what they may mean…

VIOLENT INJURY

Dreams: In one version, a part of your body might get stabbed. On another night, that same body part might get branded with a hot iron. In yet a third dream, that part of your body may be shot. Although the method of injury may change, the body part you dream about remains the same.

What it means: You may be developing a health problem in that part of your body.

What to do: If the dream is a recurring one about a particular part of your body, ask your doctor for an exam.

EATING ROTTEN FOOD

Dreams: You eat food that is spoiled or has bugs all over it.

What it means: You may be overindulging in "junk food" or developing a problem that involves digestion.

What to do: Ask yourself if you are under excessive stress. If you are, try to change the stressful situation or take better care of yourself by getting more rest, eating a healthful diet and exercising.

SICK ANIMALS

Dreams: Your pet, former pet or a stray has become ill or received a violent injury.

What it means: Our pets are dream symbols of ourselves. This dream often means that some part of you is suffering. People who are in abusive relationships often have this dream. It also can mean that you have been abusing your own body by neglecting your health.

What to do: If you are in an abusive relationship, seek help from the authorities and/or a mental health professional. If you are not, take stock of your lifestyle and try to find a way to improve your diet and/or get more exercise.

COLLAPSING HOUSE

Dreams: The floor in your house is collapsing, most commonly due to termites. Or perhaps the walls are crumbling. Or the stairs can't hold your weight.

What it means: Something is giving way or losing ground in your life, or you have a chronic health condition that might be worsening. For example, a woman who has scoliosis (curvature of the spine) dreamed of a problem with a spiral staircase in her house at a time when her back was flaring up.

What to do: Ask your doctor what therapies may be available for your condition. For example, people who have chronic ailments often think that they must live with them. In some cases, there are treatments available that can relieve your symptoms.

CANCER DIAGNOSIS

Dreams: You go to the doctor and are told that you have cancer and have only a short time to live.

What it means: This is a very common dream, and it does not necessarily mean that you have cancer. It almost always means that you simply are overextending yourself and are anxious about it.

What to do: Reflect on what is causing anxiety in your life. If you are overloaded, delegate as much as you can to others. If you suspect cancer or have a family history of the disease, see your doctor.

8

Family Health

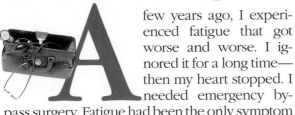

Common Symptoms You Should Never Ignore

A few years ago, I experienced fatigue that got worse and worse. I ignored it for a long time—then my heart stopped. I needed emergency bypass surgery. Fatigue had been the only symptom of a serious heart condition.

Symptoms we all experience occasionally, such as upset stomach or headache, are rarely cause for concern. Yet even mild symptoms may be a sign of serious underlying illness. The challenge is knowing when you can treat yourself and when you need medical attention.

Common symptoms—and when they may be dangerous...

ABDOMINAL PAIN

This is one of the most difficult symptoms to evaluate because it can be caused by hundreds of conditions.

Usual causes: Gas, stress, viral or bacterial infections (such as food poisoning).

Warning: Abdominal pain that lasts more than a day or two...causes severe cramps...or is accompanied by other symptoms, such as persistent nausea or vomiting, should be evaluated by a physician. *The problem could be...*

● **Appendicitis.** Patients often experience fever or nausea as well as intense stomach pain. The pain typically begins around the navel and shifts to the lower-right abdomen over six to 12 hours. If the appendix isn't surgically removed before it ruptures, it can cause a life-threatening infection called *peritonitis.*

● **Gallbladder disease, gallstones, ulcers and stomach cancer** can cause abdominal pain ranging from sharp and intermittent to dull and constant.

J. Edward Hill, MD, president, American Medical Association, and editor, *American Medical Association Family Medical Guide.* Wiley. He is a family physician at North Mississippi Medical Center and a faculty member at Family Medicine Residency Center, both in Tupelo.

BACK PAIN

Back pain is a leading cause of lost work days. Even minor back injuries can sometimes cause excruciating pain.

Usual causes: Muscle pulls or spasms cause 90% of back pain.

Apply an ice pack as often as possible during the first 24 hours after pain starts…switch to heat after 24 hours…and take a *nonsteroidal anti-inflammatory drug* (NSAID), such as aspirin or ibuprofen, to control pain and swelling.

If back pain does not improve after a week, see your doctor.

Warning: Back pain that is accompanied by fever and neurological symptoms, such as tingling, numbness or shooting pains down one or both legs, is potentially serious. These symptoms may indicate a spinal infection, which is relatively rare but can cause permanent damage. See your doctor or go to an emergency room immediately.

CHEST PAIN

Any pain that is in the chest should be taken seriously because it is a common symptom of heart attack.

Usual causes: Musculoskeletal injury that is caused by overexertion. Working all day in the yard or pushing yourself too hard at the gym can result in a muscle pull between the ribs or in the upper chest. This may cause a dull ache or shooting pains.

If pain occurs only when you move your body in a certain way, it is probably caused by a strained muscle or inflammation in the ribs (costochondritis). The pain usually subsides in a day or two.

Warning: Suspect a heart attack if the pain is accompanied by a pressing or crushing sensation, radiates out from the chest to other parts of the body (such as the breastbone, jaw, arms or neck) and/or is accompanied by heavy sweating, nausea or vomiting. Call 911 immediately. Then take an aspirin, unlock your door and wait for help to arrive.

Severe chest pain that occurs in patients who have had surgery recently or have been bedridden due to illness or injury may be caused by a *pulmonary embolism* (a blood clot in the lung). Again, get medical assistance immediately.

CONSTIPATION

The frequency of bowel movements is highly variable—from twice a day to several times a week may be normal. Any change in your usual habits deserves attention.

Usual causes: Most constipation is due to insufficient fiber and/or water in the diet.

Try to get at least 25 grams (g) of fiber daily. Start the day with a high-fiber cereal, such as oatmeal…snack on fresh fruits…and eat more beans, whole grains and vegetables. Drink two quarts of liquid daily—water is best.

Also, exercise for at least 20 minutes most days of the week. Exercise stimulates intestinal contractions that promote bowel movements.

Warning: Sudden constipation or alternating bouts of diarrhea and constipation may be a sign of colon cancer. Call your doctor—you may need a colonoscopy to determine if cancer is present.

FATIGUE

It's normal to be exhausted after a hard day, but persistent fatigue is not normal, especially when it suddenly worsens.

Usual causes: A combination of inadequate sleep and bad diet, such as loading up on coffee or junk food, can cause fatigue. Caffeine is a stimulant—but after the initial stimulation, people often experience *rebound fatigue*. Junk food is usually high in carbohydrates, which can cause a surge in blood sugar followed by a drop, resulting in fatigue.

Limit your intake of caffeinated beverages to one or two servings daily. Go to bed and get up at the same times most days of the week. Eat nutritious meals and exercise regularly—it promotes deeper sleep.

Warning: Fatigue can be a symptom of almost all acute and chronic diseases, but people who experience significantly more fatigue than usual—in the absence of any lifestyle changes—should suspect underlying heart disease and get an immediate checkup. This is especially true for women because fatigue, not chest pain, often is the first symptom.

HEADACHE

Anyone who gets headaches more often than once a month or is incapacitated by a headache needs to go to a doctor for a complete medical workup immediately.

Usual causes: Approximately 90% of headaches are tension headaches, caused by fatigue or emotional stress.

Aspirin, ibuprofen and acetaminophen are effective at relieving pain—see which works best for you. Stress-reduction techniques, such as yoga, can also help.

Migraine headaches are more severe, but they usually can be controlled or prevented by using ibuprofen or prescription drugs, such as *sumatriptan* (Imitrex).

Warning: Headaches that increase in frequency...are unusually severe...or are accompanied by other symptoms, such as nausea, slurred speech or vision changes, should be brought to a doctor's attention immediately. They could be a sign of stroke, infection in a brain blood vessel, meningitis or even a brain tumor.

Important: Call 911 if you suspect a stroke or experience an excruciating headache that comes out of the blue. This is known as a *thunderclap* headache, and it may be due to a potentially fatal ruptured blood vessel in the brain.

HEARTBURN

Most of us have experienced this burning sensation behind the breastbone.

Usual causes: Indigestion, often from eating fatty or spicy foods.

Warning: *Gastroesophageal reflux disease* (GERD) is a common cause of heartburn. Mild cases can be treated with antacids, but GERD that occurs more than once a week can cause serious damage to the esophagus. There also is an association between chronic GERD and esophagus cancer.

Patients usually require acid-blocking medications, such as *omeprazole* (Prilosec) or *ranitidine* (Zantac).

Helpful: If you need antacids more than once or twice a week, see your doctor.

Deadly! Flu Shots Contain Mercury

Mark A. Stengler, ND, naturopathic physician, La Jolla Whole Health Clinic, La Jolla, CA, and associate clinical professor, the National College of Naturopathic Medicine, Portland, OR. He is author of numerous books on natural healing, including *The Natural Physician's Healing Therapies*. Bottom Line. *www.bottomlinesecrets.com.*

Every flu season, the government and much of the medical community promote flu vaccinations for millions of Americans. Should you get the vaccine? *Here's what you need to know to make your decision...*

There are two types of vaccines...

The flu shot contains *inactive* (killed) virus. The Centers for Disease Control and Prevention (CDC) says that it can be given to anyone older than six months of age, including healthy people, pregnant and nursing women and those who have chronic medical conditions.

The other form is a nasal-spray vaccine called FluMist. It contains *attenuated* (weakened) live viruses and should be used only by healthy people. Because FluMist involves live viruses, it should not be used by those who come in contact with people who have severely suppressed immune systems (such as transplant recipients or AIDS patients).

In addition, according to the CDC, the nasal-spray vaccine should not be used by...

●**Children younger than five years of age.**

●**People age 50 and older.**

●**People who have a medical condition that places them at high risk for complications** from influenza, including those who have chronic heart or lung disease, such as asthma or reactive airway disease...those who have diabetes or kidney failure...those who have illnesses that weaken the immune system...or anyone who takes medications that can weaken the immune system.

●**Children or adolescents taking aspirin.**

●**People who have a history of Guillain-Barré syndrome,** a rare nervous system disorder.

●**Pregnant or nursing women.**

●**People who have a history of allergy to any components of the vaccine or to eggs.**

One of my biggest problems with the flu shot is that it contains *thimerosal*, a preservative that contains mercury.

Mercury is a known immune-system suppressant and is toxic to the nervous system. In my opinion, it can be particularly harmful to pregnant women because it exposes the fetus to mercury. Infants are not able to detoxify mercury effectively, and it can cause nerve and brain damage in children.

Some scientific evidence shows that thimerosal in vaccines leads to health problems, so in 1999 the US Public Health Service and the American Academy of Pediatrics—along with vaccine manufacturers—agreed that thimerosal should be reduced or eliminated from vaccines as a precaution. It has since been removed from childhood vaccines, yet manufacturers still are using thimerosal in the adult flu vaccine.

However, a preservative-free vaccine in a single-dose syringe is available. It contains only trace amounts of thimerosal—a residual from early manufacturing steps. Thimerosal is used as a preservative in an amount less than 1 microgram (mcg) of mercury per 0.5 milliliter (mL) dose. The regular injectable version contains 25 mcg mercury/0.5 mL dose. Ask your doctor about it if you are getting a shot.

For people who have a choice between types of flu vaccine, I recommend FluMist, which contains no mercury and is often available at pharmacies without a prescription.

The flu can be life-threatening for some people. For that reason, if you have risk factors for developing complications from the flu (see below) and aren't eligible to use FluMist, I recommend that you consider getting a preservative-free flu shot in October or November. *If a preservative-free vaccine is not available to you, you should still get a flu shot if you fall into any of the following groups...*

●**Anyone age 65 and older.**

●**Residents of nursing homes** or other long-term-care facilities that house people of any age who have chronic medical conditions.

●**Anyone who has chronic disorders of the pulmonary or cardiovascular system.**

●**Anyone who has required hospitalization or regular medical follow-up during the preceding year** because of chronic metabolic diseases (including diabetes), renal dysfunction, blood cell disorders or immunosuppression (including that caused by medications or by human immunodeficiency virus, also known as HIV).

●**Children and adolescents ages six months to 18 years who are receiving long-term aspirin therapy** and, therefore, might be at risk for experiencing Reye's syndrome after influenza infection.

●**Children ages six months to 23 months.**

●**Women who will be pregnant during the influenza season.**

For my healthy patients, I recommend focusing on powerful, natural cold-and-flu-fighting strategies rather than vaccination.

THE POSSIBILITY OF A FLU PANDEMIC

Experts are concerned about a global flu epidemic (pandemic) that could kill millions around the world—and it is quite possible. *Consider the three influenza pandemics of the 20th century...*

The Spanish flu of 1918 affected 20% to 40% of the world's population and killed more than 50 million people—675,000 people died in the US alone. The 1957 Asian flu pandemic resulted in approximately 70,000 deaths, and many still remember the 1968 Hong Kong flu that took the lives of more than 34,000 Americans.

In August 2004, Tommy G. Thompson, then Secretary of the US Department of Health and Human Services, unveiled the department's Pandemic Influenza Response and Preparedness Plan, which outlines a coordinated national strategy to prepare for and respond to an influenza pandemic. "This plan will serve as our road map on how we, as a nation and as a member of the global health community, respond to the next pandemic influenza outbreak, whenever that may be," he said at the time.

Recently, the US has been stockpiling flu vaccines, yet these are not likely to be of much help. Influenza (and other viruses) constantly change their structure just enough so that the immune system doesn't recognize them. The mutation of viruses makes it difficult for manufacturers to predict which flu strain (out of the many hundreds) will make its way to the US.

Flu vaccines are manufactured several months before flu season actually begins, so they may not be accurate at all for the incoming influenza strain. With a pandemic influenza virus, there is a sudden change in the structure of the virus, making the manufacture of a vaccine nearly impossible.

According to a Department of Health and Human Services press release, "Pandemic virus will likely be unaffected by currently available flu vaccines that are modified each year to match the strains of the virus that are known to be in circulation among humans around the world."

Normally, changes occur gradually in the influenza viruses that appear. A pandemic influenza virus is particularly dangerous due to the major, sudden shift that is seen in the virus's structure. This increases the pandemic influenza virus's ability to cause illness in a large proportion of the population.

What is your best defense? A supercharged immune system that's ready to do battle with these viral intruders.

Vitamin C...Hot Tea And Other Crazy Myths About Colds

William Schaffner, MD, chairman, department of preventive medicine, Vanderbilt University School of Medicine, Nashville. He is a fellow of the Infectious Diseases Society of America, a liaison member of the Advisory Committee on Immunization Practices, Centers for Disease Control and Prevention, and an associate editor of *Journal of Infectious Diseases.*

The average American gets more than 100 colds in his/her lifetime, and scientists have amassed a great deal of information about the common cold. But misinformation is still widely circulated as fact. *Take the following quiz to see how much you really know about the common cold...*

●**True or False? Colds are mainly spread by coughs and sneezes.**

False: The viruses that cause colds are usually spread by hand-to-hand, hand-to-nose or hand-to-object contact. The *rhinovirus*, the most common cold virus, flourishes in mucus membranes.

Someone who is infected with the virus rubs his nose or eyes, picking up the virus on his fingers. He then touches you or deposits the virus on a doorknob, telephone, etc. The virus can survive for 24 to 48 hours, so it can easily be picked up by the next person who comes along.

●**True or False? People who have colds are highly contagious before they experience symptoms.**

True: You're most contagious in the 24 hours before symptoms start. You may feel healthy, but the virus is incubating—and spreading. Colds often are transmitted during this period because people who are infected aren't yet staying home—and other people aren't avoiding them the way they would someone who is coughing or sneezing.

●**True or False? Antimicrobial soap kills cold viruses.**

False: Antimicrobial soap kills bacteria, not the viruses that cause colds. The best protection against colds is to wash your hands often using warm, soapy water. It takes approximately one minute of handwashing to remove viruses.

Waterless alcohol-based hand sanitizers can be helpful when soap and water aren't available. Hand sanitizers such as Purell and Nexcare kill cold viruses, as do disposable alcohol towelettes.

●**True or False? Being cold increases the risk of getting a cold.**

False: Generations of moms have said, *Bundle up or you'll catch a cold,* but the best current evidence indicates that Mom was wrong.

In one well-regarded study, scientists divided volunteers into a "warm" group and a group that was damp and chilled. They exposed people in both groups to cold viruses. There was no difference in the incidence of subsequent colds between the two groups.

Opposing view: In a study recently reported in *Journal of Family Practice,* scientists did find an increase in the number of colds in volunteers who soaked their feet in icy water for 20 minutes. This wasn't a controlled experiment, however. The scientists didn't know, for example, if the volunteers who got sick had more contact with people who already had colds than those who didn't get sick.

Cold weather brings an increase in colds, but being cold doesn't seem to be a factor.

●**True or False? Vitamin C has been proven to reduce the duration and/or severity of colds.**

False: Ever since the publication of Linus Pauling's book *Vitamin C and the Common Cold*, millions of Americans have attempted to prevent and/or treat colds by taking enormous amounts of vitamin C—as much as 1,000 milligrams (mg) every few hours.

Since then, many studies have looked at the connection between colds and vitamin C. Most have been inconclusive—and many showed no benefit at all.

In large doses, vitamin C inhibits the effects of *histamine*, a body chemical that causes sniffles and other cold symptoms. Yet there's no evidence that reducing histamine in this way has any effect on cold symptoms—and studies have not shown that it prevents colds.

Caution: Vitamin C is cleared through the kidneys. Taking large amounts can cause the vitamin to crystallize and result in kidney stones. Drink more water than usual if you decide to take extra vitamin C—and don't exceed 250 to 500 mg daily.

●**True or False? Yellow or green mucus indicates a serious infection.**

False: People who develop yellow or greenish mucus often rush to their doctors to ask for antibiotics because they believe that discolored mucus indicates a serious bacterial infection.

Colds can cause either clear, watery mucus or mucus that's thick and discolored. The coloration means that there's inflammation and more white blood cells. These immune cells are present in both viral and bacterial infections.

Discolored mucus isn't a useful way to distinguish one from the other—and it doesn't mean that your cold is more serious or that it will last any longer.

●**True or False? We get fewer colds as we get older.**

True: There are approximately 200 different viruses that cause colds. Each time your immune system is exposed to one of these viruses, it develops antibodies that make you immune to that particular strain. By the time you reach your 60s or 70s and have a lifetime of colds behind you, you have developed immunity to many—but not all—of the circulating cold viruses.

●**True or False? Stress increases the likelihood of getting a cold.**

False: There are theoretical reasons to think that stress could raise the risk of getting a cold, but it has never been shown conclusively.

Studies have shown that chronic stress decreases the immune system's ability to suppress infections. But stress is ubiquitous—nearly everyone reports having stress in the days or weeks before a survey—so it's difficult to link it with illness.

●**True or False? Drinking hot tea eases cold symptoms.**

True: Black and green tea both contain *theophylline*, a mild bronchodilator. Drinking tea when you have a cold may open the airways and make it easier to breathe. The heat and steam from the liquid also thin mucus and ease congestion.

Chicken soup is also a traditional remedy for colds—but don't expect too much. Though it provides extra fluids and the steam eases congestion, chicken soup cannot cure a cold.

Fever Myths Even Your Doctor May Believe

Mary E. Frank, MD, associate clinical professor of ambulatory and community medicine, University of California, San Francisco, and president, American Academy of Family Physicians.

If you've always believed that you can detect a fever by touching someone's forehead, then think again.

The abdomen is actually more likely to feel warm when someone has a fever. However, a thermometer is the only way to accurately measure body temperature.

Here are six other common—and potentially dangerous—myths about fever...

Myth 1: **All adults have a normal body temperature of 98.6°F.** "Normal" body temperature is conventionally said to be 98.6°F, but it actually varies. For some people, 98°F is normal, and for others, it could be 99°F. Body temperature usually rises during the course of the day—your temperature may be 98.2°F in the morning and rise to 99.4°F in the late afternoon.

Normal temperature tends to decline as you age. According to a study conducted at Yeshiva University in New York City, the average oral temperature of 150 healthy people age 65 and older was 97.5°F. Because their normal body temperature tends to be lower, some older adults may be seriously ill—they may have pneumonia or a widespread infection—yet appear to have no fever at all.

Myth 2: **A fever always means that you have an infection.** Not necessarily. Bacterial pneumonia or a bladder infection is typically accompanied by a fever. Elevated body temperature also occurs during a number of viral illnesses, such as influenza, gastroenteritis (stomach flu)—even the common cold.

However, a fever can also signal an allergic reaction…dehydration…inflammation…a hormone disorder, such as hyperthyroidism…or an autoimmune disease, such as rheumatoid arthritis. Medications, such as antibiotics, narcotics, barbiturates and antihistamines, can trigger a fever as well. Cancer, especially leukemia or lymphoma, can cause a persistent fever of 100°F to 101°F.

Myth 3: **Fever should always be treated.** Most of the time, you don't need to do anything to reduce a fever. Unless it goes quite high (above 104°F in an adult), it causes no permanent damage—but you will feel uncomfortable. Some doctors suggest letting a fever run its course. That way, you won't undermine your body's natural defense process.

If you choose to let a fever run its course, drink lots of fluids to avoid becoming dehydrated by the increased metabolism that accompanies fever.

Even if you're not thirsty, keep a glass of water or juice at your bedside and take sips often. Eat soups and suck on popsicles. Take lukewarm baths or showers.

Myth 4: **Aspirin is the best medicine for a fever.** The most common *antipyretics*—fever reducers—are available over-the-counter. They include *acetaminophen* (Tylenol) and *aspirin* and other nonsteroidal anti-inflammatory drugs (NSAIDs), such as *ibuprofen* (Advil) and *naproxen* (Aleve).

As far as effectiveness goes, there's little difference among them—no solid evidence shows that any of these drugs works faster or better than the others at reducing fever.

Important: Never exceed the dosage recommendations without first discussing it with your physician.

Choose the best fever-reducer on the basis of your own medical profile and the medication's potential side effects…

If you take daily aspirin therapy: Take acetaminophen. NSAIDs can sometimes undermine the benefits of aspirin therapy, according to the latest studies.

If you have high blood pressure: Take acetaminophen. Aspirin and other NSAIDs can raise blood pressure.

If you have kidney disease: Take acetaminophen. Aspirin and other NSAIDs can damage the kidneys.

If you're susceptible to gastrointestinal problems: Take acetaminophen. Aspirin and other NSAIDs can irritate the digestive system and cause bleeding.

If you have asthma: Take acetaminophen. Aspirin and other NSAIDs may trigger an attack.

If you have liver disease or drink more than three alcoholic beverages a day: Take aspirin or another NSAID. Acetaminophen can harm the liver in some people.

Important: Don't give aspirin to anyone younger than age 15—it can cause *Reye's syndrome*, a potentially life-threatening condition that causes swelling of the brain and degeneration of the liver.

Myth 5: **A fever means you're contagious.** Not so. A person who has an upper respiratory tract infection may be contagious early on, when he/she has a runny nose but no fever. On the other hand, a person who has a bacterial infection can still be running a fever after several days of antibiotic treatment but no longer be contagious.

***Myth 6:* All thermometers are equally accurate.** Glass mercury thermometers are the most accurate but are being phased out because of the potential exposure to mercury if the glass breaks. Digital oral and digital rectal thermometers are both accurate. Ear thermometers are slightly less accurate. Forehead thermometers (plastic strips that are pressed against the forehead) are not reliable for exact measurements.

Important: Always inform your doctor what type of thermometer you are using to take your temperature.

■ ■ ■ ■

What Is a Fever?

Apart of the brain called the *hypothalamus* regulates body temperature. To fight infection and other illnesses, the hypothalamus increases body temperature (fever). Fever is defined as 100°F and higher as measured by an oral thermometer.

■ ■ ■ ■

Natural Remedies That Fight Fever

Holistic treatments work with the healing properties of a fever to help fight infection or injury.* *The following remedies are available at health-food stores...*

●**Ferrum phosphoricum** is a homeopathic remedy that promotes the beneficial effects of fever. *Take two pellets of a 30C potency four times daily along with one of these herbal remedies...*

●Ginger is particularly helpful for people who have a sore throat and chills. Take a 500-milligram (mg) capsule or 2 milliliters (mL) of the tincture with 6 ounces of water four times daily. Even better, drink one cup of fresh ginger tea four times every day.

●Elderberry is excellent for flu-related fever. Take 10 mL of the tincture with 6 ounces of water three times daily.

Mark Stengler, ND, naturopathic physician, La Jolla Whole Health Clinic, La Jolla, CA.

*Before trying a natural remedy, check with your physician if you are taking medication.

4-in-1 Childhood Vaccine— Helpful or Harmful?

Henry Shinefield, MD, clinical professor of pediatrics and dermatology, University of California, San Francisco School of Medicine.

Barbara Loe Fisher, cofounder and president, National Vaccine Information Center.

Merck press release.

Anew single-shot vaccine that protects children against measles, mumps, rubella and chicken pox could mean one less shot and one less doctor visit, advocates say.

The US Food and Drug Administration (FDA) has approved the vaccine after testing in more than 5,000 children. It is called Proquad and is manufactured by Merck.

The vaccine—which is a combination of the company's measles, mumps, rubella (MMR II) vaccine and its chicken pox shot—is designed for children from 12 months to 12 years of age.

Proquad is the first and only vaccine that is approved in the United States to help protect against these four diseases in one single shot, according to Merck.

ADVANTAGES

"The advantage of putting two vaccines together has been recognized by medical authorities," says Dr. Henry Shinefield, a clinical professor of pediatrics and dermatology at the University of California, San Francisco, School of Medicine, and a consultant to Merck.

"There is an obvious advantage to the children," Shinefield says. "They only get one shot." The advantage to doctors is they can limit the number of different vaccines they have on hand, he says.

Shinefield notes that the four-in-one vaccine also benefits the community. Having to get only one shot instead of two may mean that more children get vaccinated, he says. "The community benefits by having less disease."

"Based on the public health benefits realized following the introduction of other combination vaccines, such as MMR II, we expect Proquad to become a primary option for the prevention of measles, mumps, rubella and chicken pox," says Dr. Mark Feinberg, vice president of policy, public health and medical affairs in Merck's Vaccine Division.

Proquad can help reduce the gap that exists in the United States between vaccination rates for chickenpox—which were an estimated 87.5% in 2004—and vaccination rates for measles, mumps and rubella—which were an estimated 93% in 2004, Feinberg says. "The main goal for any vaccine is to help eliminate disease, and this is possible when very high vaccination rates are achieved in the community."

> *There is an obvious advantage to the children. They only get one shot.*
>
> *Henry Shinefield, MD*

In terms of potential side effects, Shinefield doesn't see any more danger than there is with the current two vaccines. "It is important that children and parents be made aware of every side effect," he says. "The side effects with this vaccine are in line with what we see with other vaccines," he notes.

CONCERNS

However, some experts are cautious about the use of this new vaccine.

"The FDA should have required far larger studies," says Barbara Loe Fisher, cofounder and president of the National Vaccine Information Center. "You are combining four live viruses into one vaccine, which has never been done before."

Fisher notes that there are still unanswered questions about the long-term adverse effects of these vaccines when they are given separately.

And she believes it has not been examined sufficiently because it has only been tested against other vaccines and not against a placebo. "With a new vaccine like this, you should be comparing it against placebo to find out the true adverse reaction rate," Fisher says.

info The American Academy of Pediatrics can provide more information about childhood vaccines at *www.cispimmunize.org*.

Vaccine May End Ear Infections

Allan S. Lieberthal, MD, pediatrician, Kaiser Permanente, Panorama City, CA, and cochairman of the American Academy of Pediatrics' and the American Academy of Family Physicians' subcommittee on the management of acute otitis media.
The Lancet.

Researchers from the Czech Republic report a successful trial of a vaccine for acute *otitis media*, the inner ear condition that is the most common bacterial infection in children.

The vaccine contains proteins from 11 different strains of the bacterium *Streptococcus pneumoniae* that are attached to a protein from another infectious agent, *Haemophilus influenzae*. Thus, the vaccine protects against the two main causes of middle ear infections, the researchers say.

THE STUDY

The study included nearly 4,700 infants, ages three to 15 months, who were followed-up until the end of their second year. Half of the infants got the vaccine and half were given a hepatitis A vaccine to serve as a control group.

The researchers found 333 cases of acute otitis media in the group that received the vaccine compared with 499 ear infection cases in the control group.

Therefore, the incidence of ear infections in the children who were given the vaccine was one-third lower than in those who didn't receive it, according to doctors at the University of Defence in Prague.

TESTING CONTINUES

The study results are "very exciting" but still preliminary, says Dr. Allan S. Lieberthal, a pediatrician at Kaiser Permanente in California and cochairman of the American Academy of Pediatrics' and American Academy of Family Physicians' subcommittee on the management of acute otitis media.

Lieberthal says he is cautious because of the criteria used in the study to define acute otitis media. He was a member of the committee that drew up criteria to distinguish an ear infection that requires antibiotics from otitis media with *effusion*, or an accumulation of fluid in the middle ear, a condition that usually clears up on its own.

While the committee criteria for an ear infection requires an onset of symptoms within 48 hours, the Czech study accepted cases that were diagnosed as late as 14 days afterward, Lieberthal says. In addition, the study did not require signs of inflammation, another criterion set by the committee.

"If this is reproduced in other studies and the vaccine is safe, it would suggest that the vaccine would decrease infection by those bacteria and possibly result in a reduction of acute otitis media," Lieberthal says. "But before you say 'this is an acute otitis media vaccine,' you have to do studies using a better definition of acute otitis media," he adds.

Still, Lieberthal's caution is coupled with enthusiasm. The trial results "strongly suggest" that the vaccine protects against infection, and he says, "I think it is a very important vaccine."

Drug maker GlaxoSmithKline plans to market the shot as Streptorix. The vaccine is undergoing Phase 3 trials, the final set of tests that is needed to seek approval for marketing a pharmaceutical product.

Breakthrough Vaccines: Meningitis, Whooping Cough

David Neumann, executive director, National Partnership for Immunization.

Paul Offit, MD, chief of infectious diseases, The Children's Hospital of Philadelphia.

Health experts are recommending that children receive breakthrough vaccines for meningitis as well as for whooping cough (*pertussis*).

Both vaccines are safe enough to be used by 11-year-old children, providing youngsters with protection that they have not had up until this point, doctors say.

Vaccines have eradicated smallpox globally, and in the United States, they have eliminated wild polio virus and significantly reduced the number of cases of measles, diphtheria, rubella and other diseases, according to the National Partnership for Immunization. However, tens of thousands of Americans still die from vaccine-preventable diseases.

More frustrating to doctors, is that 15% of adults do not believe inoculations are necessary to prevent certain diseases. And a persistent rumor linking vaccination with autism has led some parents to choose not to immunize their children.

You can be fine one minute, and dead four hours later.

Paul Offit, MD

If diseases such as measles, diphtheria and whooping cough were to resurface unchecked, thousands of American children would die.

"We are pretty complacent about vaccine-preventable diseases, primarily because the vaccines are so effective we rarely see the diseases," says David Neumann, executive director of the National Partnership for Immunization. "It's kind of out-of-sight, out-of-mind."

MENINGITIS VACCINE

The new meningococcal vaccine is important because it is effective over a longer period of time than the old vaccine was, says Dr. Paul Offit, chief of infectious diseases at The Children's Hospital of Philadelphia.

"The problem was the earlier vaccines didn't provide long-lasting immunity," Offit says. "Frequent boosting was required."

Meningitis is a viral or bacterial infection of the membranes and cerebrospinal fluid that surround the brain and spinal cord. It is spread by coughing, sneezing, kissing or sharing drinking glasses, experts say.

Symptoms include a fever of 101°F or higher, a stiff neck, a purple rash, vomiting and headache. Meningitis can result in long-term permanent disabilities such as hearing loss and brain damage. The most serious type of meningitis is caused by the *meningococcus* bacteria, for which the vaccine was developed. According to the Centers for Disease Control and Prevention (CDC), approximately 3,000 cases of meningococcal disease occur in the United States every year. The overall fatality rate is approximately 10%, but it is sometimes higher in young people.

The most dangerous result from the meningococcal bacteria is *sepsis*, or blood infection, Offit says. "You can be fine one minute, and dead four hours later," he says.

The CDC recommends giving the new vaccine to children at age 11 or at age 15, if they have not received the vaccine before; and to college students living in the close quarters of dormitories.

PERTUSSIS VACCINE

The new pertussis vaccine also comes as a relief to doctors, as whooping cough is the only vaccine-preventable disease that has not been quelled. In 1998, there were 7,405 reported cases in the United States. That figure rose to 9,771 in 2002.

"The problem with the original vaccine is that when it was given to kids over seven, it caused some pretty severe reactions," Offit says. So children would receive as many as five combination diphtheria-tetanus-pertussis (DTP) shots by age seven, but only receive a diphtheria-tetanus booster after age seven. Therefore, their protection from pertussis was good, but not perfect, because the vaccine's effectiveness deteriorated after five years.

This new form of the vaccine is safe for children ages 10 to 18.

"The public health community is very excited by this new booster shot," Neumann says. "We're optimistic that the incidence rates will be driven back down. The challenge will be to get those 11-year-olds back in [to the doctors' offices] for their booster shot."

VACCINE CONTROVERSY

Another challenge is convincing parents of the importance of vaccines. A 1998 article cited studies of 12 children who had pervasive developmental disorder, primarily autism. The parents and doctors of eight of the children said this began after they received the measles-mumps-rubella (MMR) vaccine.

A later report from the Institute of Medicine collected all of the available evidence and found no connection between vaccines and autism. However, that has made little difference to many parents, Neumann says.

"We see no evidence for the alleged effects that have been linked with vaccines," he says. "Unfortunately, people who have heard the allegations about vaccines have discounted the science, [and] the rumors persist."

info To learn more about vaccines, visit the National Partnership for Immunization at *www.partnersforimmunization.org.*

Pacifier May Prevent SIDS

Fern R. Hauck, MD, MS, associate professor of family medicine and public health sciences, University of Virginia Health System, Charlottesville, and member, American Academy of Pediatrics Task Force on Sudden Infant Death Syndrome.

Dan Polk, MD, vice chairman, division of neonatology, Children's Memorial Hospital, Chicago.

Rachel Moon, MD, pediatrician and SIDS researcher, Children's National Medical Center, Washington, DC, and member, American Academy of Pediatrics Task Force on Sudden Infant Death Syndrome.

American Academy of Pediatrics National Conference and Exhibition, Washington, DC.

Pediatrics.

Giving a baby a pacifier before bed may help reduce the risk of *sudden infant death syndrome* (SIDS), according to a review of studies done on pacifier use. And the evidence was compelling enough for the American Academy of Pediatrics (AAP) to include a recommendation about pacifier use in its updated SIDS guidelines.

THE NEWEST STUDY

Study author Dr. Fern R. Hauck, an associate professor of family medicine and public health sciences at the University of Virginia Health System in Charlottesville, and her colleagues reviewed seven studies that looked at the link between pacifier use and SIDS. They concluded that approximately one SIDS death could be prevented for every 2,733 babies if they used a pacifier while they slept.

"When we looked at the last time the baby was placed for sleep, there was a consistent protective effect for SIDS from pacifier use," says Hauck. "There was a 61% reduction in SIDS risk."

BENEFIT OUTWEIGHS RISK

That benefit outweighs any potential risks of pacifier use, including dental problems, a slightly increased risk of ear infections and breast-feeding difficulties, Hauck says.

Although she doesn't know why pacifier use might protect against SIDS, Hauck says there are several theories. One is that sucking on a pacifier brings the tongue forward, forcing the airway to open more. Another theory is that when babies suck on a pacifier, they may be more easily aroused from sleep.

Dr. Dan Polk, vice chairman of the division of neonatology at Children's Memorial Hospital in Chicago, says this study's findings may be reassuring to parents who already give their infant a pacifier, but they prove only an association between pacifier use and a reduced incidence of SIDS, not necessarily a cause-and-effect relationship. The findings do not prove that pacifier use can actually reduce SIDS, he says.

SIDS GUIDELINES

Whatever the reason for the apparent protective effect, the AAP is recommending offering infants a pacifier at bedtime and naptime for the first year of life. The pacifier doesn't need to be reinserted if it falls out during sleep, and parents should not coat the pacifier with any sweet substances to entice the baby to take it. Breast-fed infants should not be given a pacifier until breast-feeding is well-established, usually at one month, the Academy says.

Along with endorsing pacifier use, other big changes in the AAP SIDS guidelines include recommending that babies sleep in the same room as the parents, but not in the same bed, and that parents not put babies to sleep on their sides.

"There's been a lot of new information on SIDS in the past five years, which is why the committee revised the SIDS guidelines," explains Dr. Rachel Moon, a pediatrician and SIDS researcher at Children's National Medical Center in Washington DC.

Other key recommendations for preventing SIDS include...

●**Place infants to sleep on their backs** every time they go to sleep.

●**Only use firm sleep surfaces** and keep soft objects, such as pillows and heavy blankets, out of the baby's crib.

●**Give the baby a smoke-free environment** both before and after pregnancy.

●**Don't share your bed with your baby,** but if possible, keep the baby in a crib in your bedroom.

●**Avoid overheating your baby.** Babies shouldn't feel hot to the touch. Keep the room warm enough so a lightly clothed adult would be comfortable.

The AAP committee also recommends that parents not use commercial products that are marketed as reducing the risk of SIDS. There is no evidence that such products actually provide any benefit.

Also, the committee recommends that babies be given plenty of *tummy time* when they are awake to avoid the development of a flat spot on the back of the head from always sleeping in the same position.

"Parents need to make sure that everyone caring for the baby is aware of the guidelines. The babysitter, the grandparents—everybody needs to know," says Moon.

"Since we don't know the cause of SIDS, the best we can do is try to control the markers," says Polk. "Just do the best you can, but that doesn't guarantee you've eliminated the risk of SIDS," he adds.

info For more advice on how you might be able to prevent SIDS, visit the American SIDS Institute at *www.sids.org*.

High Humidity—Is It the Best Way to Ease Croup?

Dennis Scolnik, MB, ChB, associate professor of pediatrics, Hospital for Sick Children and University of Toronto, Ontario, Canada.

Mehmet Karliyil, MD, pediatric emergency physician, Nyack Hospital, Nyack, NY.

The Journal of the American Medical Association.

A time-honored treatment to ease the seal-like bark of croup is to bring a child into a steamy bathroom or run a cool-mist vaporizer until symptoms subside. The theory behind this treatment is that the moisture from the steam soothes the irritated airway and thins mucus secretions, making breathing easier. However, a new study suggests that these measures probably don't help very much.

THE STUDY

Dennis Scolnik, an associate professor of pediatrics at the Hospital for Sick Children and the University of Toronto in Canada, and his colleagues randomly divided a group of 140 children who had been diagnosed with moderate to severe croup into three treatment groups. The control group received "blow-by" humidity, which is variable and often equivalent to room air. A second group received a consistent 40% humidity, and the third group was given 100% humidity.

> *The illness has a tendency to get better, and if it gets better while you're giving humidity, you'll think it was due to the humidity.*
>
> *Dennis Scolnik, MB, ChB*

Symptoms were assessed at 30 minutes and 60 minutes after treatment. The researchers found no statistically significant differences between the groups.

"The use of humidity failed to show any improvement in croup symptoms," Scolnik reports.

WHAT'S WORKING IF NOT THE HUMIDITY?

Without good scientific evidence to support the use of humidity, why do so many people believe that it is effective in treating croup?

"The illness has a tendency to get better, and if it gets better while you're giving humidity, you'll think it was due to the humidity," he says.

Another possible reason for an improvement in symptoms is that parents often sit with children while administering humidity and try to calm them. As the child calms down, some of the coughing and crying stop. And because the worst symptoms of croup probably have some component of airway spasm, calming a child helps relieve those spasms, making breathing easier, Skolnik says.

HUMIDITY, PLUS OTHER TREATMENTS

Not everyone is convinced, however, that humidity should not be used in croup treatment.

"This is a good study, but it's not going to change anything here," says Dr. Mehmet Karliyil, a pediatric emergency physician at Nyack Hospital in Nyack, NY.

"Humidity is useful. What this study shows is that 40% humidity isn't any more effective than 100%," says Karliyil. The study has just shown that more humidity isn't necessarily better.

Both Scolnik and Karliyil note that other treatments are available for croup, such as breathing in cold air to help shrink swollen airways. Doctors can also prescribe steroid medications or inhaled *epinephrine* to lessen inflammation, Scolnik says.

■ ■ ■ ■

What Is Croup?

Croup, which is the swelling of the tissues around the voice box, is actually a response to a viral or bacterial infection rather than a distinct illness.

The inflammation can sometimes be severe enough to obstruct the airway, and in fact, is one of the most common causes of upper airway blockage in youngsters, affecting as many as 5% of children younger than six years old.

Croup is characterized by a cough that often sounds like the bark of a seal.

info To learn more about croup, visit the US National Library of Medicine's MedlinePlus Web site at *www.medlineplus.gov*. Click on "Medical Encyclopedia."

■ ■ ■ ■

Better Cough Suppressant

A compound found in cocoa, *theobromine*, was more effective at calming coughs than *codeine*, the active ingredient in many over-the-counter (OTC) and prescription cough medicines.

Helpful: Drink a cup of hot chocolate or a glass of cold chocolate milk to soothe a cough.

Important: If coughing persists for more than five days, see your doctor.

Peter J. Barnes, MD, head of respiratory medicine, Imperial College London, England.

Attention Parents: When Bottle-Feeding Is Bad for Your Baby

Jane Brotanek, MD, MPH, assistant professor of pediatrics, Medical College of Wisconsin, Milwaukee.

Ruth Lawrence, MD, professor of pediatrics, University of Rochester School of Medicine, NY, and member, executive committee, section on breast-feeding, American Academy of Pediatrics.

Archives of Pediatrics & Adolescent Medicine.

Bottle-fed toddlers have a high risk of iron deficiency, which can lead to anemia and learning problems, according to the results of a new study.

THE STUDY

In the study, lead author Dr. Jane Brotanek, an assistant professor of pediatrics at the Medical College of Wisconsin, and her team collected data on 2,121 children, ages one to three years old, who participated in the National Health and Nutrition Examination Survey III.

The researchers found that the prevalence of iron deficiency was 6% among Caucasian children, 8% among African-American children and 17% among Mexican-American children.

The study also found that the longer the duration of bottle-feeding, the higher the prevalence of iron deficiency among all children.

For those children who were bottle-fed less than 12 months, 3.8% were iron-deficient; of the children bottle-fed between 13 and 23 months, 11.5% were iron-deficient; and 12.4% of the children were iron-deficient if they were bottle-fed between 24 and 48 months.

"The more milk the children drank, the more they used the bottle for a longer period of time, the greater their likelihood for anemia," Brotanek says.

At 24 to 48 months of age, 36.8% of Mexican-American children were still bottle-fed, compared with 16.9% of Caucasian and 13.8% of African-American children, the researchers report.

"We found that prolonged bottle-feeding among Mexican-American children puts them at higher risk for iron deficiency," says Brotanek.

IMPLICATIONS

According to Dr. Ruth Lawrence, a professor of pediatrics at the University of Rochester School of Medicine, and a member of the executive committee of the section on breast-feeding at the American Academy of Pediatrics, lack of iron in children's diets has been a concern for 25 years. This new study shows that the problem has not gone away. "It's pretty interesting that there are substantial numbers of children who are still iron-deficient," she says.

Although Lawrence is not surprised by the findings, she questions what was in the bottles of the children in the study. "Were they using milk, or Coke or juice? That might be the cause of the problem.

> *We have known that infants who drink too much milk after the age of one usually don't have much else in their diet.*
>
> *Ruth Lawrence, MD*

"In addition, we have known that infants who drink too much milk after the age of one usually don't have much else in their diet, and therefore, don't have any iron-containing food in their diet," Lawrence adds.

WHAT PARENTS CAN DO

"Parents need to know that bottle-feeding their child too long can put the child at risk for iron deficiency and anemia," Brotanek explains.

"Iron deficiency and anemia are problems because they are associated with behavior and cognitive delays, and cause a fall in IQ scores, impaired learning and decreased school achievement," she says.

Right now, there are an estimated 3.8 million American children at risk for iron deficiency and anemia because they are being bottle-fed past 12 months of age, Brotanek says.

"It is important for parents to transition their child to the cup early on, preferably at nine months of age, so that by 12 months of age their child can be completely weaned from the bottle," Brotanek advises.

She notes that while milk is important for toddlers, "Parents of toddlers older than 12 months should make sure that they drink no more than two cups of regular milk a day, since drinking more decreases a child's appetite."

Parents also need to be aware that it is important to give toddlers iron-rich foods, Brotanek says. "These are important for growth and well-being. They include beans, meat, fortified cereals, eggs and green leafy vegetables," she says.

Uncanny Canines Sense Oncoming Seizures

Cheryl and Taylor Huey, Monroe, LA.
Jennifer Arnold, founder, Canine Assistants, Alpharetta, GA.

One recent morning at 4 am, Cheryl Huey of Monroe, Louisiana, felt her two-year-old female golden retriever, Chelsea, pawing at her arm.

Huey and her 16-year-old son, Taylor, had just brought the dog home the day before, and thought she needed to go out. However, the dog was alerting Huey to her son's oncoming epileptic seizure.

"About 10 minutes later we were out in the parking lot," Huey recalls, "and Taylor started having a seizure."

Chelsea's ability to sense the onset of an attack—even while Taylor was sleeping—was extraordinary, Huey says. "At the time, I just couldn't believe it."

A SIXTH SENSE?

Chelsea is one of the dogs born and raised at Canine Assistants, a nonprofit organization that trains dogs to help individuals who have epilepsy as well as other disorders such as Parkinson's disease, multiple sclerosis, muscular dystrophy and *amyotrophic lateral sclerosis* (ALS, or Lou Gehrig's disease).

Seizure-alert dogs, like Chelsea, are trained to alert epileptics to seizures before they happen. Even from across a room, seizure-alert dogs seem to be able to pick up on extremely subtle physiological changes—minute alterations in odor or

movement—that may begin anywhere from 45 to five or 10 minutes before an attack occurs.

This ability to sense these changes can be invaluable, since getting an early warning of a seizure's onset helps people who have epilepsy find a safe environment or take precautionary measures.

These dogs can also be taught to push a button to dial 911, tug open doors to run and get help, and even use their mouths to bring the person in need a cordless phone or medication.

How do dogs have that instinct that lying on the ground is safer? We have no idea.

Jennifer Arnold

Jennifer Arnold, founder and operator of Canine Assistants, says the ability of these canines to sense many hidden health dangers is emerging. "There are already dogs that have been anecdotally reported to be able to pick up on dangerously low blood sugar," she says.

"And a service dog alerted his owner in the middle of the night that he was having a heart attack in his sleep—and then did it again for a stranger in a mall," Arnold adds.

While the results are encouraging, the mechanism behind them is still unknown. "More research needs to be done," Arnold says. "We don't exactly know right now what the dogs are responding to."

TRAINING AND INSTINCT

The dogs trained by the experts at Canine Assistants begin their 18 months of instruction at just two days' old, learning over 90 standard commands.

More mysteriously, some protective measures seem to come to the dogs instinctively, Arnold says. For example, when sensing an oncoming seizure, "they tend to want their person to lie on the ground," she says.

As any person who has epilepsy knows, that's the most sensible action an individual can take before a seizure, since falling is the leading cause of serious injury during an attack.

"It's fascinating! Dogs who have never seen anyone have a seizure will tug at their person's sleeve—they want you on the ground," Arnold says. "How do they have that instinct that lying on the ground is safer? We have no idea."

Huey bears witness to this phenomenon. After Taylor's seizure, Huey told Chelsea, "Stay." Huey says, "Chelsea crawled across Taylor's body and lay on top of him as I ran inside to get help. When I came out again, she was still across his body. Part of her training is to protect and stay with him," Huey says.

EARLY WARNING SYSTEM

For people who have epilepsy, having a four-legged, early warning system that can be taken everywhere gives them a sense of security and independence many haven't had before.

And Chelsea's arrival means Cheryl Huey can finally let her teenager go off on his own without as much worry. "Seeing Chelsea's reaction that first time, the response she had, I now have confidence that in the event of a seizure, she's going to be in charge," Huey says.

 Learn more about Canine Assistants at *www.canineassistants.org.*

Petting Zoos Breed Bacteria

Amy E. Belflower, MPH, epidemiologist, South Carolina Department of Health and Environmental Control.
Marcy McMillian, MPH, epidemiologist, Tennessee Department of Health.
Philip M. Tierno, Jr., PhD, director, Clinical Microbiology and Immunology, New York University Medical Center, New York City.
David L. Katz, MD, MPH, associate professor of public health, and director, Prevention Research Center, Yale University School of Medicine, New Haven, CT.
International Conference on Emerging Infectious Diseases, Atlanta.

Petting zoos may be fun for kids, but they are breeding grounds for bacteria that can cause severe gastrointestinal illness, new research contends. Most people are not aware that simple measures, such as handwashing, could prevent infection, and some people do things that might even increase their risk, according to three studies.

Bacterial infection can result from touching anything that has come into contact with animal feces, including the animals themselves and the surfaces that people have touched after petting the animals. Eating or drinking while petting or feeding the animals can also transmit infection, the researchers note.

THE FIRST STUDY

The first study looked at two previous outbreaks of *E. coli O157:H7* at Florida petting zoos that sickened at least 34 people. The researchers, from the Centers for Disease Control and Prevention (CDC) and the Florida Department of Health, interviewed petting-zoo visitors to find out what behaviors caused people to get an infection.

The behaviors most strongly associated with E. coli were feeding a cow or goat, touching a goat and stepping in manure or having manure on your shoes. Indirect contact that also led to illness included drying hands on clothes after washing them at the zoo.

People who washed their hands after visiting the petting zoo, including lathering with soap and washing them again before eating, did not get sick, the researchers report.

THE SECOND STUDY

In the second study, a team led by Amy E. Belflower, an epidemiologist at the South Carolina Department of Health and Environmental Control, watched 227 people in a petting zoo to see how many of them engaged in risky behaviors and how many washed their hands.

The petting zoos followed the guidelines for safe practices to avoid infection. "They had the animals in pens, had signs about not bringing food and drink in, and lots of signs about washing your hands, and had good handwashing stations," Belflower says.

"But even with all those precautions, we still saw people engaging in risky behavior," she adds. "The top three were bringing food into the area, bringing a stroller into the area and picking stuff like pet food off the ground. We also saw that 28% of the people who exited the petting area did not wash their hands."

THE THIRD STUDY

Researchers from the Tennessee Department of Health and the US Department of Agriculture (USDA) also looked at how people behave in petting zoos.

Among 991 visitors to six petting zoos in Tennessee, 49% touched their faces while in the petting zoo; 87% came into contact with environmental surfaces, such as handrails or benches; 22% ate or drank while in the area; and 62% did not wash their hands after leaving the petting zoo.

"There is a lot that can be done to educate zoo operators and the public," says lead author Marcy McMillian, an epidemiologist at the Tennessee Department of Health.

"People need to know that they have to do handwashing, and that when they touch environmental surfaces and the animals, they are potentially exposing themselves to pathogens," McMillian says.

ARE PETTING ZOOS WORTH IT?

Philip M. Tierno, Jr., director of Clinical Microbiology and Immunology at New York University Medical Center, questions the logic of petting zoos. "You have too many pathogens that can create problems in people. It's not worth it," he says. "The problem is that the public is not aware of the dynamic of infection. It's not just on your hands. So, even if you wash your hands, you are not assured that you [haven't] picked it up."

Dr. David L. Katz, an associate professor of public health and director of the Prevention Research Center at Yale University School of Medicine, thinks petting zoos are fine if visitors take the proper precautions. "Children shouldn't be denied the joy of petting zoos," he says. "After all, fraternizing with other people is also a potential source of bacterial contamination and potentially serious infection."

PRECAUTIONS

Tierno warns against eating while in the petting zoo. If you are eating, you may directly ingest E. coli, he says. "Even if you think that you have washed your hands correctly, you may not have."

To effectively eliminate pathogens, you must wash your hands for the amount of time that it takes to sing *Happy Birthday* twice, Tierno

advises. "You have to wash in between your fingers, the top of your hands and under the nail beds," he adds.

info The Centers for Disease Control and Prevention can tell you more about safety at petting zoos at *www.cdc.gov/healthypets/spot light_an_exhbts.htm.*

Child's Growth Pattern Predicts Heart Problems

David J.P. Barker, MD, PhD, professor of medicine, Heart Research Center, Oregon Health and Science University, Portland.
The New England Journal of Medicine.

Researchers say they've identified a pattern of growth in children that is strongly linked to an increased risk of cardiovascular trouble decades later.

A CLEAR PATTERN

A review of the medical histories of 357 men and 87 women who were born in Helsinki, Finland, between 1934 and 1944, and who developed coronary heart disease as adults by 2003 showed a clear pattern, explains Dr. David J.P. Barker, who led the study while at the University of Southampton in the United Kingdom.

"The people who developed coronary heart disease were born small and did not thrive in the first two years after birth for one reason or another," he says. "Then, after the first two years, they put on weight more rapidly, putting on fat rather than muscle between [ages] 2 and 13."

Children who exhibited this pattern were at nearly three times the risk of developing heart disease compared with those who had a more standard growth pattern. They were also likely to develop insulin resistance, a known risk factor for heart disease.

Children at the highest risk of developing heart disease weighed less than 3 kilograms (6.6 pounds) at birth, had body mass indices (BMIs) lower than 16 at age two and higher than 17.5 at age 11. (For reference, a 5-foot 2-inch child weighing 95 pounds has a BMI of 17.5.)

WHO IS AT RISK?

The new study differs from others that focused on links between childhood growth and adult heart disease risk. These studies have shown that low birth weight increases coronary risk later in life. Others have shown a link between youthful obesity and adult coronary disease. But this study suggests that youngsters who are not obese may still be at an increased risk.

"The group of children at risk is identified by their current stage [of growth] in comparison to where they were earlier," says Barker.

While the study singled out children of low birth weight, the finding "potentially applies to anyone," Barker says. "If they don't grow normally in the first two years after birth—for whatever reason—then put on fat rather than muscle, they end up with a body that is high in fat and low in muscle."

Such children "are vulnerable, but they are not doomed," he says. Their risk can be reduced by an emphasis on improving their diet and exercise patterns.

The study's finding indicates that the growth of children should be monitored "in relation to where they were, rather than in relation to all other children," Barker says.

info For suggestions on how to keep kids heart-healthy, visit *www.nhlbi.nih.gov/health/public/heart/obesity/wecan*, the Web site of the national program, Ways to Enhance Children's Activity & Nutrition (We Can!).

SUVs No Safer for Kids Than Cars

Dennis R. Durbin, MD, MSCE, emergency room physician and clinical epidemiologist, The Children's Hospital of Philadelphia.
Bella Dinh-Zarr, PhD, national director, Traffic Safety Policy, American Automobile Association.
Pediatrics.

Despite the public perception that sports utility vehicles (SUVs) are safer than passenger cars, a new report shows that when accidents happen, the bigger vehicles are no better at preventing injuries to children.

THE STUDY

In a review of car crashes involving nearly 4,000 children ranging in age from infancy to 15, study coauthor Dr. Dennis R. Durbin, an emergency room doctor at The Children's Hospital of Philadelphia, and his colleagues found that rollovers occurred twice as frequently in SUVs as in passenger cars, and that children involved in rollover crashes were three times more likely to be injured than children involved in crashes in which the vehicle did not roll over.

Many people assume the weight and size of an SUV make them safer, but the potential benefits are canceled by the increased likelihood of rolling over.

Dennis R. Durbin, MD, MSCE

Further, when rollover accidents occurred, the children who weren't appropriately restrained in SUVs had a 25 times greater risk of injury compared with children who were appropriately restrained. Nearly half of these unrestrained children were seriously injured, compared with only 3% of the children who were properly restrained.

PERCEPTION VS. REALITY

The study findings are important, Durbin says, because although passenger cars are still the vehicle of choice for most families—61.8% of the children in the study were in passenger cars compared with 38.2% who were in SUVs—SUVs are becoming increasingly popular. The number of SUV registrations rose by 250% between 1995 and 2002. Part of their popularity is due to the perception that they are safer, Durbin notes.

"Many people just assume that the extra weight and size of an SUV make them safer, but what we found was that the potential benefits were canceled by the SUVs' increased likelihood of rolling over," adds Durbin.

Bella Dinh-Zarr, national director of Traffic Safety Policy for the American Automobile Association (AAA), says this study contains new and interesting information. "We've all been curious whether the size and weight of SUVs overcame the rollover risk."

"Most previous research on SUV safety was focused on adults, and this [analysis] demonstrates the burden that rollovers have on children," Durbin says.

THE MESSAGE FOR PARENTS

"The message for parents is that SUVs are no safer, and that they should know the importance of ensuring that their children are properly restrained for their age on every trip in the car," Durbin adds.

Because SUVs are no safer than passenger cars, the focus of child safety in all vehicles should be on safe seating, Dinh-Zarr says.

"No matter what vehicle you transport your children in, keep them in the back seat and properly restrain them in age-appropriate seatbelts," she advises.

Durbin says motor vehicle crashes are a leading cause of death in children, and with 1.5 million children in car crashes every year, "it is a significant public health problem."

■ ■ ■ ■

Safe Seating Recommendations

Among the recommendations for safe seating in a vehicle are…

•**Children younger than one year old who weigh 20 pounds or less** should be in a backward-facing car seat in the back seat.

•**Older children should be in a forward-facing car seat in the back,** and can then graduate to a booster seat as they grow. (They can sit safely without a booster seat when they are tall enough to sit on the regular car seat with their back flush with the back of the seat and their knees bent naturally at the front of the seat.)

•**The seatbelt should cross children at the shoulder,** not the neck.

•**Children should ride in the back seat until they are 13,** as the back seat is much safer than the front seat.

Because of the problem of rollovers in SUVs, in 2005 Congress passed a transportation bill that requires the National Highway Traffic Safety Administration to establish standards to reduce vehicle rollover crashes for SUVs and other passenger cars.

info For help in choosing and installing the right car seat for your child, go to The Children's Hospital of Philadelphia Web site at *www.chop.edu.* Click on "Specialties and Services" under "Patient Care and Family Services." Partners for Child Passenger Safety can be found under "Programs and Services."

Preschoolers Missing Out On Hours of Sleep

Christine Acebo, PhD, sleep researcher and assistant director, Bradley Hospital Sleep and Chronobiology Research Laboratory, and assistant professor, Brown Medical School, Providence, RI.
Irwin Benuck, MD, pediatrician, Children's Memorial Hospital, and professor of clinical pediatrics, Northwestern University Medical School, both in Chicago.
Sleep.

While the sleep problems that often plague teens and adults are widely known, a new study has found that many young children may not be getting enough sleep either.

Approximately 12 to 15 hours of sleep is usually recommended for children ages one to five, according to Christine Acebo, an assistant professor at Brown University Medical School. But the children in her study fell short of that goal.

THE STUDY

Acebo's team visited the homes of 169 children between ages one and five to interview the mothers and put *actigraphs*, or activity monitors, on the children's ankles or wrists that helped the researchers evaluate when they slept. The mothers also logged their children's sleep habits in diaries.

During the week-long study, the researchers telephoned the mothers to ask about any problems or illnesses. A second home visit was done at the end of the week to collect the diaries and the actigraphs, which contained downloadable records of activity.

"When we looked at the full 24 hours [including naps], the older kids got less than 9.5 hours" of sleep, reports Acebo, who is also assistant director of the Bradley Hospital Sleep and Chronobiology Research Laboratory, in Providence,

Rhode Island. "The one-year-olds and the two-year-olds got 10.5 to 11" hours of sleep.

"It's less than usually recommended—12 to 15 hours is pretty standard," she says.

She calls the new research "one of the first studies in a long time to look at the amount of sleep kids this age are getting, using objectives measured in the home other than surveys. They're not getting as much sleep as we think they should."

IMPLICATIONS

Previous studies have shown that not enough sleep in older children, teenagers and adults may lead to physical and cognitive problems, including decreased physical performance, lower academic performance and other daytime problems. And several studies in adults have linked a lack of sleep to "neuroendocrine abnormalities" that may lead to overeating and obesity, according to the researchers.

"We are concerned that the problem of too little sleep extends even to the youngest members of families, though we do not know if this puts them at risk for problems down the line," Acebo says.

Acebo acknowledges that the sleep needs of young children haven't been studied adequately, and that the 12- to 15-hour recommendation is based on what experts think is the best amount to foster normal growth and development. "We don't really know how much sleep kids this age need. Those studies have not been done."

PARENTS SHOULDN'T BE ALARMED

Another expert, Dr. Irwin Benuck, a pediatrician at Children's Memorial Hospital and a professor of clinical pediatrics at Northwestern University Medical School, says the findings don't surprise him, but parents should not be alarmed. "I think we have a lot to learn about sleep in kids and how much sleep they need. I think it's a new area that is evolving right now," he says.

The key, he says, is for parents to pay attention to their child during waking hours to determine if he or she is getting enough sleep.

"The bottom line is how your kid is performing during the day," Benuck says. If you have a five-year-old and hook him up to a monitor and

he is sleeping 8.5 hours at night and has a great day, participates in kindergarten and all his activities and is not moody and sleepy, that child is probably doing fine, he says.

"If you have a kid who is moody during the day and not functioning to his ability, I think it's worth looking at what goes on at night," he adds. "If you have a child who has restless sleep and is snoring, take it up with your pediatrician."

In some cases, children have enlarged tonsils and when they are removed, the sleep quality improves, Benuck says.

info To learn more about children and sleep, visit the National Sleep Foundation at *www.sleepfoundation.org*. Click on "Children & Sleep."

■ ■ ■ ■

The Best Bedtime Snack

The right bedtime snack can help you sleep better. A recent study found that a tryptophan-rich snack at bedtime helped participants sleep better and be more alert the next morning. Foods that contain tryptophan include bananas, dairy, peanuts and almonds, tuna, chicken, eggs and soybeans.

Andrew L. Rubman, ND, medical director, Southbury Clinic for Traditional Medicines, Southbury, CT.

Scientists Create Artificial Penis

Ira Sharlip, MD, clinical professor of urology, University of California, San Francisco, and spokesman, American Urological Association.
American Urological Association annual meeting, Atlanta.

Success in rabbits suggests that an artificial penis made from a patient's own penile cells might someday help men who have impotence that is difficult to treat.

THE STUDY

In the study, Wake Forest University researchers first used standard biopsy techniques to harvest smooth-muscle and blood-vessel cells from the penises of healthy adult male rabbits. The researchers then added these cells to a nutrient-rich collagen matrix, which caused the cells to multiply and grow into new penile tissue.

Next, the team surgically removed all of the natural spongy tissue from the penises of the donor rabbits and grafted in the engineered tissue.

If we could regrow and replace worn-out tissue in other body parts, that would have tremendous implications.

Ira Sharlip, MD

The rabbits' penile growth and function were tracked over the next one, three and six months. The researchers found that the new penises were similar in structure to natural rabbit penises, and that they achieved and maintained erectile pressures equal to that found in normal rabbits.

The real test was to see if the rabbits that had received the new penises could impregnate female rabbits.

"Mating activity in the animals with the engineered [penis] resumed by one month after implantation," the researchers report. "The presence of sperm was confirmed in the female partners, and all females conceived and delivered healthy pups."

IMPLICATIONS

"This is very exciting. The researchers have been working on this for a long time in a variety of different organs. It's not yet clinically available, but if it works and proves safe and effective, it would be a tremendous advance," says Dr. Ira Sharlip, a spokesman for the American Urological Association and a clinical professor of urology at the University of California, San Francisco.

Sharlip cautions that this is a preliminary study involving animals. But he says, "Rabbit tissue is fairly similar to human tissue. If it can be done in rabbits, it probably can be done in humans."

Sharlip was not involved in the study, which was led by Dr. Anthony Atala, director of the Institute for Regenerative Medicine at Wake Forest University in Winston-Salem, North Carolina,

who is studying not just penile tissue, but tissue from other organs as well.

Success in tissue engineering has implications "not only for the treatment of erectile dysfunction but in the world of medicine in general. If we could regrow and replace worn-out tissue [in other body parts], that would have tremendous implications," Sharlip says.

PRACTICAL APPLICATION

Cialis, Levitra and Viagra have revolutionized the treatment of impotence for millions of men over the past decade.

However, some forms of erectile dysfunction, such as *corporal fibrosis*, remain very difficult to treat, and an artificial penis may be helpful in treating these disorders.

Corporal fibrosis occurs when the penis' spongy-tissue cells, which maintain an erection, don't get the oxygen they need to survive, usually because of a chronic reduction in blood flow. The spongy tissue is gradually replaced by inactive, fibrous scar tissue.

"It's relatively common in men with diabetes and various forms of vascular disease, or men who've previously had infections—usually infections of a penile prosthesis," Sharlip says.

However, even if men who have corporal fibrosis could get an artificial penis, doctors would still need to treat the underlying cause of the fibrosis itself.

"There's the question of how you restore that needed blood supply," Sharlip says. "You may be able to restore the natural spongy tissue of these erection chambers, but in a patient with severe corporal fibrosis you also have to get the blood supply to come back into the new, restored tissue." Without a steady source of oxygen, any implant might meet the same fate as the tissue it had replaced, he says.

Still, the advance does mark one of the few breakthroughs against the disorder in years, Sharlip says.

info For more information on erectile dysfunction, visit the Web site of the American Urological Association at *www.urology health.org/adult*. Click on "Sexual Function & Infertility."

Testosterone—
Is Yours Too Low?

Culley Carson, MD, Rhodes Distinguished Professor and chief of urology, University of North Carolina Medical Center, Chapel Hill, and editor in chief, *Contemporary Urology.*

I f you're a middle-aged or older man and are feeling irritable, depressed or fatigued…are having trouble concentrating…losing muscle mass and strength and/or putting on more body fat…losing bone density, as indicated by a bone-density test…or experiencing a decreased sex drive or difficulty achieving or maintaining an erection…then you might be one of the estimated 5 million men in the US with abnormally low testosterone levels, or *hypogonadism.*

It's estimated that only one out of 20 men who has low testosterone is currently being treated.

Good news: All it takes is a simple blood test to determine if you have low testosterone. If you do have low testosterone, the latest form of *testosterone replacement therapy* (TRT), in which the hormone is applied to the skin as a gel, is safe and effective and can begin to reverse all of the above symptoms almost immediately.

WHY IS TESTOSTERONE IMPORTANT?

Testosterone, the most powerful of a group of male hormones known as *androgens,* is largely responsible for men's growth of facial and pubic hair and deepening of the voice, as well as increased muscle and bone mass, sex drive and, to some extent, aggressiveness. Although testosterone is present in both sexes, women typically have only one-tenth the amount of testosterone that men do.

In men, a normal blood testosterone level is generally considered to be between 300 and 1,000 nanograms per deciliter (ng/dL). Testosterone levels tend to be highest in the early morning hours, and then go down somewhat as the day progresses.

As men get older, however, testosterone levels gradually decline. This occurs most acutely after age 65, but the decline can also be noticeable among men in their 50s and even 40s. Testosterone levels vary greatly from patient to patient,

and drops are relative to each patient's starting level—which is usually not known.

There can be many causes for decreasing levels, but the most common is testicular failure—the testicles "wear out" and fail to produce enough testosterone.

Low testosterone has long been associated with decreased sex drive, but researchers are now discovering that low testosterone levels can cause numerous other negative health effects (in addition to those already mentioned), including reduced fertility, loss of body hair, reduced muscle mass and strength, problems sleeping and an increased risk of depression.

In addition, men who have several chronic conditions are also much more likely to have low testosterone levels. These conditions include type 2 diabetes, cardiovascular disease, chronic renal failure, obesity, hypertension, insulin resistance (prediabetes) and HIV/AIDS. If you have any of these conditions, it's important to get treatment for the underlying medical problem and a blood testosterone test to see if you might benefit from TRT as well.

DIAGNOSIS AND TREATMENT

You can visit your doctor specifically to get a screening testosterone level blood test, or you can request to have it done as part of your annual checkup.

The accuracy of lab tests is far better than it used to be, and testing of free circulating testosterone (not the testosterone that is bound to protein in the body) is also now available. Your doctor may also do this test if your levels in the screening test indicate a problem. Among men who have low testosterone, what we typically see are levels in the 150 ng/dL range—approximately half of what is considered the minimum normal level. These men are prime candidates for TRT to bring blood levels into the normal range (higher than 300 ng/dL).

In addition to ordering a blood test, your primary-care doctor can also prescribe TRT treatments. If he/she is unfamiliar or uncomfortable using TRT, however, you should consider seeing a urologist or endocrinologist for treatment.

One reason doctors have been reluctant in the past to check the testosterone levels of male patients who are depressed, overweight or lacking in energy is that they had no good tools for treating low testosterone. One older treatment, injection therapy, requires frequent visits to the doctor for shots and produces uneven testosterone levels, which spike drastically after injection, and then decline steadily afterward. Testosterone pills carry a high risk of liver damage because of the strain put on the liver as it breaks down the testosterone. And the earliest testosterone treatment—patches, introduced in the early 1990s—were safer than pills but caused skin irritation in many patients.

On the other hand, the latest testosterone treatment—gels—have proven to be very safe and nonirritating. They are effective at raising testosterone levels back into the normal range.

Gels are more effective than patches, which are rarely used anymore, and have fewer side effects. An added benefit of these gels is that, when applied in the morning, they come close to mimicking the normal daily fluctuations in testosterone levels—high in the morning, lower at night.

There are currently two FDA-approved gels. AndroGel is scent-free, but takes up to two hours to dry completely. Testim has a slightly musky scent and dries a little more quickly on the skin.

The recommended method is to apply a 5-gram packet of gel (approximately the size of a fast-food ketchup packet) containing 50 milligrams (mg) of testosterone in the morning to the shoulders, upper arms and/or abdomen. After applying, wash hands carefully, cover the treated area with clothing and avoid bathing or swimming for six hours.

After applying either type of gel, avoid skin-to-skin contact of that area with your partner or any other family members until the gel has dried completely. Otherwise, they may experience elevated testosterone levels as well. (If your female partner experiences any unusual acne or body hair growth, she should see her doctor immediately.)

What to expect: The initial benefits of TRT tend to be seen quickly, particularly improvements in libido, mood and mental sharpness.

Example: One of my patients, a university professor, had been depressed and very forgetful, and was convinced that he had early Alzheimer's. After his blood test showed a testosterone level of 100 ng/dL, he was placed on TRT—and found that within a few weeks his mood and his mental abilities were fully restored.

Increases in muscle and bone mass occur more slowly and can be enhanced by strength training (for muscle and bone development), calcium/vitamin D supplements (for bone growth) and, if necessary, osteoporosis medication.

No long-term studies have been done on TRT—the longest was three years. But, in the three-year study, there was no indication of any risks or side effects.

Prostate alert: While TRT does not appear to increase the risk of prostate cancer or *benign prostatic hyperplasia* (BPH), testosterone supplements may spur the growth of existing prostate tumors. For this reason, TRT should never be taken by anyone who has been diagnosed with prostate cancer.

Men on TRT should be given both a *prostate-specific antigen* (PSA) test for prostate cancer and a *digital rectal exam* (DRE) twice a year. As testosterone levels move from low to normal, it's typical to experience a slight rise in PSA levels and a slight increase in prostate size, but these changes usually present no problem.

■ ■ ■ ■

Estrogen Affects Men, Too

Both men and women produce varying degrees of estrogen and testosterone. There's some evidence that men who are *low* in estrogen or related hormones may have an increased risk of osteoporosis and cardiovascular disease. *Elevated* estrogen may increase the risk of *benign prostatic hyperplasia* (prostate gland enlargement) as well as prostate cancer.

Important: Men who are at high risk for prostate disease—due to an elevated prostate-specific antigen (PSA) test or an abnormally sized or shaped prostate—or those experiencing low energy, a decrease in libido or other symptoms associated with a hormonal imbalance, should ask their doctors to include estrogen as part of a wide-spectrum hormonal screening test.

Andrew L. Rubman, ND, medical director, Southbury Clinic for Traditional Medicines, Southbury, CT.

Not All Hernias Need Surgery

Robert J. Fitzgibbons, Jr., MD, professor of surgery, Creighton University, Omaha.

Olga Jonasson, MD, professor of surgery, University of Illinois at Chicago.

David R. Flum, MD, MPH, associate professor of surgery, University of Washington, Seattle.

Robert Bell, MD, assistant professor of surgery, Yale University School of Medicine, New Haven, CT.

The Journal of the American Medical Association.

Men who have a hernia that does not cause pain or discomfort may not need surgery, a new study has found.

Hernias occur when a portion of an organ (the intestine, for example) protrudes through an abnormal opening in the muscle wall, often as the result of a muscle tear injury. Sometimes the organ can become *incarcerated*, or caught, in this opening, and *strangulated* if its blood supply is cut off.

THE STUDY

Researchers compared the pain, physical function and other outcomes in 720 men who had asymptomatic or minimally symptomatic *inguinal* hernias, which are the most common type and occur near the groin.

Some of the participants were randomly selected to have their hernia repaired, while others did not have surgery.

After two years, the research team measured pain levels for both groups of men and found a similar number of patients in each group had pain that was significant enough to interfere with daily activities.

IMPLICATIONS

The finding "changes the traditional teaching that's been taught for hundreds of years," says lead author Dr. Robert J. Fitzgibbons, Jr., a professor of surgery at Creighton University in Omaha. "Patients should understand that they don't have to have their hernias fixed, if they can live with it.

"In the past, doctors have told men that they have to fix hernias because of the danger of incarceration leading to gangrene," says Fitzgib-bons. "Those data were based on historical times when medical care wasn't immediately available," he adds.

"For men who have little or no symptoms from a hernia, it is safe to defer having an operation until they do have symptoms," says study coauthor Dr. Olga Jonasson, a professor of surgery at the University of Illinois at Chicago.

COMPLICATIONS FROM SURGERY

Jonasson notes that hernia surgery can cause complications. "The main complication is that after having a hernia repaired, many men will have chronic groin pain that will last for years," she says.

"There are men who have had hernias for 40 years, and it doesn't bother them and they don't bother it," Jonasson says.

Dr. David R. Flum, an associate professor of surgery at the University of Washington in Seattle, agrees that surgery is not always necessary. "There are tons of people who have hernias who don't even know they have them," he says.

> *There are men who have had hernias for 40 years, and it doesn't bother them and they don't bother it.*
>
> *Olga Jonasson, MD*

The major risk of not having hernia surgery is strangulation, and according to Flum, this risk is very small.

"If you operate on people preventively, before they have symptoms, they don't do any better or any worse than the group of people who decide they are going to watch and wait, and if it becomes symptomatic fix it," he says.

"I have been practicing this way for years," agrees Dr. Robert Bell, an assistant professor of surgery at Yale University School of Medicine. "I tell patients, 'If it doesn't bother you, you don't need to get it fixed. If it ever does bother you, you know where to find me. If it even bothers you psychologically, we will go ahead and fix it.' "

info For more information on hernias, visit the National Digestive Diseases Information Clearinghouse at *http://digestive.niddk.nih.gov/ddiseases/pubs/inguinalhernia.*

How to Avoid Unnecessary Surgery

Charles B. Inlander, health-care consultant and president, People's Medical Society, a nonprofit consumer health advocacy group, Allentown, PA. He is author of more than 20 books, including *Take This Book to the Hospital with You: A Consumer Guide to Surviving Your Hospital Stay.* St. Martin's.

F ew things are worse than having an unnecessary surgical procedure. Yet every year, millions of Americans have operations that they do not need. In fact, the Congressional Committee on Energy and Commerce reports that 20% of all surgeries performed in the US are unnecessary. *Surgeries you may not need...*

•**Prostate removal.** The most common treatment for prostate cancer is removal of the prostate gland, but clinical studies show that the operation is of little benefit to men who have a life expectancy of 10 years or less because the cancer grows very slowly. This means that most men older than 75 have nothing to gain and may have side effects after sugery, such as incontinence and infection. Regardless of a man's age, he should seek several medical opinions (including that of a urologist who does not perform surgery).

•**Cataract removal.** More than a decade ago, the Agency for Healthcare Policy and Research warned that many of the operations performed to remove a cataract were not necessary. The National Institutes for Health suggests that cataract removal is best performed if your vision has been reduced to at least 20/150—even with glasses. Yet each year, hundreds of thousands of Americans whose eyesight is far better than 20/150 have the surgery. In many cases, surgery will not improve sight and can cause infection. For a more impartial view, get a second opinion from an optometrist (a health-care provider licensed to provide a broad range of eye-care services), rather than a surgical ophthalmologist (a medical doctor who specializes in eye disease).

•**Gallbladder removal.** Since the late 1980s, the number of gallbladder surgeries has increased by 40%. The reason is the advent of minimally invasive *laparoscopic* surgery. This procedure can be done in an outpatient setting —conventional surgery typically requires three days in the hospital—is more convenient and more profitable for doctors. But it is often not necessary. Before agreeing to gallbladder removal, consult an experienced internist about nonsurgical options, such as a special diet or the gallstone-dissolving medication *ursodiol* (Actigall).

•**Wisdom tooth extraction.** This one is the granddaddy of all unnecessary surgeries—approximately half of all wisdom tooth extractions are unnecessary. For decades, major dental organizations and journals have criticized the removal of wisdom teeth that are symptom-free. To protect yourself, any time a dentist recommends having your wisdom teeth removed, get a second opinion from another dentist. If wisdom teeth are impacted, infected or are causing other teeth to shift, surgery may be necessary. But many times they will not cause any problems, and you can save yourself a lot of time, money and pain.

Hidden Dangers of Gastric Bypass Surgery

Edward Livingston, MD, Hudson-Penn Chair in Surgery, professor and chairman of gastrointestinal and endocrine surgery, University of Texas Southwestern School of Medicine, Dallas, and chairman of the bariatric surgery work group, Department of Veterans Affairs' national health care system.

David Zingmond, MD, PhD, assistant professor of medicine, Center for Surgical Outcomes and Quality, David Geffen School of Medicine, University of California at Los Angeles.

The Journal of the American Medical Association.

B ecause it is very difficult to lose weight through diet and exercise, it's not surprising that more people are turning to *bariatric*, or gastric bypass, surgery to treat their weight problems.

But several new studies point out the risks that are associated with this procedure.

STUDY FINDINGS

One study conducted by researchers at the University of Chicago and the University of California, Irvine, found that the number of bariatric surgeries being performed in the United States have increased dramatically, from 13,365 in 1998 to an estimated 102,794 in 2003.

Another study found that rehospitalization rates one year following the surgery were 19.3%. In contrast, in the year prior to the surgery, hospitalization rates were only 7.9%. The most common reasons for being admitted to the hospital prior to the surgery were obesity-related problems. After the surgery, the most common reasons for hospitalization were surgery-related problems, such as a hernia.

A University of Washington study found the death rate for Medicare recipients 30 days after gastric bypass surgery was 2%. After 90 days, that rate was 2.8% and after one year, the death rate for bariatric surgery patients receiving Medicare benefits was 4.6%. This study also found that when the surgery was performed by a surgeon who had not done many of these procedures the death rate was 1.6 times higher than when the procedure was done by a more experienced surgeon.

REACTION

"I was not surprised by these findings. These studies are really a very small piece of the overall picture for bariatric surgery," says Dr. Edward Livingston, chairman of gastrointestinal and endocrine surgery at the University of Texas Southwestern School of Medicine and chairman of the bariatric surgery work group for the Department of Veterans Affairs' national health care system.

"Bariatric surgeries result in weight loss, but they can [also] result in complications and death. They can improve the complications of obesity and the quality of life, and they may increase longevity," says Livingston. However, the decision about whether to have the surgery is a complicated one and needs to be made on a case-by-case basis, he adds

"These findings indicate more morbidity in the initial three years after surgery. People should be aware when they're making this decision that this is a possibility," says study author Dr. David Zingmond, an assistant professor of medicine at the David Geffen School of Medicine at the University of California at Los Angeles' Center for Surgical Outcomes and Quality.

■ ■ ■ ■

What Is Bariatric Surgery?

The most commonly performed inpatient bariatric surgery is called the Roux-en-Y gastric bypass. In this procedure, the stomach is made smaller and a part of the small intestine is bypassed so that fewer calories and nutrients are absorbed, according to the National Institute for Diabetes and Digestive and Kidney Diseases (NIDDK). Among the risks from this procedure are infection, hernia and long-term nutritional deficiencies.

Generally, people who are considered candidates for bariatric surgery have a body mass index (BMI) higher than 40, which means they are approximately 100 pounds overweight if they are male and 80 pounds overweight if they are female, according to the NIDDK. People who have lower BMIs may also be considered candidates for the surgery if they have obesity-related health problems, such as type 2 diabetes, severe sleep apnea or heart disease.

A majority of the procedures are done on women (84%) and those who have private insurance (83%), according to the study.

info To learn more about surgery for obesity, visit the National Institute of Diabetes and Digestive and Kidney Diseases's Weight-control Information Network at *http://win.niddk. nih.gov/publications/gastric.htm.*

■ ■ ■ ■

Families that Stay Together...

Hospitals are letting patients' families stay during emergencies and some procedures. A growing body of evidence indicates that patients and family members benefit by staying close to one another during stressful situations.
The Wall Street Journal.

Chewing Gum Speeds Surgery Recovery

The Western Pennsylvania Hospital news release.

Patients who chew gum have shorter hospital stays after laparoscopic colon surgery than those who don't chew gum, according to a recent study.

In laparoscopic surgery, surgeons use video-equipped tools inserted through a tiny incision to operate in a specific area.

"We know that patients who undergo laparoscopic surgery have a faster recovery and less pain than with traditional techniques. We wanted to see if we could do even better. People today want to get home as soon as possible, back to their lives and families," says Dr. James McCormick, a laparoscopic surgeon at The Western Pennsylvania Hospital in Pittsburgh and a lead investigator in this study. "Something as simple as chewing gum can help make that a reality," he says.

THE STUDY

In the study, 102 patients undergoing elective colon resection surgery were divided into two groups. Those in the control group received the standard fare after abdominal surgery—sips of clear liquid. Patients in the other group were given gum to chew at mealtimes in addition to the clear liquid.

The sooner the body thinks it is normal, the sooner it will act normally.

James McCormick, MD

On average, patients who chewed gum went home one day sooner than those who didn't chew gum, the researchers report.

The study authors say chewing gum after surgery can prevent or reduce postoperative *ileus*, a condition in which the digestive system becomes inactive for a period of time. Ileus is a major cause of postoperative problems and prolonged hospital stays, and costs up to $1 billion a year in the United States, the researchers say.

SHAM FEEDING

"There are a few scientific theories which attempt to explain why this approach works. Most prevalent is the concept of 'sham feeding,' " McCormick says.

"It is normal to sit down at meal time and chew and swallow for 15 minutes," he explains. "Gum chewing simulates that activity nicely. The sooner the body thinks it is normal, the sooner it will act normally. And the sooner you get to go home."

info The Nemours Foundation has a helpful article, "What's It Like to Have Surgery?" at *http://kidshealth.org/teen/question.*

■ ■ ■ ■

Better Homecomings

Going home after a hospital stay can be unnerving. It's a good idea to coordinate as much as possible before your return.

Here are some pointers from the Naval Hospital in Camp Pendleton, California…

●**Make sure that you have written instructions** regarding your discharge and at-home medical routine.

●**Take all prescribed medications** at the assigned time.

●**Ensure your home environment is conducive to your recovery.**

●**Avoid using steps** unless you are instructed otherwise.

●**Choose a bedroom that's close to a bathroom** if you are staying in bed.

●**Keep a phone and phone numbers handy** for emergencies and medical questions.

Oxygen Reduces Risk of Infection

Jimmy Windsor, MD, anesthesiologist and critical-care physician, Ochsner Clinic Foundation, New Orleans.

Daniel I. Sessler, MD, chairman, department of outcomes research, The Cleveland Clinic Foundation, and L&S Weakley Professor of Anesthesiology, University of Louisville, KY.
The Journal of the American Medical Association.

Giving higher concentrations of supplemental oxygen during elective colorectal surgery reduces the risk of surgical site infections, according to a new study. And the practice comes with very little down side, if any, the authors of the study report.

THE STUDY

For the new study, researchers in Spain randomly selected 300 patients ages 18 to 80 who were undergoing elective colorectal surgery in

14 Spanish hospitals. Each patient received either 80% oxygen or 30% oxygen during the procedure and for six hours after.

Almost one-quarter (24.4%) of the patients receiving 30% oxygen developed surgical site infections, compared with only 14.9% of those receiving the purer mix. The 80% mixture resulted in an absolute risk reduction of 6%, according to the study authors.

Supplemental oxygen costs only a few cents per patient and is essentially risk-free.

Daniel I. Sessler, MD

Oxygen kills bacteria by activating the immune system's *neutrophils*, white blood cells that are among the first to arrive at an infection site.

EARLIER STUDIES

The role of supplemental oxygen in preventing these infections has been the subject of debate. One study, conducted in 2000, showed that providing 80% oxygen throughout the surgery and for two hours afterward cut infection risk by half, compared with patients who got 30% oxygen. A less rigorous study, however, conducted in 2004, found that supplemental oxygen doubled the risk of infection.

"This helps to settle [the debate]," says Dr. Jimmy Windsor, an anesthesiologist and critical-care physician at the Ochsner Clinic Foundation in New Orleans. Although Windsor was not involved in the study, he had already been using supplemental oxygen. "These low-risk interventions are probably very, very effective but are not being practiced," he says. "People aren't doing the simple things they could be doing. We need to pay attention to the small details."

LITTLE RISK

"Wound infections are among the most common serious complications of surgery. Supplemental oxygen costs only a few cents per patient and is essentially risk-free. Providing extra oxygen halves the risk of infection and should be used in most patients," says study coauthor Dr. Daniel I. Sessler, chairman of the department of outcomes research at The Cleveland Clinic Foundation. "Now that two large studies, with a total of 800 patients, clearly indicate that supplemental

oxygen is beneficial, we expect that it will become common practice. Consequently, fewer patients will suffer wound infections."

Windsor agrees that there is little risk to the practice. However, if a patient has damaged lungs, he suggests using the lowest possible amount of oxygen. Even then, the oxygen would have to be given for many hours—or even days—to pose any real danger.

Sessler concurs. "The major potential risk of supplemental oxygen is collapse of lung spaces or *atelectasis*," he says. "However, we have shown in a previous study, [which has been] confirmed by others, that 80% oxygen does not cause any pulmonary problems whatsoever. Basically, the drug is inexpensive, risk-free and highly effective."

Wound infections prolong hospitalization by an average of one week and double the risk of death, the researchers say. To prevent such infections doctors recommend antibiotics given at appropriate times, clipping rather than shaving hair and maintaining normal body temperature during the operation.

info The Institute for Healthcare Improvement has more information on surgical site infections at *www.ihi.org*. Click on "Patient Safety" under "Topics," and look for "Surgical Site Infections."

▪ ▪ ▪ ▪

Wise Words on Wound Care

When cuts or other wounds happen, taking some simple steps can help speed the body's natural healing process. *Experts writing in the Mayo Clinic Women's HealthSource offer the following suggestions...*

•**Cover, press, clean.** Cover the wound with a sterile dressing and apply pressure to stop the bleeding. Use tap/bottled water or sterile saline to wash the wound. Seek medical help if you think you need stitches, you can't clean the wound or if the injury was caused by an animal or human bite. You should also seek medical attention if it has been 10 years or longer since your last tetanus shot.

•**Medicate.** Apply a topical antibiotic ointment to the wound. Cover with a heavy lubricant such as Vaseline or Aquaphor to create a barrier to keep the wound moist. Don't use betadine, alcohol or hydrogen peroxide because they all interfere with healing.

●**Keep the area moist.** Experts have turned their back on older advice to keep wounds dry and exposed to the open air. Instead, they now recommend covering the wound with a sterile dressing to create a warm, moist environment, which is best for wound healing. This kind of environment decreases pain, infection and the likelihood of re-injury.

●**Dress the wound.** The best kind of dressing is one that keeps the wound moist and the surrounding tissue dry. Use a nonstick dressing and gently change it every day or two. Try to keep the wet scab intact. Wounds should normally stay covered for approximately five days or until the surface layers have healed. Don't use plain gauze to cover the wound. It can stick to the scab and cause reinjury when it's removed.

●**Don't scratch.** Scratching the wound that is healing can reopen it. Remember, itching is a normal (albeit, frustrating) part of the healing process.

●**Eat right, don't smoke.** Healthy lifestyles promote wound healing.

●**Watch it.** If the wound shows signs of infection (redness, increased pain or swelling, yellow or green discharge), seek medical attention.

info The American Academy of Family Physicians has more information on caring for wounds at *http://familydoctor.org/041.xml*.

Mayo Clinic news release.

■ ■ ■ ■

The Healing Power of Honey

The combination of the sugar and antibacterial components in honey kills germs when applied topically. Honey's thickness also creates a protective barrier over the wounded area, and its antioxidants stop damaging inflammation. Raw honey has better antibacterial properties than processed honey.

Peter Molan, PhD, director, honey research unit, University of Waikato, New Zealand.

Drug Clears Psoriasis in Up to 80% of Patients

Joel M. Gelfand, MD, assistant professor of dermatology, associate scholar, Center for Clinical Epidemiology and Biostatistics, and medical director, clinical studies unit, department of dermatology, University of Pennsylvania, Philadelphia.

Until recently, there were few effective treatment options for the 1.5 million people who have moderate to severe *psoriasis*, the skin condition characterized by red, scaly patches.

Now: Drugs known as *biologics*, made from the proteins of living cells, inhibit the immune cells that trigger psoriasis flare-ups.

Result: Reduced skin-cell buildups and inflammation in patients who have extensive psoriasis—and fewer side effects compared with older treatments.

Here's what you should know...

CAUSES

Psoriasis results from genetic abnormalities in the immune system. The disease occurs when killer immune cells, called *T cells*, target healthy skin cells rather than foreign pathogens. The attacks trigger the release of *cytokines*, proteins that cause the rapid proliferation of skin cells. Because sunlight has a protective effect against flare-ups, psoriasis symptoms often worsen during late fall and early winter.

TOPICAL TREATMENTS

Prescription topical creams and ointments are used when psoriasis affects less than 10% of the skin surface. *They also can be applied to control mild flare-ups...*

●**Steroids** are the most effective topical drugs. They're applied twice daily. When used long-term, strong steroids can thin the skin and cause stretch marks.

●**Topical retinoids,** such as *tazarotene* (Tazorac), usually are used in combination with steroids, allowing for a lower steroid dose to be effective and reducing the risk of side effects. Retinoids can be irritating to the skin.

Warning: Topical or oral retinoids are not recommended for women who are pregnant or planning to become pregnant because they can cause serious birth defects.

•**Vitamin D analogues,** such as *calcipotriene* (Dovonex), are synthetic forms of vitamin D. These creams, typically used along with a steroid, reduce skin inflammation and inhibit cell proliferation.

PHOTOTHERAPY

Ultraviolet light (UV) from the sun or artificial sources can slow cell proliferation and reduce inflammation. Light therapy is a good choice for psoriasis that doesn't respond to—or is too extensive for—topical treatment.

•**Narrow-band ultraviolet B (UVB) phototherapy** delivers light wavelengths that treat psoriasis while minimizing the rays that cause burning. Patients usually get three treatments per week. Skin clearing takes at least four to eight weeks.

Narrow-band light therapy can result in total skin clearing in some cases, but skin lesions typically return approximately four to 12 weeks after the treatments are discontinued.

•**Psoralen UVA (PUVA) therapy** uses ultraviolet A light and a medication (*psoralen*) that makes the skin more sensitive to light. PUVA is effective against severe psoriasis, but it's usually a last resort. Patients given PUVA long-term are seven to 10 times more likely to develop squamous-cell carcinoma (cancer of the upper layers of the skin).

•**Combination light therapy.** This particular approach combines UVB light with an oral retinoid, such as *acitretin* (Soriatane). It's effective in 70% to 80% of cases.

SYSTEMIC DRUGS

Patients who do not respond to topical treatments or phototherapy—or whose psoriasis is severe—may need oral drugs such as *methotrexate* (Trexall), *cyclosporine* (Neoral) or acitretin, which suppress the immune system and inhibit rapid cell division. These medications are cheaper than some of the newer psoriasis medications.

Drawback: They have a high risk of serious side effects, including organ damage. However, the damage can be managed if your physician closely monitors you.

Methotrexate can cause liver damage and a reduced white blood cell count. A patient taking methotrexate should have his/her liver biopsied every one to two years to check for liver damage. Cyclosporine can cause high blood pressure, infections and decreased kidney function. Because of the potential for kidney damage, cyclosporine is typically used for only one year. Acitretin, the only oral retinoid approved by the US Food and Drug Administration (FDA) to treat psoriasis, can thin the hair, cause dry skin and lips, cause bone abnormalities and affect liver function. Because of the risk of birth defects, women of childbearing years should not take it.

BIOLOGICS

These drugs are a new option for moderate to severe psoriasis.

•**TNF inhibitors.** Drugs such as *etanercept* (Enbrel) block the action of *tumor necrosis factor* (TNF), an immune system chemical that triggers rapid cell division. *Adalimumab* (Humira) and *infliximab* (Remicade) are approved by the FDA to treat rheumatoid arthritis but are often prescribed "off-label" to treat psoriasis. Approximately 50% to 80% of patients taking TNF inhibitors experience almost total clearing of their skin.

Drawbacks: TNF inhibitors are given only by injection. Side effects are rare but may include an increased risk of infection, lymphoma, neurological problems and exacerbation of heart failure.

•**T-cell inhibitors.** *Alefacept* (Amevive) slows skin cell division by blocking the effects of the T cells. Approximately 20% of patients experience almost total skin clearing.

Drawbacks: Alefacept is given by intramuscular injection in the doctor's office. Side effects are rare but may include liver function abnormalities.

•**Efalizumab** (Raptiva) is the newest biologic. It prevents T cells from triggering scaling and/or inflammation. It's injected *subcutaneously* (just under the skin) by patients. Approximately 30% experience almost total clearing of the skin.

Drawbacks: Side effects include flu-like symptoms and low blood platelet counts. Also, psoriasis may worsen when efalizumab is stopped. Patients taking alefacept or efalizumab require regular blood tests to determine if T-cell levels have dropped, which can lead to increased risk of infection.

info For more information, you can contact the National Psoriasis Foundation, 800-723-9166, *www.psoriasis.org*.

■ ■ ■ ■

What Is Psoriasis?

This chronic skin disease causes red, scaly patches on the trunk, knees, elbows, palms and/or scalp. It is due to an abnormality in the skin cell growth cycle—a process that includes the division of cells and their migration to the skin surface, where they slowly die and flake off.

Rosacea: Millions Have This Skin Disease and Don't Know It

James Del Rosso, DO, clinical assistant professor of dermatology, University of Nevada School of Medicine, and spokesman, National Rosacea Society. *www.rosacea.org.*

Rosacea, a chronic skin condition, affects at least 15 million Americans. Its primary symptom is facial redness, often accompanied by red bumps and visibly dilated blood vessels on the face. It leads to both physical discomfort and social embarrassment.

For the more than 40% of rosacea patients who develop the ailment in their 30s and 40s, this is a chronic disease, so they will have to deal with it for years. Some of the afflicted first seek treatment after age 50.

Reason for the delay: Research has found that 78% of Americans are not aware of the symptoms of rosacea, and therefore, many people tend to ignore the problem until symptoms become advanced.

The biggest news in the rosacea field is that we are learning more about the biochemical substances and microorganisms that are associated with rosacea symptoms—which will hopefully lead to more effective medical treatments.

While various factors are known to trigger rosacea flare-ups, the condition's underlying cause is still unknown. Though it can occur in all ethnic groups, it is most prevalent among fair-skinned people of Celtic or Scandinavian origin.

Rosacea cannot be cured, and the symptoms may grow worse if not treated.

Good news: In most cases, rosacea symptoms can be effectively controlled through a combination of lifestyle changes and medical treatment.

WHAT ARE THE SIGNS?

There is no lab test for rosacea. Instead, diagnosis is based on a visual inspection by a dermatologist who is familiar with the spectrum of symptoms. Early signs of rosacea include a flushing or redness in the cheeks, chin, nose and/or forehead that comes and goes.

Over time, this redness persists for increasingly longer periods until, eventually, it is always present. Fine, dilated blood vessels may also appear in the face, and red bumps and pus bumps ("pimples") can develop as well.

Sometimes patients may also experience a burning, stinging or itching sensation in the affected areas. In severe cases, the skin may become thick and swollen, especially around the nose. Actor W.C. Fields had a classic case of this type of advanced rosacea called *rhinophyma.* Rosacea also may cause watery, bloodshot or irritated eyes, a condition known as *ocular rosacea.* Someone who has ocular rosacea may feel as though there is a foreign body or something gritty in his/her eyes. He may also have feelings of burning, stinging, itching or dryness similar to eye allergies.

ENVIRONMENTAL TRIGGERS

Once rosacea has been diagnosed, the next step is to begin identifying any environmental factors that may be triggering outbreaks. Your doctor might ask you to keep a diary recording foods consumed and other daily details, such as your exposure to light, heat and wind…stressful events or situations…and what skin-care products you used. *While different individuals will have different environmental triggers, common ones include…*

●**Ultraviolet (UV) light.** Cumulative exposure to sunlight creates changes in the skin—such as the production of a substance called *vascular endothelial growth factor* (VEGF), which dilates blood vessels—and damages the structural integrity of the skin, predisposing it to redness and dilated blood vessels.

To protect against ultraviolet damage:
Always apply sunscreen (SPF 15 or higher) to your face when you are out in the sun, and wear a wide-brimmed hat that shades your face before going out for extended periods (when playing golf or tennis or when you are at the beach, for example).

●**Heat.** Flare-ups of rosacea are often triggered by exposure to heat, including drinking hot beverages.

Prevention: Limit the amount of time you spend outdoors in hot weather, avoid steam-rooms and saunas, and keep your showers as short as possible. Also, drink coffee and other heated beverages warm, not hot.

●**Skin-care products.** Because many people who have rosacea have sensitive skin, rosacea flare-ups are often triggered by excessively harsh soaps and other skin-care products.

Prevention: Use only facial cleansers formulated for sensitive skin, such as Cetaphil liquid cleanser...Dove Sensitive Skin Bar...or the gentle-care products of Neutrogena, Purpose, Aveeno and Oil of Olay. You can also ask your dermatologist for recommendations. Wash your face gently in the morning and evening using lukewarm water and blot your face dry with a soft cotton towel to avoid irritation.

Also use a moisturizer designed for sensitive skin, such as one offered by the brands listed above. Make sure it contains no fragrances or the potentially irritating ingredients *alpha-hydroxy acid, retinol* or *salicylic acid.*

Other potential triggers include spicy foods, stress, wind and humidity.

Rosacea is not a sign of heavy alcohol use. However, because consuming alcohol causes blood vessels to dilate, it may temporarily intensify existing symptoms.

Certain medications can also cause rosacea-like symptoms. Vasodilators and topical steroids have been known to cause rosacea outbreaks.

ROSACEA MEDICATIONS

While patients often experience significantly less redness once they switch from soap to a mild cleanser and make the other changes suggested above, many will also need to use medication to bring their symptoms fully under control.

A variety of topical rosacea medications can help reduce bumps and pimples and, to some extent, redness. These include *metronidazole* 0.75% gel (including MetroGel as well as other brands)...*azelaic acid* 15% gel (Finacea)...and *sulfacetamide-sulfur* (including Rosac, which also contains SPF 18 sunscreen, and other brands). Sulfur-based prescription cleansers such as Plexion and Rosanil can also be helpful. Metronidazole gel is an antibiotic—but it is prescribed here for its anti-inflammatory properties rather than its antibiotic effects.

Your dermatologist will choose the medication to try based on his evaluation of you. A combination of two different topical medications may also be prescribed. Their effectiveness varies from person to person—some patients will see dramatic results, and others only a slight reduction in symptoms. It's important to apply medication consistently as directed, and recognize that it may take two to three months to see substantial improvement.

To eliminate bumps and pimples, rosacea patients may also be put on oral antibiotics, such as *tetracycline, doxycycline* or *minocycline.* Doxycycline in very low doses (20 milligrams [mg] of Periostat twice daily) is actually *subantimicrobial*, meaning that there is no antibiotic effect, but inflammation is still reduced, and therefore, signs and symptoms improve.

Reason: Rosacea's bumps and pimples are due to inflammation, possibly caused by microscopic skin mites that live in everyone's facial skin but that are found in greater numbers in the skin of rosacea patients. Typically, oral medication is used together with topical medication for three to six months. The oral medication is then tapered off, while topical medication is continued as part of a long-term maintenance regimen.

Whatever approach is used, the types and dosages of the medications may need some adjustment at first. For this reason, it's important to alert your doctor if you experience any new skin irritation or other problems after starting treatment.

LASER AND LIGHT TREATMENTS

Despite medication and changes in lifestyle, some patients may still have persistent facial redness and dilated blood vessels. In these cases, laser treatments and light treatments, such as *intense pulsed light* (IPL), can help eliminate the enlarged blood vessels and redness.

Caution: These treatments should be performed by a highly skilled dermatologist. If not done properly, they can lead to complications. Since these treatments typically are not covered by insurance, it is also a good idea to establish the cost of the treatments in advance.

Restless Legs Syndrome Can Be Cured 70% Of the Time

Clete Kushida, MD, PhD, neurologist; director, Center for Human Sleep Research, Stanford University, Palo Alto, CA (*www.med.stanford.edu/school/psychiatry/human sleep*); associate professor, department of psychiatry and behavioral sciences, Stanford University Medical Center; and member, medical advisory board, Restless Legs Syndrome Foundation. *www.rls.org.*

An estimated one in 10 adults experiences some degree of *restless legs syndrome* (RLS), but fewer than 10% of patients who tell their physicians about their symptoms are diagnosed with RLS.

RLS symptoms are vague and hard to describe —patients use words like "tingling," "crawling" and "creeping" to explain uncomfortable sensations and/or pain in the legs and, in some cases, arms. Sensations mainly occur (or worsen) at night. A neurologist or sleep specialist can diagnose and treat RLS.

Latest development: The US Food and Drug Administration (FDA) recently approved *ropinirole* (Requip), the first drug specifically to treat RLS. It can eliminate or greatly reduce symptoms in 70% of patients—without the relapses that often occur when using other drugs.

CAUSES

RLS is believed to be caused by low levels or the impaired transmission of *dopamine*, a neurotransmitter that controls muscle movement. The majority of RLS patients have the *idiopathic*

form, which has no known cause. *Less commonly, RLS is a secondary disorder caused by...*

• **Iron deficiency.** Low levels of iron may inhibit dopamine production. If you are diagnosed with RLS, have your iron levels checked.

Recommended: If your iron (*serum ferritin*) level is below 50 micrograms per liter (mcg/L), ask your doctor about taking 325 milligrams (mg) of iron and 200 mg of vitamin C (to enhance iron absorption) daily. It may take months for iron supplementation to improve this type of RLS. Treatment should be monitored by a doctor to prevent iron overload.

• **Peripheral neuropathy.** This nerve damage, which often triggers pain in the legs and/ or arms, is caused by chronic diseases, such as diabetes (which constricts the blood vessels that supply the nerves) or alcoholism (because of its toxic effects on the nerves and often an accompanying vitamin deficiency due to poor dietary habits).

Recommended: If you have a history of diabetes, alcoholism or another condition that can cause nerve damage and you have RLS, ask your doctor about getting an *electromyogram* (EMG). This test assesses the electrical activity in the muscles. It is usually combined with a *nerve conduction velocity test*, in which a nerve is stimulated by a mild electrical impulse and the speed at which the nerve carries the impulse is recorded. Together, these tests can determine whether RLS may be due to nerve damage. Peripheral neuropathy may be reversed by treating the underlying disorder. Antidepressants, analgesics and antiseizure drugs help reduce RLS symptoms linked to neuropathy.

• **Pregnancy.** This is a common cause of RLS. The exact mechanism is unknown, but iron-deficiency anemia, hormonal changes and poor circulation may be culprits.

Recommended: Ferritin levels should be checked to rule out iron-deficiency anemia. No drugs to treat RLS are considered by the FDA to be completely safe during pregnancy...and symptoms usually disappear within one month of delivery.

TREATING PRIMARY RLS

Until recently, the main treatment for unexplained RLS was the Parkinson's drug *levodopa*

(Larodopa). It is effective initially, but approximately 80% of patients experience *augmentation*, or a worsening of symptoms, within a few months of starting the medication.

When it helps: Levodopa is a short-acting drug that's good for patients who experience RLS episodically—on planes, for example, or a few times a week at home. Because of the high risk for augmentation, levodopa is usually taken only intermittenly as needed.

New approach: Studies show that ropinirole, approved by the FDA in May 2005, can significantly improve symptoms.

Ropinirole is a *dopamine agonist*, a class of drugs that stimulate the brain's dopamine receptors and make dopamine work more efficiently. Dopamine agonists are currently the best treatment for RLS. Others include *pramipexole* (Mirapex) and *pergolide* (Permax).

Dopamine agonists typically relieve symptoms in less than one month and are effective for more than two-thirds of RLS patients. Unlike levodopa, dopamine agonists are not associated with augmentation and appear to remain effective for as long as they're taken. They are typically well-tolerated, but side effects may include nausea, dizziness, sleepiness, fainting and low blood pressure.

Some patients don't respond to ropinirole or other dopamine agonists, or their symptoms are not severe enough to justify taking these drugs for life. *Other choices…*

●**Opioids,** such as *codeine* and *hydrocodone*, relieve RLS in most patients. Because opioids can be addictive, they are recommended only for patients who need occasional relief or when symptoms aren't relieved by other treatments. Side effects include drowsiness, stomach upset and constipation.

●**Anticonvulsants,** such as *gabapentin* (Neurontin), *phenytoin* (Dilantin) and *carbamazepine* (Tegretol), inhibit abnormal increases in brain activity and reduce involuntary muscle sensations. Side effects include drowsiness, headache, blurred vision, tremor and anxiety.

●**Sedatives,** such as *clonazepam* (Klonopin), help patients fall asleep and make RLS symptoms less noticeable. However, it is unclear whether they directly improve RLS. Because of

side effects (drowsiness and the risk of addiction), these drugs are usually used for patients who need occasional relief or who don't respond to other treatments.

FDA Advisers Reject Safety Report on Dental Fillings

Ron R. Zentz, DDS, senior director, Council on Scientific Affairs, American Dental Association.
Michael Bender, director, Mercury Policy Project, Montpelier, VT.
ADA statement.
International Academy of Oral Medicine and Toxicology news release.
Associated Press.

I n the first public hearings on the subject in more than a decade, federal health advisers have rejected a government report suggesting that mercury-containing amalgam dental fillings are safe.

However, this decision by the US Food and Drug Administration (FDA) advisory panel is not a declaration that the widely used fillings are *unsafe*. Instead, in a 13 to 7 vote, the panel said that a large federal review of data fails to clearly and objectively present the current body of knowledge on the subject and that further study is needed.

The FDA is not compelled to act on the advice of its advisory committees, although it frequently does.

BACKGROUND

Dental amalgam contains elemental mercury combined with other metals such as silver, copper, tin and zinc. The fillings, which are approximately 50% mercury, have been used for generations to stabilize decaying teeth. Dental experts contend that when mercury is bound to the other metals it is encapsulated and does not pose a health risk.

Consumer groups, however, contend that mercury, a known neurotoxin, leaks out from the amalgam in the form of mercury vapor and then gets into the bloodstream.

According to the American Dental Association (ADA), the use of amalgam is declining. In 1990, dental amalgams comprised 67.6% of all dental restorations, by 1999 45.3% used amalgams, and in 2003, an estimated 30% of dental restorations used amalgam. Cavities that previously would have been treated using dental amalgam are now usually filled with a resin composite.

Several countries, including Canada, Norway, Sweden, Britain, Germany and Denmark, currently advise dentists against using mercury fillings for pregnant women. However, the ADA contends that this recommendation was made despite the lack of scientific evidence of systemic health problems or toxic effects and maintains its position that dental amalgam should remain an option for patients.

ADA POSITION

"Our position is one of looking at the scientific evidence and believing it's safe and effective and that dentists and patients should have the option," says Dr. Ron R. Zentz, senior director of the ADA Council on Scientific Affairs.

Zentz points to two studies (the Children's Amalgam Trials), in particular, that compared the use of amalgam with composite dental fillings in children. The studies found no differences in IQ, memory, attention, kidney function or other measures between the children who had amalgam fillings and the children who had composite fillings.

Officials at the FDA also asked committee members to carefully review findings from an internal agency meta-analysis of 34 recent studies that found "no significant new information" that might change the FDA's conclusion that amalgam fillings are safe.

Michael Aschner, a professor of pediatrics and pharmacology at Vanderbilt University, notes, "Just by looking at this paper, we are in a sense really limiting ourselves. I am not convinced we are doing justice to the topic at hand."

REACTION

A consortium of organizations including Consumers for Dental Choice, the Mercury Policy Project and the International Academy of Oral Medicine and Toxicology filed a petition to the FDA to immediately ban mercury fillings for pregnant women so as to protect their unborn children. The FDA has six months to respond to the petition.

"We're doing this primarily as a precautionary measure to protect unborn children from unnecessary exposure to mercury," says Michael Bender, director of the Mercury Policy Project, located in Montpelier, Vermont. "We're very concerned that our government is not doing what it should to protect the unborn.

"Why isn't the FDA joining Health Canada and the other countries in banning the placement [of mercury fillings] in expectant mothers?" he asks. "FDA silence over mercury is the same kind of silence our government once had for tobacco."

Still, any ban could have consequences. A study by dentist Howard Bailit and colleagues at the University of Connecticut found that a ban on amalgam fillings would raise costs, cut down on the number of cavities filled and hurt the oral health of most Americans.

info To learn more about amalgam fillings, visit the Web site of International Health News at *www.yourhealthbase.com/amalgams.html.*

9

Heart Disease

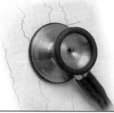

More than 40% of Heart Attacks Go Undiagnosed

More than four in 10 heart attacks go undiagnosed at the time they occur, a new European study reports. And these so-called "silent heart attacks" occur more often in women than in men.

THE STUDY

For the study, researchers analyzed more than 4,000 men and women older than 55 who were participating in the Rotterdam Study. A baseline *electrocardiographic screening* (ECG) and medical examination showed no evidence that any of the participants had had a heart attack. The subjects then underwent at least one follow-up examination several years later.

In total, 43% of the heart attacks went unrecognized by the patients themselves and by doctors, including one-third in men and more than one-half in women, the researchers found.

The results for women are particularly troubling. "Clearly heart attacks are being missed in women, and these are women who were in the health-care system," says Dr. Nieca Goldberg, former chief of women's cardiac care at Lenox Hill Hospital in New York City, and author of *The Women's Healthy Heart Program.*

Previous studies that have been conducted have indicated that up to 44% of ischemic heart attacks are clinically unrecognized, but the data have been limited and contradictory.

Although the study was conducted in the Netherlands, the researchers believe the results would apply to any other developed country.

IMPLICATIONS

"There is quite a proportion of myocardial infarctions [heart attacks] that is clinically unrecognized by the patient him- or herself, and

Nieca Goldberg, MD, former chief, women's cardiac care, Lenox Hill Hospital, New York City, spokeswoman, American Heart Association, and author of *The Women's Healthy Heart Program.* Ballantine.

Eric Boersma, PhD, associate professor of clinical cardiovascular epidemiology, Erasmus Medical Centre, Rotterdam, the Netherlands.
European Heart Journal.

also by the medical system," says study coauthor Eric Boersma, an associate professor of clinical cardiovascular epidemiology at Erasmus Medical Centre in Rotterdam, the Netherlands.

Atypical symptoms, different symptoms in women and men, as well as in the elderly and diabetics, may explain why heart attacks often go unnoticed. However, it's important to identify people who have had silent heart attacks because they are at a higher risk of experiencing additional cardiovascular complications.

We know from other research that unattended myocardial infarctions do have prognostic implications in the sense of lower life expectancy.

Eric Boersma, PhD

"We know from other research that unattended myocardial infarctions do have prognostic implications in the sense of lower life expectancy," Boersma says.

The study authors suggest that periodic, repeat ECGs be performed to find out if there is any evidence of silent heart attacks that had previously gone unnoticed, and patients could then be treated accordingly, with aspirin, beta-blockers, statins and lifestyle changes.

7 Ways to Make Sure You Survive a Heart Attack

Marjory Abrams, publisher, newsletters, Boardroom Inc., 281 Tresser Blvd., Stamford, CT 06901.

Choosing the right hospital can be the key to surviving a heart attack, according to cardiologist Dr. Richard Stein, the director of preventive cardiology at Beth Israel Medical Center in New York City and author of *Outliving Heart Disease.*

To find the best hospital in your area, he advises checking the Hospital Compare heart attack statistics at *www.hospitalcompare.hhs.gov.* Do it now *before* an emergency. In addition, call the cardiology departments of several hospitals

to find out which perform emergency angioplasty to open blocked arteries and if it is done less than 90 minutes after arrival at the hospital. (Medication can be used instead, but angioplasty is generally more effective if it's done soon after arrival.) If possible, pick a hospital where your doctor has admitting privileges.

HEART ATTACK SURVIVAL CHECKLIST

●**Know the symptoms.** The classic heart attack symptoms are chest pain or discomfort that may also be felt in the neck or left arm and may be accompanied by nausea. Women are more likely than men to have atypical symptoms—shortness of breath, profound fatigue, sweating, racing heart, burning stomach.

●**Call 911** for an ambulance to take you to the hospital immediately if you experience symptoms. Don't let embarrassment or concern that it is something minor prevent you from getting it checked out.

●**Chew two full-strength aspirin.**

●**Tell ambulance and hospital staff that you think you are having a heart attack.** Don't minimize your symptoms.

●**Have the appropriate tests,** including an electrocardiogram (EKG) and blood tests to measure certain cardiac enzymes. Stein notes that women who experience the atypical symptoms cited above (or their health advocates) may need to be assertive to get these tests.

According to Stein, accurate diagnosis may require several EKGs and/or blood tests within the first few hours.

In 2000, Vice President Dick Cheney experienced chest and shoulder pain. The initial EKG and blood tests showed no evidence of a heart attack. However, several hours later, the second set of tests revealed that he had indeed had a minor heart attack.

●**Get the proper treatment.** *The following treatment should begin even before all of the test results are in…*

●Aspirin immediately if you did not take it at home.

●A beta-blocker, such as *metoprolol* (Lopressor) or *propranolol* (Inderal) to reduce the heart's need for oxygen-rich blood and to minimize heart damage.

●Nitroglycerin to dilate blood vessels if the heart is short of blood or the patient is experiencing chest pain.

●An ACE inhibitor to decrease blood pressure and the heart's workload.

●Clot-busting treatments, which can include the drug *tissue plasminogen activator* (tPA), and/or angioplasty.

●**Save this article so you can take it with you to the ER.** I hope that you will never need it, but if you do, it may save your life.

■ ■ ■ ■

Aggressive vs. Conservative Treatment

Aggressive treatment for a heart attack is almost always better than a more conservative approach.

Recent study: People who had coronary angioplasty and stents had a 50% lower rate of death, new heart attacks or other coronary events within one year than people who underwent more conservative treatments.

Key: Coronary intervention should occur as early as possible.

Michael Mogadam, MD, clinical associate professor of medicine, George Washington University School of Medicine, Washington, DC.

■ ■ ■ ■

Depression May Hamper Recovery After Heart Attack

Depression after a heart attack can be particularly dangerous.

Recent study: Depressed people are twice as likely as others to die or have another heart attack within two years of the first one.

Self-defense: People who have heart disease —or who are at high risk for it—and are depressed should consult their cardiologists about the most appropriate treatment, which might include antidepressants and psychotherapy.

Stephen J. Bunker, PhD, RN, manager, cardiac rehabilitation, National Heart Foundation, West Melbourne, Victoria, Australia.

Factors that Make Hospital Heart Care Great

Harlan J. Krumholz, MD, professor of medicine, Health Management Program, Yale University School of Medicine, New Haven, CT.
Elizabeth H. Bradley, PhD, director, Health Management Program, Yale University School of Medicine, New Haven, CT.
Circulation.

Researchers have identified the key factors that help hospitals treat heart attack patients as quickly as possible.

THE STUDY

"In order to understand what makes great places great, you have to get on the ground and talk to people to learn how they achieve things that are beyond the reach of other places," says Dr. Harlan J. Krumholz, lead researcher and a professor of medicine at Yale University School of Medicine's Health Management Program. "When we look at large numbers, we often miss what we can learn by talking to a very small number of places to find out what they are doing."

For this reason, Krumholz's study focused on just 11 hospitals that were able to consistently restore blood flow to damaged hearts in 90 minutes or less.

The hospitals were not identified in the study, but they are all listed in a national registry of heart attack treatment. And despite some major differences among them—for example, one had 111 beds; another had 870—what they did have in common was getting heart attack patients artery-opening balloon angioplasty very quickly. Time-to-treat ranged from an average of just 55.5 minutes at one hospital to 87 at another.

COMMON CHARACTERISTICS

The researchers found that these hospitals shared eight characteristics...

●**Commitment** to the explicit goal of providing the fastest treatment possible.

●**Support** from senior management.

●**Innovative protocols.**

●**Flexibility** to change protocols if it becomes necessary.

●**Uncompromising leaders.**

- **Teamwork.**
- **Quick data retrieval** to identify problems.
- **An organizational culture that could learn from its mistakes.**

Most surprising to Elizabeth H. Bradley, director of the Yale Health Management Program as well as a member of the research team, was the give-and-take between the team leaders and the team members.

"In every organization there are conflicts," Bradley says. "These organizations were able to balance two things—intense data feedback, but in a blame-free way that could allow changes in rigid protocols."

The common denominator in all the hospitals was "amazing people who are so devoted," Bradley says. "There were a lot of impressive leaders, but also impressive team members."

THE NEXT STEP

The research group now is working with national organizations to translate the findings into action that can help improve hospital performance everywhere, Krumholz says.

"We are in the midst of developing a national campaign by the American College of Cardiology," Krumholz says, with educational materials for hospitals across the country.

However, simply providing a set of instructions is not enough, Bradley cautions. "You need a whole cultural commitment to making these changes, and that takes a lot more than what you do when you read a book," she says.

■ ■ ■ ■

Smoking-Ban Benefit

Heart attack rates have declined in cities that have banned smoking in public places.

Example: After Pueblo, Colorado, banned smoking in restaurants, bars and other public places, the number of heart attacks decreased by almost 30%.

Approximately 35,000 Americans die of heart disease that is caused by exposure to second-hand smoke.

Centers for Disease Control and Prevention.

Best Time to Get Statin Drugs to Save Your Life

Gregg C. Fonarow, MD, professor of cardiology, University of California at Los Angeles.
R. Scott Wright, MD, cardiologist, Mayo Clinic, Rochester, MN.
American Journal of Cardiology.

Patients who get a statin drug in the critical first hours after a heart attack are much more likely to leave the hospital alive than those who do not get the cholesterol-lowering medication, new research has found.

The benefits of the statin therapy carry on for several years beyond discharge.

R. Scott Wright, MD

Previous studies have shown that giving statins during a hospital stay for a heart attack reduces the long-term death rate. This study—the largest of its kind—shows that *when* the drug is administered plays a significant role in improving survival.

THE STUDY

The study looked at the records of 170,000 people who were admitted to hospitals because of heart attacks. Study author Dr. Gregg C. Fonarow, a cardiology professor at the University of California at Los Angeles (UCLA), found that the people who had been taking statins before going to the hospital and who were given these drugs within 24 hours after admission had a 54% lower risk of dying during their hospital stay.

Patients who had not been taking a statin but were started on one within 24 hours of hospital admission were 58% less likely to die in the hospital than those who did not receive the drugs.

"There was not only less mortality, but also fewer complications, such as severe arrhythmias and shock," Fonarow says. "This is a truly new and very important clinical finding."

IMPLICATIONS

Although the study was not a controlled trial, "it may lead to a recommendation for changes in the guidelines," Fonarow says.

"The current guidelines say that statin therapy should start before hospital discharge," Fonarow says. "This study indicates that it should be started at once, just as aspirin therapy."

Such changes have already been instituted at UCLA, where heart attack patients are started on statin therapy in the emergency department, along with aspirin and other recommended drugs, he says.

The same is true at the Mayo Clinic, according to Dr. R. Scott Wright, a cardiologist who participated in the study.

"The evidence isn't 100% certain, but we think the preponderance of it is such that we have put these drugs on our acute myocardial infarction order set," the list of things that are absolutely necessary for heart attack patients, he says.

And while the current study reports only on survival in the hospital, analysis of the data "shows enhanced long-term survival," Wright says. "The benefits of the therapy carry on for several years beyond discharge."

Ultra-Low Cholesterol Levels More than Safe— Healthier, Too!

Christopher P. Cannon, MD, cardiologist, Brigham and Women's Hospital, Boston.

Eric J. Topol, MD, chairman, department of cardiovascular medicine and chief academic officer, The Cleveland Clinic.

Journal of the American College of Cardiology.

Very low levels of *low-density lipoprotein* (LDL) cholesterol, the so-called "bad" cholesterol, seem to be safe for heart patients who are taking statins, researchers report.

Patients who are taking high doses of statins can see their LDL cholesterol drop from more than 200 milligrams per deciliter (mg/dL) past a target goal of 70 to 80 mg/dL to as low as 40 mg/dL. Whether such low cholesterol levels are safe has been the subject of debate.

"We looked at patients who got to ultra-low [LDL] cholesterol levels, and wanted to make sure that was safe," says study coauthor Dr. Christopher P. Cannon, a cardiologist at Brigham and Women's Hospital in Boston.

"We found that it was not only safe, but it was better to have your [LDL] cholesterol down in the range of 40 or 50 mg/dL than 70 or 80 mg/dL," Cannon says.

THE STUDY

In their study, Cannon and his team collected data on 1,825 patients who had experienced a heart attack or unstable angina and were taking 80 mg of Lipitor daily.

We can feel comfortable using high-dose statins even if LDL cholesterol ends up at 40 mg/dL. That's actually a good thing.

Christopher P. Cannon, MD

After four months of therapy, LDL cholesterol dropped below 100 mg/dL for 91% of the patients. Of these, 11% saw their LDL cholesterol drop below 40 mg/dL, according to the report.

Compared with other groups, the patients who had cholesterol levels lower than 40 mg/dL and those whose cholesterol was between 40 and 60 mg/dL had fewer heart attacks, strokes, cardiac death, chest pain and additional heart procedures, the researchers found.

Moreover, there were no significant differences in adverse side effects from statins, such as muscle or liver abnormalities or death.

'A GOOD THING'

"We can feel comfortable using high-dose statins in all high-risk patients, even if their [LDL] cholesterol ends up at 40 mg/dL. That's actually a good thing," Cannon says. "The message is that lower is better and safe."

Dr. Eric J. Topol, chairman of the department of cardiovascular medicine and chief academic officer at The Cleveland Clinic, believes that these results will lower current cholesterol goals. "I think this is an important direction of our therapy for the future—lowering the bar," he says. "And this study helps, validating [statins'] remarkable safety."

CRP Not the Best Heart Disease Predictor After All

University of Maryland Medical Center news release.

Recent research is challenging the widespread use of the *C-reactive protein* (CRP) test for assessing heart disease risk.

STUDY FINDINGS

The University of Maryland Medical School study of more than 15,000 adults found that elevated blood levels of CRP are closely connected with traditional heart disease risk factors, such as obesity, smoking, high blood pressure and elevated cholesterol. Elevated CRP levels rarely occur in the absence of these traditional risk factors, the researchers say.

> *The CRP test turned out to be one of the greatest myths in cardiovascular medicine.*
>
> Michael Miller, MD

"We believe that high C-reactive protein is truly related to the company it keeps," says principal investigator Dr. Michael Miller, director of preventive cardiology at the University of Maryland Medical Center, and is not an independent risk factor for cardiovascular disease.

CRP is released by the liver in response to inflammation that is triggered by injury, infection or health conditions such as arthritis. Inflammation has been associated with the start and progression of cardiovascular disease.

THE 'GREATEST MYTH'

"The CRP test gained popularity in the late 1990s when it was believed that only 50% of heart attacks could be explained by traditional risk factors. However, this turned out to be one of the greatest myths in cardiovascular medicine, as recent studies have affirmed that more than 90% of heart attacks can be accounted for by traditional risk factors, as well as poor diet, sedentary lifestyle and mental stress," Miller says.

"If you exercise, don't smoke, have normal levels of blood pressure, cholesterol and glucose and are not overweight, the likelihood of having a high CRP is only one in 2,000," Miller says.

Rather than using CRP screening to test for heart disease, Miller suggests that health experts "work more intensively to reduce the known culprits, such as obesity and diabetes, which are growing to epidemic proportions and have become major public health concerns in the US."

Lifesaving Drug Increases Survival

Rory Collins, MD, professor of medicine and epidemiology, University of Oxford, England.
Marc S. Sabatine, MD, associate physician, cardiovascular division, Brigham and Women's Hospital, Boston.
The Lancet.

Adding the clot-preventing drug *clopidogrel* (Plavix) to the emergency treatment of heart attack patients saves lives and reduces the incidence of second heart attacks and stroke, a major study has found.

THE STUDY

The study included more than 45,800 patients who were treated at the onset of a heart attack at 1,250 hospitals. Half of the patients were given the standard treatment, including aspirin, while the other half received aspirin along with clopidogrel.

The death rate was 7% lower in the patients who got clopidogrel compared with those who received only aspirin. During the treatment period, the incidence of second heart attacks for the clopidogrel group was 14% lower, and the overall incidence of repeat heart attacks, stroke and death was 9% lower than for the aspirin-only group.

The results also showed that clopidogrel did not increase bleeding. There have been fears that clopidogrel may cause dangerous bleeding because the drug prevents platelets from banding together to form blood clots.

IMPLICATIONS

"A [previous] study looked at the effect of clopidogrel on whether the artery remained open," says Dr. Rory Collins, a professor of medicine and epidemiology at the University of

Oxford in England. "What our study shows is that that translates into an increase in survival and a reduction of second heart attacks."

The study could change medical practice, Collins says. "At the moment, clopidogrel is used for people having a stent put into an artery or [for those] who have unstable angina, but it is not used routinely in the emergency treatment of heart attack," he says. "This study argues strongly for clopidogrel to be used routinely for patients having a heart attack."

Dr. Marc S. Sabatine, an associate physician in the cardiovascular division of Brigham and Women's Hospital in Boston, says there has been a trend toward using clopidogrel early in the treatment of a heart attack, and that these new study results should accelerate that trend.

"This larger trial gives larger, definitive data. I suspect that, based on these results, the treatment will be adopted by physicians," Sabatine says.

Previous studies have also shown the value of clopidogrel in cardiac care. One such study found a 50% reduction in complications and deaths in heart attack patients who got clopidogrel before, rather than during, artery-opening angioplasty.

Just Revealed: Aspirin–Plavix Combo Could Be Deadly

Eric J. Topol, MD, chairman, department of cardiovascular medicine and chief academic officer, The Cleveland Clinic.

David D. Waters, MD, chief of cardiology, San Francisco General Hospital, and professor of medicine, University of California, San Francisco.

Byron Cryer, MD, associate professor of medicine, University of Texas Southwestern Medical School, Dallas.

55th annual scientific sessions of the American College of Cardiology, Atlanta.

The New England Journal of Medicine.

A startling new study has doctors rethinking the practice of prescribing the blood thinner *clopidogrel* (Plavix) in combination with low-dose aspirin to patients who are at risk of having a first heart attack or stroke. The

international study included more than 15,000 patients who had heart disease or risk factors for heart disease.

The conclusion: The tandem drug therapy was of some benefit to those who had diagnosed heart disease, but it nearly doubled the risk of death, heart attack or stroke in patients who only had risk factors for heart disease, such as high cholesterol and high blood pressure.

THE STUDY

In the trial, called CHARISMA (Clopidogrel for High Atherothrombotic Risk and Ischemic Stabilization, Management and Avoidance), 15,603 patients in 32 countries who had either cardiovascular disease or risk factors for it were randomly selected to receive Plavix plus low-dose aspirin or a placebo plus low-dose aspirin. The patients were then followed-up for 28 months.

The researchers found that in the group taking Plavix and aspirin, 6.6% died or had a heart attack or stroke, compared with 5.5% of the patients taking aspirin alone.

Among those receiving Plavix and aspirin, 3.9% died of cardiovascular disease, compared with 2.2% of those receiving aspirin alone, according to the study authors.

However, among the patients who had diagnosed heart disease at the start of the trial, 6.9% of those receiving Plavix plus aspirin died or had a second heart attack or stroke, compared with 7.9% of those taking aspirin alone.

Study coauthor Dr. Eric Topol, a professor of genetics at Case Western Reserve University in Cleveland and a leading heart expert, says, "Plavix didn't do well for patients in primary prevention. For patients with established vascular disease, there was some benefit. Among these patients, there was nearly a 20% reduction of death, heart attack or stroke."

RECOMMENDATIONS

Topol is urging doctors to stop prescribing Plavix plus aspirin to patients who have not had a previous heart attack or stroke. However, the researchers say that the Plavix-plus-aspirin combination still has a place in preventing a second heart attack or stroke.

"This trial was a big surprise," according to Topol. "We never thought that in primary prevention the Plavix–aspirin combination would backfire in high-risk patients. Any physician who is using Plavix and aspirin as a primary prevention shouldn't do that," he stresses, adding that he suspects many doctors are using the drug combination in this way.

> *If you don't have symptomatic coronary disease yet, Plavix probably causes more harm than good.*
>
> David D. Waters, MD

Topol notes that when taken alone, aspirin and Plavix have approximately the same benefit in preventing a first heart attack or stroke. But aspirin is much less expensive, he notes.

MORE HARM THAN GOOD

"CHARISMA strongly suggests that if you do not have symptomatic coronary disease yet, [Plavix] probably causes more harm than good," says Dr. David D. Waters, chief of cardiology at San Francisco General Hospital and a professor of medicine at the University of California, San Francisco. "There are other useful treatments for high-risk primary prevention—aspirin and statins, for example. So, we should focus on those and forget about clopidogrel for these patients," he advises.

"Last year we learned that Plavix has a greater risk for gastrointestinal bleeding than previously thought," says Dr. Byron Cryer, an associate professor of medicine at the University of Texas Southwestern Medical School, Dallas. "This year we learned that the combination of Plavix plus aspirin is not as effective for the prevention of cardiovascular events as we previously thought. In sum, this means that the benefit-to-risk ratio of Plavix has become even narrower," he says.

"Physicians will need to be even more selective in choosing appropriate patients for the aspirin–Plavix combination," Cryer adds.

Funding for the trial was provided by the makers and distributors of Plavix, Sanofi-Aventis and Bristol-Myers Squibb.

info You can learn more about clopidogrel by visiting the US National Library of Medicine's MedlinePlus Web site at *www.medlineplus. gov.* Click on "Drugs & Supplements."

■ ■ ■ ■

Should You Be Taking Aspirin?

A new study suggests that some people who are age 70 and older may be better off not using aspirin to protect themselves against cardiovascular disease. Theoretical calculations show that aspirin therapy could cause 57% more life-threatening hemorrhages in this age group.

However, older people who have diabetes, high blood pressure or other major cardiovascular risk factors are likely to benefit from aspirin therapy.

Bottom line: If you are currently on aspirin therapy, talk with your physician about whether you should continue taking aspirin daily.

Mark R. Nelson, MD, professor and chair of general practice, University of Tasmania School of Medicine, Hobart, Tasmania, Australia.

Aspirin Before Bypass Surgery Boosts Survival Rates

R. Scott Wright, MD, cardiologist, Mayo Clinic, Rochester, MN.
Eric J. Topol, MD, chairman, department of cardiovascular medicine and chief academic officer, The Cleveland Clinic.
Circulation.

People who are taking low-dose aspirin to help their hearts benefit substantially if they continue to take it in the days prior to bypass surgery, a Mayo Clinic study indicates.

THE STUDY

The researchers looked at more than 1,600 people who had bypass operations at the Mayo Clinic, and found that the in-hospital death rate for those who took aspirin in the five days before surgery was 1.7%, compared with 4.4% for those who did not take aspirin.

Some surgeons have patients stop taking aspirin before bypass surgery because of the fear of excessive bleeding. But the study found no increased incidence of re-operation because of internal bleeding, according to the lead author of the report, Dr. R. Scott Wright, a Mayo Clinic cardiologist.

The incidence of death and stroke was significantly lower in patients taking aspirin, Wright reports. "And in those who took aspirin, there was a reduced need for postoperative blood products."

The aspirin did what it was supposed to do—prevent heart attacks and other cardiac events by making blood flow more freely, he explains.

"We know that many of the deaths that occur after the operation are due to ischemic heart disease," in which a coronary blood vessel is blocked, Wright says.

Although the study supports the findings of smaller studies done in other countries, the case for giving aspirin before bypass surgery is still not definitively proved, he says.

"This is level two evidence—an observational study," Wright says. "A randomized trial is needed for definitive evidence. The data from this study would justify carrying out a randomized trial in patients getting bypass surgery."

THE CASE FOR ASPIRIN

"These new data from the Mayo Clinic certainly help support the case for using aspirin before surgery," says Dr. Eric Topol, chairman of the department of cardiovascular medicine at The Cleveland Clinic.

The case for using aspirin immediately after bypass surgery has been proven by a number of studies showing major benefits, Topol says, but there has been a debate about its use before surgery because the data has been mixed about whether aspirin creates a bleeding hazard.

The Mayo study shows that "the bleeding hazard doesn't appear to be in any way prohibitive," Topol says.

In practice, surgeons at The Cleveland Clinic generally continue aspirin therapy if the bypass patient has been taking it, he says. However, it is not yet standard procedure to start a patient on aspirin in the days before surgery, unless there are unusual circumstances, such as a high risk of a heart attack, Topol says.

"Patients who have heart disease and are not taking aspirin should ask themselves—and their doctors—'Why not?'" he adds.

Chilling Fact: More Heart Attack Patients Die in December

Robert A. Kloner, MD, PhD, director of research, Heart Institute, Good Samaritan Hospital, and professor of medicine, cardiovascular division, Keck School of Medicine, University of Southern California, both in Los Angeles.
Annals of Internal Medicine.

People who have heart attacks in December are more likely to die than those who have heart attacks in other months, according to a new study.

Previous studies that have come to similar conclusions have blamed reduced health-care staff because of the holidays, cold weather or uneven care for this anomaly. However, the researchers who conducted the current study took these factors into account and still found that more patients died in December compared with other months.

THE STUDY

In the study, a research team led by Dr. James Jollis, a cardiologist at Duke University Medical Center, collected data on 127,959 Medicare patients who were hospitalized for heart attacks between January 1994 and February 1996.

The researchers found that, while treatment was essentially the same for all of the patients, 21.7% of those admitted to the hospital in December died, compared with 20.1% of those admitted to hospitals in other months.

"We found that the 30-day mortality of patients hospitalized with acute MI [*myocardial infarction*, or heart attack] in December was higher than in other months, even after adjusting for patient, physician and hospital characteristics," the researchers report.

MORE RESEARCH NEEDED

"Our findings highlight the need for further research into the mechanism of increased mortality in patients hospitalized in December, while ensuring continued emphasis on standardized care during holiday seasons for patients with acute MI," the researchers conclude.

"This paper is at least reassuring that standards of care do not diminish during the month of December," says Dr. Robert A. Kloner, director of research at the Heart Institute at Good Samaritan Hospital and professor of medicine in the cardiovascular division at the Keck School of Medicine at the University of Southern California.

"The study further confirms our observation of increased cardiovascular mortality during the winter months," Kloner adds. "Still, we are left with an unexplained higher mortality rate during the month of December."

WHAT PATIENTS CAN DO

Kloner agrees that there is a need for more research into the mechanism of higher cardiac mortality in December. However, "until we have definitive answers, there are some common-sense approaches" physicians and patients can take, he says.

"Physicians can remind their patients not to delay seeking medical attention if they develop symptoms. Patients should also avoid running out of medications, overindulgence in food, salt, fatty foods and alcohol, exposure to extreme cold, and exposure to particulate pollutants, which can be generated from wood-burning fireplaces—often common during the holiday season," Kloner says.

info The American Heart Association can tell you more about heart attack warning signs at *www.americanheart.org*.

■ ■ ■ ■

Winter Heart Attack Danger

A study has found that rapid decreases in barometric pressure (usually associated with precipitation, especially during winter) are linked to heart attacks. In a review of 1,300 hospital admissions of heart attack patients over a three-year period, when the pressure dropped one unit on the barometer, heart attack risk was 10% greater during the next 24 hours...a two-unit drop per hour resulted in a 20% increase in risk.

Theory: A rapid drop in barometric pressure causes inflamed atherosclerotic plaque to break off and trigger a heart attack.

Philip D. Houck, MD, associate professor of internal medicine, Texas A&M University, Temple.

■ ■ ■ ■

The Most Dangerous Time of Year

More people die of natural causes between Christmas and New Year's than at any other time of year.

Possible reason: People delay seeking medical care due to the holidays.

David Phillips, PhD, professor of sociology, University of California, San Diego.

High-Risk Patients Not Getting the Care They Need

Douglas S. Lee, MD, PhD, research fellow, University of Toronto, Ontario, Canada.
Frederick Masoudi, MD, associate professor of medicine, Denver Health Medical Center.
The Journal of the American Medical Association.

Heart failure patients for whom drug therapy is essential after release from the hospital are the least likely to get it, a Canadian study has found.

And a likely explanation is that doctors may not be devoting the time that is needed to care for these higher-risk patients, says lead researcher Dr. Douglas S. Lee, a research fellow at the University of Toronto.

THE STUDY

In a study of more than 1,400 Ontario residents who were hospitalized for heart failure, those judged to be at the greatest risk of dying within a year after release were significantly less likely to be prescribed front-line medications for the condition.

The risk assessment was based on a number of factors, including age (older people are at higher risk), kidney function and the presence of other medical problems.

Those in the highest risk category had a 50% chance of dying within one year, Lee says. Yet only 60% of them were prescribed ACE inhibitor drugs to treat their condition, compared with 73% of the people in the middle-risk group and 81% of those in the low-risk group.

Similarly, 24% of the high-risk patients were prescribed beta blocker medicines, compared with 33% of those classified as medium risk and 40% of those in the low-risk group.

This pattern continued outside the hospital. Within 90 days of discharge, 61% of the high-risk patients were prescribed ACE inhibitors, while 76% of the middle-risk group and 83% of the low-risk group got the same prescriptions. Post-hospital numbers were similar for other heart failure drugs as well, the study found.

> *Higher-risk patients require*
> *a lot more time and effort.*
> *That may be one of the primary*
> *reasons for the undertreatment.*
>
> Douglas S. Lee, MD, PhD

The Canadian findings "would likely also be true in the United States," says Lee, who is also a research associate with the Massachusetts-based Framingham Heart Study.

SUPPORTING STUDY

A previous study had also found consistent underuse of medications for heart failure patients. This new study adds support to those findings, says Dr. Frederick Masoudi, associate professor of medicine at the Denver Health Medical Center, and a leader of the earlier study.

POSSIBLE REASONS

"Higher-risk patients are more complicated to treat and probably require a lot more time and a lot more effort. That may be one of the primary reasons," for the undertreatment, says Lee. In medicine, as in business, time is money, and according to Lee, "Doctors are paid the same amount for treating high-risk and low-risk patients."

Because no other treatment options exist, proper drug therapy is vital for people who have heart failure, in which the heart progressively loses its ability to pump blood.

"The study shows not only that medications are underused, but also a systematic failure of physicians to calibrate their treatment to the underlying risk of the patients," Masoudi says. "The complexity of some of these patients does create additional challenges for the physicians, but the complexity shows the need for understanding the risk of individual patients and calibrating the treatment that will benefit them the most."

info You can find more information on heart failure at the American Heart Association Web site at *www.americanheart.org*. Click on "Heart Failure" under "Diseases & Conditions."

■ ■ ■ ■

Know the Difference Between Heart Attack and Heart Failure

Heart *failure* is a chronic, progressive condition in which the heart muscle is damaged and cannot pump enough blood through the body. Symptoms of heart failure include shortness of breath, swelling of the feet, ankles, legs or abdomen, weakness, coughing when lying down and impaired thinking. Heart *attack* refers to the damage that occurs to the heart muscle when a coronary artery becomes blocked. Heart attack symptoms and warning signs include chest discomfort, pain or discomfort in one or both arms, shortness of breath and breaking out in a cold sweat.

Clyde Yancy, MD, director, Congestive Heart Failure/Heart Transplant Program, University of Texas Southwestern Medical Center, Dallas.

Hard to Swallow! Patients Who Could Benefit Most Not Taking Meds

Kristin Newby, MD, associate professor of medicine, Duke University, Durham, NC.
Sidney Smith, MD, professor of medicine, University of North Carolina at Chapel Hill, and spokesman, American Heart Association.
Circulation.

Many people who have heart disease are not taking their prescribed medications as often as they should, according to some cardiologists.

During a seven-year study at Duke University, almost half of the 31,750 people treated for major heart problems acknowledged that they were not taking beta blocker drugs, aspirin and cholesterol-lowering drugs exactly as their doctors had ordered.

In fact, the patients who would gain the greatest benefit from these drugs—the elderly and those who have heart failure or other diseases—were the least likely to be using the medications as directed.

THE STUDY

The study participants had all undergone at least one heart procedure, such as bypass surgery, or had at least a 50% blockage of one coronary artery. While a majority of the patients did take the drugs occasionally, many did not take them regularly.

There were suspicions about inconsistent use of heart drugs, but it's always a surprise when you see numbers like these.

Kristin Newby, MD

For aspirin, presumably the easiest drug to take, 71% said they took it consistently as directed. The compliance rate was much lower for other medications—46% said they took beta blockers as ordered, and only 44% followed instructions for taking lipid-lowering drugs, such as statins.

Only 20% of the people who had heart failure, the progressive loss of ability to pump blood, said they took their ACE inhibitors consistently.

HEALTH-CARE WORKERS ARE KEY

"My feeling is that a number of factors are responsible," says study author Dr. Kristin Newby, an associate professor of medicine at Duke. "Cost does play a role in it, but health-care providers are the key part of the issue. That includes physicians, nurses and pharmacists."

It will take a concerted effort on the part of doctors and other medical professionals to correct the problem, Newby says.

"We have to develop algorithms for checking on medication use," she says. "It means checking every time they come in for a visit, and helping patients and their families understand the importance of taking medicine."

Although the study was not designed to show the repercussions of not taking drugs as pre-scribed, there were indications that patients who followed drug therapy instructions had a better survival rate. "This is consistent with the results we see in randomized trials," she says.

WAKE-UP CALL

"There were suspicions about inconsistent use of heart drugs," Newby says, "but it's always a surprise when you see numbers like these. The magnitude of the problem is certainly eye-opening, and it should be a wake-up call for us."

There has been some progress toward improving compliance, notes Dr. Sidney Smith, a professor of medicine at the University of North Carolina, but there is still a long way to go.

"We can't afford or justify neglect of this issue," says Smith, a spokesman for the American Heart Association. "We need a major focus in our health-care system to recognize and solve this problem."

Pooches Pump Up Heart Patients

Kathie M. Cole, RN, clinical nurse III, University of California at Los Angeles Medical Center.
American Heart Association.

Just a 12-minute visit with a dog improved the heart and lung function of heart-failure patients, a new study has found.

THE STUDY

Researchers randomly assigned 76 heart-failure patients between the ages of 18 and 80 to one of three groups. One group (26 patients) received a visit from a dog and a volunteer, the second group (25 patients) received a visit from a volunteer alone and the third group (25 patients) did not receive a visit at all.

Each visit lasted 12 minutes, during which time the dog would sit close enough to the patient for him/her to pet and/or talk to the dog.

RESULTS

Anxiety scores fell 24% for people in the group that received a visit from the dog team, but only 10% for the participants who were visited by a human volunteer. The anxiety scores for the patients who received no visit were unchanged.

There were also reductions in the stress hormone *epinephrine* in the groups that received visits. The level of epinephrine dropped an average of 17% in the group visited by the dog and 2% in the group visited by a volunteer, but rose 7% in the control group.

Systolic pulmonary artery pressure, a measure of pressure in the lungs, dropped 5% during the dog visit and another 5% after the visit. It rose in the other two groups.

IMPLICATIONS

Animal-assisted therapy has previously been shown to lower blood pressure, heart rate and cardiovascular risks. It has also been shown to reduce anxiety, isolation and fear of procedures as well as improve social interactions in hospitalized patients.

However, lead author Kathie M. Cole, a clinical nurse at the University of California at Los Angeles Medical Center, says, "There have been no randomized trials of the effects of animal-assisted therapy done in acute and critically ill patients hospitalized with heart failure."

info For more information on animal-assisted therapy, visit the Delta Society at *www.deltasociety.org.*

Short of Breath? It Could Be a Sign of Heart Trouble

Daniel S. Berman, director, cardiac imaging, Cedars-Sinai Medical Center, Los Angeles.
Alan Rozanski, MD, director of nuclear cardiology, St. Luke's-Roosevelt Hospital, New York City.
The New England Journal of Medicine.

Add *dyspnea*, or difficulty breathing, to the growing list of risk factors that could signal heart trouble.

THE STUDY

A team of researchers divided 17,991 patients into five groups based on the number and type of symptoms—no symptoms, two different forms of angina, chest pain not caused by angina, and dyspnea alone.

After an average follow-up of nearly three years, the researchers found that patients who had dyspnea but no other signs of heart problems were at more than twice the risk of death as those who had *angina*—chest pain that is the most recognized symptom of heart disease.

LESSONS LEARNED

The lesson for people is that when they visit a doctor they should be sure to mention any shortness of breath, says senior researcher Dr. Daniel S. Berman, director of cardiac imaging at Cedars-Sinai Medical Center in Los Angeles.

"The patient often doesn't think of it as a symptom," Berman notes. But when signs of a heart problem are discovered, "and we ask whether there is shortness of breath, they say 'yes.' "

Dyspnea has many causes, and physicians routinely ask people if they have trouble breathing, says Dr. Alan Rozanski, director of nuclear cardiology at St. Luke's-Roosevelt Hospital in New York City, and another member of the research team. He says that trouble breathing is often a tip-off to the physician that a patient may have some underlying lung disease, maybe even heart failure.

But until now, only a few small studies have looked at whether dyspnea is a predictor of cardiac events, Rozanski says.

The bottom line: "People who have developed shortness of breath without any obvious lung problem should consider whether it is of cardiac origin," Berman says.

A SIGN OF TROUBLE

"For years, cardiologists have focused on chest pain as the primary symptom" of heart problems, Rozanski says. They consider a variety of other factors as well, including depression, lack of sleep and fatigue. This study increases interest in looking at other factors.

"We should think of shortness of breath not only in terms of lung disease," Rozanski adds. "We might need to screen a little more deeply for coronary artery disease. Someone with dyspnea might have a heightened need to undergo stress testing or other screening."

Rozanski says the study is already affecting decisions on stress testing in his practice. Now, when evaluating the need for an individual to have a stress test, he includes such factors as age, chest pain and gender (men are more likely to be referred for the test). "If someone has an intermediate risk, the presence of shortness of breath might tip me over" to recommend a stress test, he says.

info An overview of dyspnea is provided by the US National Library of Medicine at *www.medlineplus.gov.* Click on "Medical Encyclopedia" and look under "Breathing difficulties."

Lifestyle Changes Reverse Heart Risks in Less than 30 Days

Christian Roberts, PhD, assistant researcher, physiological sciences department, University of California at Los Angeles.
Katherine Nori, MD, internist, Weight Control Center, William Beaumont Hospital, Royal Oak, MI.
Journal of Applied Physiology.

In less than one month, people can reverse serious heart disease risk factors by making significant lifestyle changes, according to researchers.

THE STUDY

The study looked at 31 overweight or obese men between the ages of 46 and 76. Of these, 15 (48%) were diagnosed with *metabolic syndrome* —a collection of health risk factors including excess fat, high cholesterol, high blood pressure and insulin resistance. All of the 31 volunteers had at least one of these risk factors. In addition, 13 (42%) of the men had type 2 diabetes.

For three weeks, the men took part in a residential diet and exercise program. Their diet was designed at the Pritikin Longevity Center and included 65% to 70% complex carbohydrates (fruits, vegetables and whole grains), 15% to 20% protein (soy, beans, nuts and occasionally fish and poultry) and 12% to 15% fat (less than half from saturated fat).

The study participants were allowed to eat unlimited quantities of fruits, vegetables and whole grains, so they wouldn't feel hungry, says Christian Roberts, an assistant researcher in the

physiological sciences department at the University of California at Los Angeles and one of the study's authors.

The men also began exercising for 45 to 60 minutes daily on a treadmill, doing both level and graded walking. Roberts says the men walked at a moderate pace, meaning they could talk while they were exercising, but if the intensity of their workout was increased slightly, talking became difficult.

You can improve your heart disease risk profile even without normalizing your body weight.

Christian Roberts, PhD

The men lost approximately two to three pounds during each week of the study, but they still remained overweight or obese at the end of the three-week period.

The researchers measured blood levels of cholesterol, insulin and markers of inflammation both before and after the study. Although 48% of the men had metabolic syndrome at the start of the study, just 19% still did after three weeks. At the start of the study, 42% of the men had diabetes, but only 23% did at the end. And the average low-density lipoprotein (LDL), or "bad," cholesterol reading decreased 25%.

IMPLICATIONS

"Our study found that when an individual partakes in a fairly intensive diet and exercise lifestyle modification, significant changes in their health can be noted in a short period of time," says Roberts.

"Most of the population is under the belief that it takes a long time to see improvement. But we found that we could reverse diabetes and metabolic syndrome within three weeks, despite the fact that these men were still obese," he says.

"I'm glad that more and more people are getting the message out that you can make a difference with lifestyle changes. Even just 10 pounds of weight loss makes a huge difference in blood sugar, blood pressure and your overall well being," says Dr. Katherine Nori, an internist at William Beaumont Hospital's Weight Control Center in Royal Oak, Michigan.

"If you have diabetes or metabolic syndrome, you need to know that they are reversible, and you can improve your heart disease risk profile [even] without normalizing your body weight," Roberts says.

DIET AND EXERCISE ARE KEY

Both Roberts and Nori say the combination of diet and exercise is the reason for these dramatic changes. Neither measure alone is as powerful as the two together. And both say you must maintain the changes in order to sustain the health benefits.

"People have the power within themselves to make a difference. Weight loss and exercise consistently improve heart disease risk, and this is something you have control over," says Nori.

info To find out more information about metabolic syndrome go to *www.medicine net.com.* Click on "Diseases & Conditions."

■ ■ ■ ■

Bacteria Linked to Dangerous Heart Rhythm

Patients who have *atrial fibrillation* (AF)—rapid, irregular rhythm in the heart's upper chambers—are 20 times more likely than others to test positive for *Helicobacter pylori* bacteria.

Self-defense: If you are diagnosed with AF, you should be checked for H. pylori. Controlling the infection using antibiotics reduces—or eliminates—the heart problem.

Annibale Sandro Montenero, MD, director, arrhythmia center, and chair of cardiology, MultiMedica General Hospital, Milan, Italy.

Overactive Thyroid Tied to Irregular Heart Rhythm

Anne R. Cappola, MD, ScM, assistant professor of medicine and epidemiology, University of Pennsylvania School of Medicine, Philadelphia.

Robert Rushakoff, MD, associate clinical professor of medicine, University of California, San Francisco.

The Journal of the American Medical Association.

People who have an overactive thyroid gland, but no symptoms of thyroid disease, are at an increased risk of *atrial fibrillation*, an abnormal heart rhythm, according to a recent study. But contrary to standard scientific thinking, the study found that an overactive or underactive thyroid is not linked to an increased risk of other heart problems or death in older patients.

THE STUDY

In the study, researchers collected data on 3,233 people ages 65 and older who had their *thyroid stimulating hormone* (TSH) levels measured in 1989 and 1990. Through June 2002, 82% of the people maintained normal thyroid function, 15% had a subclinical underactive thyroid, 1.6% had a symptomatic underactive thyroid and 1.5% had a subclinical overactive thyroid, according to the researchers.

People who had a subclinical overactive thyroid had almost twice the risk of developing atrial fibrillation, compared with those who had a normal thyroid. However, there was no increased risk for coronary heart disease, stroke or death.

> *When you actually look at the data, suddenly the answers are different from what people have thought.*
>
> Robert Rushakoff, MD

There was no difference in the risk of heart disease, stroke or death between the people who had an underactive thyroid and those who had normal thyroid.

IMPLICATIONS

"People who have subclinical underactive thyroid do not have an increased risk of cardiovascular disease, like heart attack or stroke or mortality, compared with people who have normal thyroid function," says lead author of the study, Dr. Anne R. Cappola, an assistant professor of medicine and epidemiology at the University of Pennsylvania School of Medicine.

"However, people who have subclinical overactive thyroid do have an increased risk of atrial fibrillation. They should be treated to prevent it," she says.

Dr. Robert Rushakoff, an associate clinical professor of medicine at the University of California, San Francisco, thinks that the risk of atrial fibrillation is not as great as the study suggests, and therefore, feels that even patients who have a subclinical overactive thyroid may not need treatment. "If there is no clinical issue, you don't need treatment," he says. "The evidence is pointing to that. There are also risks to treatment."

Many older people are being treated for an asymptomatic underactive thyroid in the belief that treatment will prevent heart problems, Cappola says. She thinks that's unnecessary. "We don't see any evidence that treatment is going to help the heart," she says.

In addition, Cappola believes older people do not even need to be screened for thyroid problems, since it is neither cost-effective nor likely to make a difference to their health.

"This is going against what people have been thinking," says Rushakoff. "When you actually look at the data, suddenly the answers are different from what people have thought. It's against all the recommendations right now, but that's where it's going."

info The American Academy of Otolaryngology, Head and Neck Surgery can tell you more about thyroid disease at *www.entnet.org/healthinfo*. Scroll down to "Head and Neck Surgery," and click on "Thyroid Gland." Or you can try the American Thyroid Association Web site at *www.thyroid.org*.

Robot Surgery Treats Heart 4,000 Miles Away

American College of Cardiology news release.

At a recent meeting of the Heart Rhythm Society in Boston, Dr. Carlo Pappone from the San Raffaele University Hospital in Milan, Italy, sat at a computer keyboard, flanked by onlookers, as he operated on a patient almost 4,000 miles away.

The patient, a 34-year-old man, had a history of *familial paroxysmal atrial fibrillation*, or an irregular heartbeat.

THE PROCEDURE

Via a satellite link, Pappone manipulated a special soft catheter using a magnetic navigation system and performed an ablation—a procedure

that effectively deadens cells in the heart and prevents the recurrence of the abnormal heart rhythm. The procedure lasted 50 minutes. There were no complications.

"Based on our experience with remote navigation and ablation technology, a new era in interventional electrophysiology is beginning," Pappone says. "Magnetic, very soft catheters can be navigated in the heart more precisely and safely than manual catheters without risk of major complications, even in less experienced centers," he concludes.

Pappone believes that this new procedure, coupled with the ability to operate robotically over long distances, will make this treatment available to people who could not otherwise receive it.

"People always have had a love/hate relationship with robots, but this psychological barrier must be overcome. After performing more than 10,000 procedures with manually deflectable catheters, I have become enthusiastic for this emerging field," he adds.

COST MAY BE AN OBSTACLE

The main obstacle to the widespread use of robotic surgery is cost. For example, the equipment used by Pappone cost more than $2 million. The expense of the equipment may make it prohibitive for hospitals in the developing world, where it is needed most.

Health Advice from Today's Top Cardiologists

Peter M. Okin, MD, professor of medicine and director of clinical affairs, Greenberg Division of Cardiology, Weill Medical College of Cornell University, New York City.

Wouldn't it be nice to get medical advice from a roomful of top heart specialists from around the world? Now you can.

The American College of Cardiology (ACC) held a scientific meeting that more than 28,000 physicians and scientists attended to discuss the results of more than 1,900 medical studies. *Among the most important findings for your heart health...*

NO MORE VITAMIN E

Many doctors have long believed that daily vitamin E supplements are good for the heart.

Newest finding: The National Heart, Lung, and Blood Institute's (NHLBI) Women's Health Study, an extensive 10-year research project involving nearly 40,000 healthy women ages 45 and older, showed that taking 600 international units (IU) of vitamin E every other day had no effect on a woman's risk of heart attack, stroke or death.

These results are consistent with earlier studies showing that vitamin E does not improve heart health in men.

Conclusion: There is no evidence that vitamin E supplements protect against cardiovascular disease.

Editor's note: Additional studies are under way to confirm whether vitamin E supplements help prevent other ailments, such as Alzheimer's disease, macular degeneration and certain types of cancer, such as prostate malignancies.

BEST ASPIRIN THERAPY

•**For men.** Study after study has shown that men who take aspirin regularly have a lower risk of heart attack. A new meta-analysis of 31 previous studies involving more than 190,000 patients focused on different doses of aspirin.

Newest finding: Low-dose aspirin—less than 100 milligrams (mg) per day—is just as effective as higher doses at preventing heart attack and is less likely to cause dangerous side effects, such as stomach bleeding and hemorrhagic stroke (bleeding in or around the brain). Increasing the aspirin dose—to 100 to 200 mg per day—quadrupled the risk for stomach bleeding and doubled the risk for hemorrhagic stroke.

If you take more than 100 mg of aspirin each day, ask your doctor whether a lower dose is appropriate for you. A standard aspirin tablet is 325 mg...a "baby" aspirin (the kind now packaged also for adult preventive therapy) is 81 mg.

•**For women.** Although doctors have long known that regularly taking aspirin prevents heart attack in men, the data on women have not been conclusive. Now, the most thorough study to date—the Women's Health Study—has shown that aspirin affects women differently than men.

Newest finding: In the study, women took 100 mg of aspirin or a placebo pill every other day. After 10 years, women who took aspirin had a 24% lower risk for ischemic stroke (a blood vessel blockage in the brain) and a 22% lower risk for "mini-strokes," also known as *transient ischemic attacks* (TIAs).

For reasons no one understands, aspirin did not reduce the risk for heart attack in women. Women older than age 45 who are concerned about their risk for stroke should discuss prevention strategies with their doctors—including taking low-dose aspirin. Their doctors also can recommend ways to lower heart attack risk, such as a healthful diet, exercise and smoking cessation, if necessary.

Caution: Do not take aspirin regularly without first consulting your physician. Regular aspirin use can cause gastrointestinal bleeding in some people.

NEW CHOLESTEROL TARGETS

With an abundance of recent research identifying new heart disease risk factors, many people forget that one of the most consistent and longstanding indicators of heart attack risk is low-density lipoprotein (LDL) cholesterol. Most physicians would be pleased if their patients maintained LDL levels of 100 mg/dL or below.

Newest finding: According to the Treating to New Targets study, a five-year international survey of 10,000 adults who had high cholesterol, LDL levels that are even lower than 100 mg/dL may be better. All of the participants in this study received the cholesterol-lowering medication *atorvastatin* (Lipitor) daily—half took just the minimum dose of 10 mg and the other half took the maximum dose of 80 mg.

The participants who took the low dose reduced their LDL cholesterol levels to a respectable 100 mg/dL, on average. Those who took the higher dose cut their LDL number to 77 mg/dL.

The difference in these numbers had important implications. People in the higher-dose group had a 22% lower risk of heart attack than those in the low-dose group.

As with all medications, atorvastatin and other cholesterol-lowering statins can cause side effects, such as muscle aches and potentially harmful increases in liver enzymes. Because there was a higher incidence of these side effects in the people who were taking the maximum dose, more research is needed before high doses are routinely prescribed.

PACEMAKER FOR HEART FAILURE

Every year, 550,000 Americans are diagnosed with congestive heart failure, meaning that the heart is not pumping effectively due to coronary artery disease, damage from a heart attack, high blood pressure or other factors.

As a result, the cells of the body may not receive enough oxygen, which can cause fatigue, shortness of breath, difficulty walking, reduced kidney function and even death.

In most people, the heart's pumping chambers contract in synchrony, allowing the heart to beat steadily and pump blood throughout the body.

Approximately 25% of heart failure patients have *cardiac dyssynchrony,* a problem with the synchronization of this pumping function. This means that some portion of the heart muscle is contracting later than the others, leading to a weaker pumping action.

Newest finding: The international Cardiac Resynchronization–Heart Failure (CARE-HF) study compared treatment options for heart failure patients who had synchronization problems.

These patients were randomly assigned to receive either standard drug therapy or standard drug therapy plus a pacemaker that had two electrical wires—one in the right ventricle and one in the left ventricle. This type of *biventricular pacemaker* helps restore the heart's normal beating rhythm.

Results showed that biventricular pacemakers, used in conjunction with standard drug therapy, dramatically improved quality of life and longevity. People in the pacemaker group were 37% less likely to die or have an unplanned hospitalization due to a heart problem than the drug-only group.

Based on these findings, researchers estimate that for every nine pacemakers that are implanted in heart failure patients who have synchronization problems, one death and three hospitalizations for major cardiovascular events will be prevented.

Because biventricular pacemakers are implanted during a surgical procedure, infection is a possible—but rare—associated risk.

If you have this condition, ask your cardiologist if a biventricular pacemaker is right for you.

Americans Get Unneeded Blood Transfusions

Duke University news release.

Heart patients in the United States receive more blood transfusions than heart patients in many other countries, which may indicate that doctors in this country are too liberal in recommending this procedure, researchers say.

THE RESEARCH

Researchers at Duke Clinical Research Institute in Durham, North Carolina, analyzed 24,000 patient records from 16 countries and found that transfusion rates for US heart patients were 84% higher than in Europe, 72% higher than in Canada, 70% higher than in Australia, New Zealand and Latin America, and 38% higher than in Asia. South Africa was the only country that had higher transfusion rates than the US.

Blood transfusions are not like giving a patient an aspirin or Tylenol.

Sunil Rao, MD

TRANSFUSION CONFUSION

"The old dogma in medicine has been to treat aggressively, since you can always transfuse more blood but you can't replace heart muscle. In a setting like the US, where blood is a virtually unlimited resource, physicians are more apt to reflexively transfuse their patients," according to Duke cardiologist Dr. Sunil Rao.

However, previous research at Duke and other institutions has found that blood transfusions may not be as beneficial or benign as previously believed.

"Blood transfusions are not like giving a patient an aspirin or Tylenol; they can be risky. Our message to physicians is to look at the whole patient and not just the blood count number, when considering whether or not to transfuse," Rao says.

The Duke team cautions doctors to carefully consider the ability of patients to increase blood counts without transfusions.

"If patients appear to be fine, except for an abnormal blood number, it is probably best to hold off on transfusion. The body is constantly replenishing its blood supply, so in these patients it may be best to follow them to see if they can raise their blood counts on their own. If they don't, then the physician should investigate potential underlying causes why the patient's body isn't responding," Rao says.

■ ■ ■ ■

Transfusion Danger

Heart attack patients who received a transfusion for blood loss or anemia were three times more likely to have another heart attack within the following month than those who did not get a transfusion, according to the results of a recent study.

Theory: A transfusion may trigger an immune response that can exacerbate coronary artery disease.

Self-defense: Before accepting a transfusion, heart patients should ask their doctors whether their blood counts could recover on their own.

Sunil V. Rao, MD, assistant professor of medicine, division of cardiology, Duke University Medical Center, Durham, NC.

New Heart Drug Doesn't Miss a Beat

L. Brent Mitchell, MD, director, Libin Cardiovascular Institute of Alberta, University of Calgary, Alberta, Canada.
Joseph P. Mathew, MD, associate professor of anesthesiology, Duke University Medical Center, Durham, NC.
The Journal of the American Medical Association.

A carefully controlled study has proved the value of *amiodarone* for people who are having heart surgery. Amiodarone is a drug that prevents abnormal heart rhythms such as atrial fibrillation.

THE STUDY

Comprised of 601 patients, the study was "at least twice as big as any previous trial," says study author Dr. L. Brent Mitchell, director of the Libin Cardiovascular Institute of Alberta at the University of Calgary. Most importantly, he notes, the people chosen for the study were carefully selected to represent the full range of heart surgery patients—young, old, those undergoing valve surgery and those protected by beta blockers.

Half of the participants got a 13-day course of amiodarone, starting six days before they were scheduled for heart surgery. The other half got a placebo. Researchers found that the incidence of abnormal heartbeats was 50% lower in the group receiving amiodarone than in the group getting the placebo.

"There was a substantial protective effect," Mitchell says. "It works whether a person gets a beta blocker or not."

The protective effect is especially important in high-risk patients, such as older people and those having valve surgery. "The higher the risk a patient population has, the more important the 50% reduction becomes," Mitchell says.

REACTION

The study goes "a long way to support the use of amiodarone," says Dr. Joseph P. Mathew, an associate professor of anesthesiology at Duke University Medical Center in Durham, North Carolina.

But he stops short of endorsing the drug for all heart surgery patients due to the lack of data about how many patients were started on beta blockers and then had that medication stopped.

"When patients are withdrawn from beta blockers, the risk [of atrial fibrillation] is doubled," Mathew says. "There is no information about what percentage of patients was actually withdrawn from beta blockers."

In addition, although there was no increase in the number of complications for the patients taking amiodarone, there also was no difference in readmissions to the hospital, in-hospital deaths or deaths in the year after surgery.

Mathew's recommendation is cautious: "More widespread use of amiodarone for patients undergoing elective cardiac surgery should be considered."

BACKGROUND

From 30% to 50% of the people who have valve replacement or bypass operations can experience abnormal heartbeats, which lengthen hospital stays and can be life-threatening. Some doctors have hesitated to use amiodarone "primarily because of conflicting evidence from previous studies," Mitchell says. The drug's benefits are tempered by its potential toxicity. Lung disease is one of the drug's side effects.

info More information on amiodarone is available from Drug Digest at *www.drugdigest.org*. Click on "Drugs & Vitamins" in the pull-down menu under "Drug Library."

Real Cause of In-Flight Blood Clots

Frits R. Rosendaal, MD, PhD, professor of clinical epidemiology of haemostasis and thrombosis, Leiden University Medical Centre, Leiden, the Netherlands.

Steven Deitelzweig, MD, chairman, hospital medicine, and president, medical staff, Ochsner Clinic Foundation, New Orleans.

The Lancet.

Sitting still for hours is not the only factor that puts air travelers at risk for blood clots. The low-pressure, low-oxygen environment of the plane's cabin may also play a role, new research suggests.

"Something in the environment of an airplane, for instance the low pressure, affects the clotting system of some people, particularly those with risk factors, in a way that predicts a higher risk of thrombosis," says Dr. Frits R. Rosendaal, senior author of a study and a professor of clinical epidemiology of haemostasis and thrombosis at Leiden University Medical Centre in the Netherlands.

THE STUDY

The study involved 71 men and women, 40% of whom were at a higher risk of blood clots. Concentrations of certain blood-clotting markers in the blood were measured before, during and immediately after an eight-hour flight; before, during and after eight hours of sitting in a movie theater; and during eight hours of a regular, mobile day.

Approximately 10% of the air travelers showed a change in blood that's indicative of a higher risk of clotting, and only very few who were

sitting in the theater or participating in daily life showed a similar increased risk, Rosendaal says. The 10% who were at a higher risk of clots were primarily the people who were already at high risk due to other factors, he adds.

Because the people who were sitting in the movie theater for eight hours did not exhibit a higher risk of clotting, the study concludes that there are factors in addition to forced immobilization that contribute to the increased risk of blood clots on a plane.

PROVOCATIVE FINDINGS

Although the study was small, Dr. Steven Deitelzweig, chairman of hospital medicine at the Ochsner Clinic Foundation in New Orleans, calls the finding "provocative," and one that could help develop effective prevention strategies.

While recent research has shown that air travel is related to an increased risk of blood clots, there were questions about the cause.

Frits R. Rosendaal, MD, PhD

Previous research has found that the risk of blood clots after plane travel (a phenomenon sometimes called *economy-class syndrome*) is two to four times higher than at other times. However, the mechanisms behind this phenomenon remain unclear. Data also suggest that longer flights carry a greater risk of blood clots than shorter flights.

"While recent research has shown that air travel is related to an increased risk of thrombosis [blood clots], there were questions about the cause," Rosendaal says. Was it just sitting still for a long time that increased the risk or was it also due to factors specific to air travel? "For the latter, people have suggested that the low pressure in the cabin [equal to a mountain altitude of 2,500 meters] could increase the tendency of the blood to clot," he adds.

RECOMMENDATIONS

The findings do not point to any clear change in current practice. "It doesn't change the management approach," Deitelzweig says. "People at high risk still get low-molecular heparin [an anticlotting drug]." In addition, "Everybody needs to be well-hydrated, and compression stockings may play a role" in preventing clots, he says.

Rosendaal stresses that the "indiscriminate use of aspirin, heparin or other drugs to prevent thrombosis should be discouraged, since the risks probably outweigh the benefits." However, people who are at high risk for blood clots should consider safe preventive measures, such as regular exercise and refraining from sleeping pills or excess alcohol during air travel.

info For more information on "economy-class syndrome," visit the American Heart Association Web site at *www.americanheart.org/presenter.jhtml?identifier=3010041.*

Drug-Eluting Stents Four Times Better than Others

Catheterization and Cardiovascular Interventions news release.

Drug-eluting stents improved the outcomes of patients who developed blockages in veins that had been surgically grafted onto the heart, according to a study by researchers at Cedars Sinai Medical Center in Los Angeles.

Compared with conventional bare metal stents, the drug-eluting stents—which slowly release medication to prevent the overgrowth of scar tissue inside the stent—significantly reduced the number of heart attacks and repeat procedures, both signs of *restenosis* (renarrowing) within the stent.

THE STUDY

Researchers analyzed data from 223 patients who underwent a stenting procedure to restore blood flow through clogged vein grafts. Of those patients, 139 were treated with a drug-eluting stent, and 84 were treated with a bare metal stent.

After nine months, 4% of the patients who were treated with the drug-eluting stent had had a heart attack, compared with 20% of the patients who had received a bare metal stent. Only 10% of the patients in the drug-eluting stent group required a repeat procedure, compared with 37% of those who got a bare metal stent.

"There was a fourfold reduction in the incidence of restenosis with the medicated stents, at least over the short term. That's very encouraging," says Dr. Raj Makkar, codirector of the Cardiovascular Intervention Center at Cedars Sinai Medical Center.

Overall, the combined rates of heart attack, repeat procedure and death were 10% in the drug-eluting stent group and 37% in the bare metal stent group.

The Cedars Sinai team will continue to follow the patients to study whether the drug-eluting stents offer long-term benefits.

info The US National Library of Medicine has more information about stents on their MedlinePlus Web site at *www.medlineplus.gov.* Click on "Medical Encyclopedia."

Volunteer-Operated Defibs Are Lifesavers

Riccardo Cappato, MD, professor of electrophysiology, University of Milan, Italy.
Mary F. Hazinski, RN, clinical nurse specialist, emergency and clinical care, Vanderbilt University, Nashville.
European Heart Journal.

Training volunteers in the emergency use of defibrillators does save lives, even in thinly populated rural areas, a new Italian study has shown.

Previous trials in the United States and Canada have shown that survival can be improved for people who go into cardiac arrest by making defibrillators available and providing training in how to use them.

However, this study is different because of the large, sometimes rural area studied, according to lead author Dr. Riccardo Cappato, a professor of electrophysiology at the University of Milan. "We were covering more than 1 million inhabitants in the largest county of Italy—one-sixteenth of the entire Italian [land] area," Cappato says.

THE STUDY

The trial enlisted 2,186 volunteers, each of whom got an initial five hours of training in the theory and practice of defibrillation as well as a two-hour refresher course every six months. Residents of the region were told to call a central number when someone collapsed, and the volunteer who was closest to the emergency site was dispatched. After the defibrillation, the patient was taken to the nearest hospital.

Of the 702 episodes during the two-year trial, 10% of the affected people had their circulation return, 8% survived long enough to be admitted to the hospital, 4% survived long enough to leave the hospital and 3% were still alive after one year.

WHAT THE NUMBERS MEAN

Although those numbers might not seem impressive to the untrained eye, they did impress Mary F. Hazinski, a clinical nurse specialist in emergency and clinical care at Vanderbilt University and a spokeswoman for the American Heart Association. Comparing these study results with survival statistics in the region in the two years preceding the trial, the researchers found that less than 1% of the people who experienced cardiac arrest survived for one year—meaning the availability of defibrillation tripled survival, Hazinski notes.

Because the response time was shorter and more defibrillators were available, survival was inevitably better in urban areas. In those areas, survival rose from fewer than 1.5 per 100 people to 4 per 100 in the study. In the rural areas, it rose from 0.5 to 2.5 per 100 people.

Despite these results, including rural areas is precisely why this study is important. This is "a population about which we need more information," Hazinski says. "This is the largest study of which I am aware that included rural areas."

In addition, the Italian trial looked at all causes of cardiac arrest, while most studies of defibrillators have concentrated only on the abnormal heart rhythm called ventricular fibrillation. Results from those studies also showed that defibrillators tripled survival.

HOPE FOR IMPROVEMENT

Those numbers show that "if communities can develop systems where they have trained responders, there is more hope for improvement," Hazinski says. "We have to develop community resources to provide first responders until EMS [emergency medical services] arrives."

The Italian program is being expanded, Cappato notes. "We started with 49 devices, and now we have about 180 of them," he says. "We are also educating a much larger number of volunteers and lay persons, increasing from 2,600 to more than 5,000 people being instructed."

New Drug Reduces Defibrillator Pain by 56%

Jeffrey J. Goldberger, MD, director, cardiac electrophysiology, Northwestern University, Chicago.
Robert L. Page, MD, head of cardiology, University of Washington, Seattle.
The Journal of the American Medical Association.

Implantable defibrillators save lives by shocking hearts back into a healthy rhythm, but that shock can cause physical and psychological trauma for the patient. Now, drugs used to help prevent abnormal heartbeats can reduce the need for these defibrillators to fire, according to a Canadian study.

"There can be a fair amount of psychological trauma from the shock, and it is actually fairly painful," notes Dr. Jeffrey J. Goldberger, director of cardiac electrophysiology at Northwestern University. He was not involved in the study, but has extensive experience with patients who have implanted defibrillators.

THE STUDY

The international study, led by Dr. Stuart Connolly of McMaster University in Hamilton, Ontario, included 412 heart patients who received implantable defibrillators at 39 medical centers in the United States, Canada and Europe. Some of the patients were given beta blockers, the standard treatment. Others received beta blockers plus *amiodarone*, a drug that reduces *arrhythmias,* or abnormal heartbeats. (For more information about amiodarone, see page 192.) And a third group received *sotalol*, another antiarrhythmia drug.

The risk of experiencing a shock during one year was 56% lower in the patients who got either the beta blocker–amiodarone combination or the sotalol treatment, compared with those who got a beta blocker alone. The beta blocker–amiodarone combination was the most effective, reducing the incidence of shock by 73%.

There can be a fair amount of psychological trauma from the shock, and it is actually fairly painful.

Jeffrey J. Goldberger, MD

However, some of the patients taking amiodarone reported side effects such as abnormally slow heartbeats and lung and thyroid problems, according to the researchers.

INDIVIDUALIZED APPROACH

The researchers considered whether amiodarone or sotalol should be used immediately after defibrillator implantation or some time before the first shock occurs. Their answer, based on the study's findings, was that therapeutic decisions should be made on an individual basis.

In his practice, Goldberger says, "We typically individualize each patient, and we do not routinely put patients on amiodarone." He considers treatment with anti-arrhythmia drugs "when there is a high probability of a patient having events, a lot of arrhythmias or if they already have had events."

Approximately 40% of his defibrillator patients get one of these drugs, Goldberger says.

Dr. Robert L. Page, head of cardiology at the University of Washington, agrees that treatment needs to be tailored to each patient.

Drug therapy might be used immediately after implanting the defibrillator if there has been a high frequency of abnormal heartbeats or any anxiety or intolerance of the shock in the past, Page says.

For most patients, the decision on drug therapy will be made after implantation "if there is an indication that something further is needed," he says. Page estimates that more than 50% of his patients will be taking an anti-arrhythmia drug within two years after implantation, with most getting amiodarone because it is more effective. However, he might consider sotalol for some patients because it has a lower incidence of side effects.

"Ideally, it would be great if we could prevent all [shocks]," Goldberger says. "A defibrillator is a wonderful thing; it saves lives. But the mechanism by which it saves lives is that first you must have a cardiac arrest, then the defibrillator resuscitates. A more ideal way would be to prevent the arrest from happening."

10

Natural Remedies

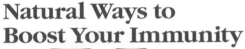

Natural Ways to Boost Your Immunity

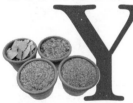

You *can* boost your immunity. With the right preparation, quick intervention and a lineup of powerful, natural virus fighters, there's a good chance that you can enjoy fall and winter without a cold or flu. This is especially important if we face a deadly avian flu pandemic.

KNOW YOUR ENEMY

Colds and flu are both caused by viruses. They are spread through the air by coughs and sneezes and through contact with contaminated objects, such as a doorknob or a hand that has been used to cover a cough.

Flu viruses are much more powerful than typical cold viruses. Cold symptoms are mainly confined to the head, neck and chest. Flu causes more general symptoms—fever, body aches, nausea, cramping, vomiting and severe fatigue. Flu also can develop into bronchitis. In the worst cases, it can lead to pneumonia and other severe respiratory diseases that are sometimes fatal, especially in seniors or other people who have weakened immune systems.

START WITH PREVENTION

●**Avoid spending time with people who already are sick,** particularly if they are coughing or sneezing. If you live with someone who is sick, sleep in separate rooms. Wash your hands frequently during cold-and-flu season, and don't share towels—assign one towel to each family member or use paper towels. Keep your hands away from your face, especially your nose, mouth and eyes.

●**Take a multivitamin/mineral supplement** that provides a base of nutrients to support a healthy immune system. A formula that I recommend in my practice as a preventive against viral infections is Wellness Formula by Source

---

Mark A. Stengler, ND, naturopathic physician, La Jolla Whole Health Clinic, La Jolla, CA, and associate clinical professor, the National College of Naturopathic Medicine, Portland, OR. He is author of numerous books on natural healing, including *The Natural Physician's Healing Therapies*. Bottom Line. *www.bottomlinesecrets.com.*

Naturals (to find a retailer near you, call 800-815-2333 or go to *www.sourcenaturals.com*). It contains vitamins A and C, which are involved in the formation of antibodies…the minerals zinc and selenium…and immune-supportive herbs, such as garlic, echinacea and astragalus, which increase the activity of virus-fighting white blood cells. The dosage used to prevent infection is two capsules daily during cold-and-flu season, along with your year-round multisupplement.

●**Reduce exposure to toxins.** You are more vulnerable to a viral infection when your body is "distracted" by having to deal with toxins that can damage or suppress the immune system. Toxins aren't necessarily exotic—they include sugar and alcohol consumed to excess, fast food and other unhealthy food laced with artificial preservatives and/or pesticides. Toxins also include small but significant amounts of metals—mercury, arsenic and lead—that are present in food, water and air pollution.

It is even more vital to eat healthfully during cold-and-flu season. Go easy on holiday sweets and other treats, and you will be less likely to get sick.

Many people cut back their exercise regimens in the winter months—a big mistake because exercise strengthens your immune system. Also consider sitting in a dry sauna once or twice a week for 20 to 30 minutes…or a wet sauna for 10 to 15 minutes. Saunas increase sweating, which excretes toxins. Be sure to check with your doctor first if you have diabetes or heart disease.

●**Be positive.** Toxic emotions can have a negative impact on your immune system. Anger, anxiety, resentment, loneliness and other chronic emotional difficulties trigger the release of hormones that suppress immune function. Seek support to overcome these problems if they linger.

RELY ON NATURE'S VIRUS KILLERS

If you start to come down with a cold or the flu, eat lightly so that your body can focus on healing. For the first 24 hours, consume filtered water, broths and soups with lots of garlic, onions and spices, such as turmeric and cayenne, which relieve congestion, promote circulation and have a natural anti-inflammatory effect. Herbal teas (especially ginger, cinnamon and peppermint) and steamed vegetables are also good choices. When you're feeling better, move toward a more normal diet.

I have found several supplements to be effective for treating colds and flu. Consider taking these when people around you are sick or when you first feel symptoms. You can use one or any combination until you feel better. These are safe for children when given in dosages of one-quarter to one-half of what I recommend for adults. The bigger the child, the higher the dose.

●**Lomatium dissectum** is a plant once used by Native Americans to fight Spanish flu. Preliminary research shows that lomatium has the ability to prevent viruses from replicating and to stimulate white blood cell activity. When used to treat colds and flu, I often see improvement within 24 hours. In my experience, the only side effect has been an allergic reaction in the form of a measles-like rash in a small percentage of users. This rash disappears a few days after lomatium is discontinued.

Eclectic Institute makes a potent product called Lomatium-Osha (800-332-4372, *www.eclecticherb. com*), which soothes the respiratory tract. This product is 50% alcohol, so take only the dosage recommended on the label. For children, add one-quarter to one-half of the adult dosage to hot water and let it sit for five minutes so that the alcohol evaporates. Women who are pregnant or nursing should not use lomatium.

●**Elderberry** can stimulate the immune system, enhance white blood cell activity and inhibit viral replication. Flu patients have reported significant improvement within 48 hours of taking elderberry. It also helps combat colds. The elderberry used in research studies is Sambucol Black Elderberry Extract from Nature's Way (to find a retailer, call 800-283-3323 or go to *www. naturesway.com*). Adults should take two teaspoons four times daily…children, one teaspoon four times daily.

●**Echinacea.** Contrary to recent media reports, extracts from this plant can be effective for treating colds and flu. Echinacea makes the body's own immune cells more efficient in attacking viruses. The key is using a product that has been processed to contain a high level of active constituents. Two potent, well-researched products are Echinamide Alcohol-Free Liquid Extract, Natural Berry Flavor and Echinamide Anti-V Formula Softgels, both from Natural Factors (to find a retailer, call 800-322-8704 or go to *www.naturalfactors.com*).

If you feel a cold or flu coming on, take 20 drops of liquid extract or two capsules every two waking hours for 24 hours, then cut back to every three waking hours until the illness has passed.

The same company makes a liquid preparation called Anti-V Formula, which contains Echinamide, lomatium and other virus fighters. It is the most aggressive product for colds and flu from the Natural Factors line and can be used instead of the other supplements. Take 1.5 milliliters (ml) every two waking hours for the first 48 hours and then every three waking hours until the illness is gone.

•**N-acetylcysteine (NAC).** This nutrient thins the mucus that accompanies colds and flu. In addition to making you feel better, NAC helps prevent sinus and more serious chest infections. It increases levels of *glutathione*, a powerful antioxidant in the body, which in turn, improves immune function. NAC is available at any health-food store and many pharmacies. If you tend to get the flu every year, take 600 milligrams (mg) twice daily when you are around people who have the flu or if you start feeling sick yourself.

•**Vitamin C** fights viral infections. Start with 5,000 mg daily in divided doses. If loose stools occur, cut back to 3,000 mg (or less).

HOMEOPATHIC REMEDIES

Homeopathy is based on the idea that "like cures like"—substances that cause certain symptoms in a healthy person can also cure those same symptoms in someone who is sick. *For the flu, I recommend the following homeopathic treatments…*

•**Homeopathic influenzinum.** Made from active flu strains, this stimulates the body's own defense system to resist infection. It can be used for the prevention or treatment of flu and has no side effects.

Take two 30C-potency pellets twice daily for two weeks at the beginning of flu season (in early November). Take two pellets four times daily when exposed to people who have the flu

or if you start to have symptoms. It is available at health-food stores and some pharmacies.

•**Oscillococcinum** is another great homeopathic remedy for flu, which is also available at health-food stores and pharmacies or by calling 800-672-4556 or visiting *www.oscillo.com*. It can be taken at the first sign of flu.

■ ■ ■ ■

Turkey May Prevent Colds

Turkey is a good source of *glutamine*, an amino acid used by cells to protect against infection. And, like other protein sources, it boosts immunity. Eat turkey often during cold season to keep protective cells functioning at their peak.

Elizabeth Ward, MS, RD, nutrition consultant, Boston.

■ ■ ■ ■

Think Before You Zinc

Zinc cold remedies should be used cautiously. There is evidence that zinc can lessen a cold's severity, but zinc products should be used only two or three times a day, primarily in the first 48 hours after symptom onset—not every three hours, as indicated on labels. Do not use zinc lozenges *and* nasal spray—choose one. High concentrations of zinc can cause nausea and diarrhea.

Neil Schachter, MD, professor of pulmonary medicine and medical director of respiratory care, Mount Sinai Medical Center, New York City.

■ ■ ■ ■

Easiest Way to Drain a Stuffy Nose

Relieve a stuffy nose by alternately thrusting your tongue against the roof of your mouth, then pressing one finger between your eyebrows. This causes the *vomer* and *ethmoid* bones to move up and down, which helps loosen congestion. After 20 seconds or so, your sinuses will start to drain.

Lisa DeStefano, DO, assistant professor, College of Osteopathic Medicine, Michigan State University, East Lansing.

Tired? Depressed? Cure May Be as Simple as Breathing

Daniel Hamner, MD, sports medicine physician, and owner and founder, Peak Energy Program, New York City. He is coauthor of *Peak Energy: The High-Oxygen Program for More Energy Now.* St. Martin's.

Every cell in the body requires oxygen to function properly. The brain alone uses at least 12% of the total oxygen inhaled.

Problem: The breathing habits of most people *don't* always provide all the oxygen that the brain and body need.

I believe oxygen deprivation is a leading cause of persistent fatigue—a condition that accounts for up to 15 million doctor visits annually, making it one of the most common health problems in the US. It also causes mental fogginess and, in some cases, depression.

My story: For years, I barely had enough energy to get through my workdays. I started reading about energy-building techniques—everything from yoga to the latest research in exercise physiology. I quickly realized that all of these techniques aim to increase oxygen levels in the body.

At the age of 47, I developed—and began practicing—a high-oxygen program. Within a matter of months, my oxygen usage rose from 42.7 milliliters of oxygen per kilogram of body weight per minute to 55 milliliters—a 30% increase. At the same time, my energy levels rose dramatically.

7 STEPS TO BETTER OXYGENATION

Nearly everyone can increase oxygen levels and experience a significant boost in energy in as little as two weeks. *Here's how...*

Step 1: Take a pro-oxygenator. The herbal supplement ginseng enhances the body's ability to utilize oxygen. A four-week study of oxygen utilization found that people taking ginseng experienced a 29% improvement in oxygen transportation to tissues and organs.

Typical dose: 400 to 600 milligrams (mg) once daily.

Caution: Do not take ginseng if you have high blood pressure. If you are taking medication, consult your physician before trying ginseng.

Step 2: Stand straight. Poor posture—rounding the shoulders, stooping forward, etc.—can inhibit oxygen intake.

People who stand straight, roll back their shoulders, push their chests out while squeezing their shoulder blades together and keep their chin up can increase lung capacity by 5%.

Helpful: To ensure proper form, practice this while looking in a full-length mirror.

Step 3: Exercise. Aerobic exercise increases pathways in the body that carry oxygen to cells. People who start an aerobic exercise program experience an immediate increase in oxygen usage and energy.

My recommendation: Walk fast, run, swim, bike, etc., for a minimum of 60 minutes three days a week.

Resistance training increases strength and endurance. Consult a physical trainer or other exercise professional for a strength-training regimen that works the muscles in your upper and lower body and your core (trunk).

My recommendation: Twenty to 30 minutes of strength training at least three times a week.

Step 4: Eat "charge-up" foods. A diet high in complex carbohydrates—fruits (such as apples and oranges)...vegetables (such as carrots and spinach)...whole grains...legumes (such as black beans)...etc.—significantly improves the blood's ability to transport oxygen to cells. A high-fat diet does the opposite—it reduces the blood's oxygen-carrying capacity.

Step 5: Practice instant-energy breathing. You can reverse fatigue almost instantly using a yoga breathing technique that floods cells with oxygen and boosts energy for 15 minutes or more. *What to do...*

●**Sit up straight and take 20 to 30 quick, panting breaths.** Only your belly should move, not your chest.

●**Take a deep breath, filling your lungs with air...and hold for 30 seconds.** This gives the blood in your lungs time to absorb as much oxygen as possible. If you can, gradually work up to holding your breath for 60 seconds.

•**Exhale completely.** Press your hand against your belly. This puts pressure on your lungs and forces out more of the used air.

After completing the exercise, walk briskly for 10 minutes, if possible. This will pull additional air into your lungs and increase the circulation of oxygen-rich blood cells.

***Step 6:* Stop smoking—and avoid second-hand smoke.** Smokers tend to have less energy and more depression than nonsmokers, in part because they get less blood and oxygen to the brain. Smoking—as well as exposure to second-hand smoke—increases blood levels of carbon monoxide, a waste chemical that increases fatigue. It also increases arterial *plaque*—fatty accumulations that inhibit circulation.

People who attend smoking-cessation programs, such as Smok-Enders, or use stop-smoking products, such as nicotine patches, are approximately twice as likely to quit the habit as those who try to stop on their own.

Important: Take 1,000 mg of vitamin C daily when trying to quit smoking. Each cigarette inactivates 25 mg of vitamin C in the body.

***Step 7:* See a doctor if you have low energy.** Fatigue is a fairly common first symptom of hundreds of medical conditions, including iron-deficiency anemia, food allergies, heart problems and cancer. Consult your doctor if you experience mental fogginess or low physical energy for more than a few weeks.

 To find out more about the benefits of oxygen, see page 165.

Enlightening Study

Steven Lockley, PhD, associate neuroscientist, Brigham and Women's Hospital, and assistant professor of medicine, Harvard Medical School, both in Boston.

Robert Vorona, MD, associate professor, department of internal medicine, Eastern Virginia Medical School, Norfolk.

Sleep.

N ew research suggests that exposure to blue light could help shift workers stay alert during the night. People who sat for more than six hours in front of a lamp emitting blue light had better reaction times and felt less sleepy than those exposed to green light, scientists report.

THE STUDY

In the study, researchers recruited eight men and eight women in their late teens and 20s, and adjusted their body clocks so they would sleep from 10 am to 6 pm, as if they were working late shifts.

> *Different colors of light can be used to change your alertness level, but blue light is better.*
>
> Steven Lockley, PhD

The researchers then attached brain-monitoring devices to the subjects and had them sit in front of specially designed blue or green lights for 6.5 hours without a break. The subjects were not allowed to do anything except sit and stay awake during the experiments.

The subjects who were exposed to blue light did better on reaction-time tests and reported being less sleepy than those who sat in front of the green lights. Brain scans also suggested that they were more alert.

IMPLICATIONS

This research shows that "different colors of light can be used to change your alertness level, but blue light is better," says lead researcher Steven Lockley, a neuroscientist at Brigham and Women's Hospital in Boston. Blue light appears to do a better job of fooling the mind into thinking that it's daylight, he says.

Therefore, it may be possible to use blue light to help workers feel alert and perform well for the duration of an entire night shift, Lockley adds.

During the past few years, scientists have developed greater insight into how light affects sleep. According to Lockley, they have found that there are light receptors in the eye that have nothing to do with vision—they work even in blind people.

These receptors let us know when it's daytime and when it's nighttime so our body clocks can adjust themselves. "Light is the major cue for enhancing wakefulness," says Dr. Robert Vorona, a sleep researcher and an associate professor of internal medicine at Eastern Virginia Medical School in Norfolk.

CAUTIONS

Vorona says the findings are interesting, but notes that the study is small.

"This may allow us to better understand the central nervous system processes that control wake and sleep," he says. In addition, the findings could provide guidance to engineers as they create lighting systems for homes and workplaces.

For now, the research supports manufacturers of light boxes that use blue light, Lockley says. People use the boxes to combat sleepiness and *seasonal affective disorder* (SAD), which can cause depression in the darker days of winter.

However, just like ultraviolet wavelengths, blue light could be dangerous to the eyes in heavy doses, Lockley warns, so it should be used with caution.

(info) Learn more about SAD at the National Mental Health Association Web site at *www.nmha.org*. Click on "Fact Sheets," and then scroll down to "Seasonal Affective Disorder" under the heading "Depression and Mood Disorders."

■ ■ ■ ■

The Health Benefits of Good Sleep

Studies now link lack of sleep with heart disease, high blood pressure, diabetes and difficulty controlling weight.

In addition, a lack of sleep boosts stress hormone levels, impairs the body's ability to process blood sugar, reduces levels of *leptin* (an appetite-depressing hormone) and increases inflammation—a factor in the development of heart disease.

In a long-term study of female nurses, the incidence of heart disease for those who slept less than five hours per night was almost double that of the nurses who slept seven to eight hours per night.

Najib T. Ayas, MD, MPH, assistant professor of medicine, Vancouver General Hospital, British Columbia, Canada.

Coffee Perks Up Short-Term Memory

Florian Koppelstatter, MD, PhD, department of radiology 2, subdivision neuroradiology, Innsbruck Medical University, Innsbruck, Austria.

Bruce Rubin, MD, assistant professor of clinical neurology, Miller School of Medicine, University of Miami.

Radiological Society of North America annual meeting, Chicago.

Coffee might sharpen your memory, an Austrian study suggests. Researchers at Innsbruck Medical University discovered that 100 milligrams (mg) of caffeine—approximately the amount in one cup of coffee—increased activity in the part of the brain that is responsible for short-term memory and improved performance on a test that measures memory function.

THE STUDY

For the study, researchers recruited 15 men between the ages of 26 and 47. On the first day of the study, each man was given 100 mg of caffeine dissolved in water. The following day, they were given just plain water. Other than the water, the men fasted during the two-day study period. Twenty minutes after having their drinks, the men underwent *functional magnetic resonance imaging* (fMRI), and then were tested to assess their working memory skills.

The fMRI showed that caffeine increased activity in the brain's *front lobe*, where part of the working memory network is located, as well as in the *anterior cingulate cortex*, the part of the brain that controls attention. None of the men showed increased activity in this area of the brain when they drank the placebo.

In an accompanying test, the men were presented with a randomized sequence of capital letters and were asked to remember whether the current letter was the same as the letter that had been presented two letters before. They were asked to respond as quickly as possible by tapping response pads with their fingers.

After consuming caffeine, all of the men studied showed a tendency toward improved reaction times on the test, compared with when they had no caffeine, according to the researchers.

The study showed that "a distinct brain area within the working memory network was more activated under caffeine compared to the placebo condition. This is the specific brain region that would be used for short-term memory function," says study author Dr. Florian Koppelstatter, a radiology fellow at the University.

These functions include being able to prioritize information in order to manage tasks efficiently, as well as plan new tasks and deal with stored information, he says. An example of this would be the process of looking up a number in a telephone book, and remembering it so you could dial the number.

HOW CAFFEINE WORKS

Dr. Bruce Rubin, a neurologist at the University of Miami's Miller School of Medicine, says this study sheds new light on how caffeine works on the brain.

He adds that previous research had shown that caffeine improves attention, and that any improved memory function identified was assumed to be the result of better focus—"You have to be attentive to remember.

"But this study showed that caffeine had a direct effect on the networks and processing of the memory," Rubin says.

Koppelstatter says the mechanism by which the caffeine acts on the brain is largely unknown, but is related to how caffeine reacts on the small blood vessels and nerve cells in the brain.

Although some coffee may improve your memory, don't think that drinking more will turn you into an intellectual, Koppelstatter says.

"The positive effects of caffeine don't increase in a linear way," he says, and too much caffeine can make you more anxious, counteracting the positive effects it can provide.

Caffeine, found in coffee, tea, soft drinks and chocolate, is the most widely used stimulant in the world, with a global per-person average of 76 mg a day. Americans consume an average of 238 mg of caffeine daily. Scandinavians have the highest daily caffeine intake—400 mg.

info To learn more about caffeine, visit the US National Library of Medicine's MedlinePlus Web site at *www.medlineplus.gov*. Click on "Health Topics," and go to "Caffeine" in the alphabetical listing.

Talk to Your Doc About Your Alternative Meds

Robert Bonakdar, MD, family physician and director of pain management, Scripps Center for Integrative Medicine, La Jolla, CA.

Janine Blackman, MD, PhD, assistant professor of family medicine and medical director, Center for Integrative Medicine, University of Maryland, Baltimore.

The popularity of complementary and alternative medicine is on the rise, with more than one-third of American adults using at least one of these treatments, according to a recent report by the Institute of Medicine.

Full disclosure enables full care.

Robert Bonakdar, MD

And if you're like most people who use these treatments, you probably don't mention them to your primary-care physician. You may think it's not important, you might just forget or you might think your doctor won't approve.

FULL DISCLOSURE

Dr. Robert Bonakdar, a family physician at the Scripps Center for Integrative Medicine in La Jolla, California, who blends conventional and alternative approaches, says it's crucial to tell your doctor about any alternative treatments that you are trying.

"Everything a patient is using is important for the doctor to know," he says. "Full disclosure enables full care."

"The best thing patients can do is be honest about what they are taking," says Dr. Janine Blackman, medical director of The Center for Integrative Medicine at the University of Maryland, Baltimore, and an assistant professor of family medicine.

Complementary and alternative medicine describes a wide variety of medical practices and products, according to the National Institutes of Health's National Center for Complementary and Alternative Medicine (NCCAM). *Complementary* describes the techniques that are used *in conjunction* with conventional medicine; *alternative* describes the techniques that can be used *in place of* conventional medicine.

STARTING THE CONVERSATION

What is the best way to approach your doctor? First, understand that your doctor may not have much background or knowledge about these approaches, Bonakdar says. Few doctors, especially older ones, studied these treatments in medical school.

"Bring it up in an open manner," he suggests, by saying, *This is something I am interested in, what do you think?*

"The patients should expect the doctor to be open and nonjudgmental in the discussion of complementary treatments," he says. "They should hear you out."

One way to facilitate the discussion is to bring as much information as you can to the appointment. If you're interested in supplements, for example, take the bottle with you so the doctor can see the exact dose, formula and manufacturer.

Your doctor "should be able to educate you from their standpoint based on whether they think it is safe, appropriate and effective," he adds. If your physician is unfamiliar with the treatment you are interested in, you should expect him/her to offer to research it to see if there is any evidence that it works, Bonakdar says.

PHYSICIANS NEED TO LEARN

In recent years, Blackman adds, more physicians have become open to alternative medicine or complementary approaches.

But a recent survey found that 84% of 302 physicians questioned thought they needed to know more about complementary and alternative medicine to address patient questions and concerns adequately. Even so, nearly half had recommended an alternative or complementary treatment to a patient.

Similarly, patients must learn that there are dangers to mixing some complementary and conventional treatments, Blackman says. For example, certain dietary supplements can increase the action of blood-thinning medications, thinning the blood to dangerous levels, she says.

If your doctor isn't comfortable with an alternative or complementary approach that you feel strongly about, you still have options, Blackman maintains. Either find a new physician or continue seeing your doctor, alerting him/her about your decision to use the complementary

or alternative approach. Then, you can consult someone else who is knowledgeable about the alternative therapy.

info To learn more about complementary and alternative medicine, visit the National Center for Complementary and Alternative Medicine at *http://nccam.nih.gov.*

Magnesium— New Medical Miracle

Carolyn Dean, MD, ND, a medical and naturopathic doctor, New York City, and author of *The Miracle of Magnesium.* Ballantine. *www.carolyndean.com.*

The mineral magnesium has amazing powers to treat and even prevent serious medical conditions.

New finding: Magnesium is a key factor in memory and learning. Adequate levels may even prevent Alzheimer's disease. Researchers at the Picower Center for Learning and Memory at the Massachusetts Institute of Technology found that magnesium affects the *synapses*—connections between brain cells—by improving their plasticity, or ability to adapt to change, which usually declines with age.

Most people don't get enough magnesium. An adult's daily nutritional requirement is 400 milligrams (mg), but a survey conducted by the Centers for Disease Control and Prevention (CDC) found that the average intake is approximately 290 mg. *Here's how magnesium can help you...*

DIABETES

We're in the midst of a diabetes epidemic— more than 18 million Americans have type 2 diabetes, a disorder of blood sugar (glucose) metabolism. Another 41 million have *insulin resistance*, a prediabetic state characterized by higher-than-normal blood levels of glucose and insulin, the hormone that regulates blood sugar. Diabetes increases the risk of heart disease and stroke and can lead to kidney failure, eye problems, nerve damage and other dangerous conditions.

Magnesium enhances insulin secretion, which facilitates sugar metabolism. Without magnesium, insulin is not able to transfer glucose into cells. Glucose and insulin build up in the blood, causing various types of tissue damage.

Proof that it works: Researchers at Harvard University tracked more than 120,000 men and women for 18 years. People who had the least dietary magnesium had a 23% higher risk of getting type 2 diabetes than people who had the greatest magnesium intake.

In another study, people who had insulin resistance took a placebo or 2,500 mg of magnesium daily (a high dose that should be taken only under a doctor's care). After three months, those taking the mineral had a 25% increase in blood levels of magnesium and a 44% decrease in insulin resistance. Those taking the placebo had no change in either.

HEART DISEASE

Magnesium helps prevent artery walls from "hardening." It relaxes blood vessels, lowering blood pressure, and keeps calcium dissolved in the blood, thus preventing artery-clogging calcium deposits.

Proof that it works: A CDC analysis of the National Health and Nutrition Examination Survey of the diets of 13,000 people found that those who had the lowest magnesium intake had a 31% higher risk of heart disease than those who had the highest magnesium intake. In a similar study of 39,633 men, researchers from Harvard found that men who took a nutritional supplement containing magnesium had a 23% lower risk of heart disease than those who didn't.

HEADACHES

Research shows that people who get migraine, tension and cluster (bouts of frequent attacks) headaches often have a magnesium deficiency. Magnesium relaxes blood vessels and muscles, regulates neurotransmitters and thins the blood—which can defuse headaches.

Proof that it works: Doctors at the State University of New York in Brooklyn gave 1 gram (g) of magnesium intravenously to each of 40 patients who were experiencing migraine, tension or cluster headaches. Thirty-two of the patients reported complete pain relief within 15 minutes. People who had migraines also experienced complete relief of symptoms such as light sensitivity and nausea. All of the patients who got relief had low blood levels of magnesium before the treatment.

RESTLESS LEGS SYNDROME

You're desperate to move your legs. They have a creepy, crawly sensation, usually at bedtime, preventing you from falling asleep. This is *restless legs syndrome* (RLS), a condition that afflicts an estimated 8% of Americans and can lead to chronic insomnia.

No one knows what causes RLS. The only drug approved by the US Food and Drug Administration (FDA) for the problem is *ropinirole* (Requip), which is also used to treat Parkinson's disease. The drug's side effects include intense drowsiness, and over time, you can develop a tolerance so that you need higher and higher doses. If you try to stop taking it, you may find that your restless legs get worse, a problem called *rebound syndrome.*

Magnesium is a natural muscle relaxant, calming spasms and twitches that either cause or aggravate RLS.

Proof that it works: For six weeks, German researchers administered magnesium to 10 RLS patients at bedtime and then monitored their sleep. Patients went from being disturbed by RLS an average of 17 times per hour to seven times per hour. Their sleep efficiency—the time spent sleeping—rose from 75% to 85%.

KIDNEY STONES

Magnesium's ability to keep calcium dissolved in the blood helps prevent painful kidney stones.

Proof that it works: In a 14-year study, researchers found that men who got the most dietary magnesium had a 29% lower risk of kidney stones than men who got the least magnesium.

CRAMPS AND MUSCLE PAIN

Magnesium relaxes muscles and relieves back and neck pain as well as fibromyalgia, a chronic condition that is characterized by fatigue and widespread pain. Magnesium also relieves nighttime leg cramps.

Proof that it works: Patients taking 300 mg of magnesium daily for six weeks at bedtime saw their average number of nighttime cramps decrease from nine to five.

In another study, 82 patients who had chronic low back pain were given a multimineral supplement that included magnesium. After four weeks, 72 patients had significant pain reduction.

Natural Healing Remedies...Without Dangerous Side Effects

Earl Mindell, RPh, PhD, emeritus professor of nutrition, Pacific Western University, Los Angeles, and a director of the corporate board, Illinois College of Physicians and Surgeons. He is author of *Natural Remedies for 150 Ailments* (Basic Health) and *Bottom Line's Prescription Alternatives* (Bottom Line).

It's a little-known fact that an estimated 50% of hospital admissions are the result of adverse reactions to prescription and over-the-counter (OTC) drugs.

But aren't drugs the only option for treating some medical conditions? Certainly—but not as often as you might think.

Many natural remedies are effective, inexpensive *and* safe. Dietary supplements, herbs and simple lifestyle changes are available for most health problems.*

Important: Some natural remedies can bring immediate relief, but others may take weeks. Be prepared to wait up to one month before you feel the full effect.

To see what works best for you, try one of the following remedies, available in health-food stores, for two weeks. If you don't begin to see a beneficial effect during that time, try a different remedy for the condition.

FATIGUE

A persistent lack of energy is common in our culture of too little sleep, too much stress, lack of exercise and inadequate nutrition.

Natural approach: The dietary supplement *coenzyme Q10* (60 milligrams [mg] daily) fights fatigue by strengthening the heart muscle...*dehydroepiandrosterone* (DHEA), taken as a supplement first thing in the morning (25 mg for women and 50 mg for men daily), increases energy, because levels of this hormone naturally decline after age 40. If you are older than 40, ask

*To find a naturopathic physician in your area who can monitor your use of natural remedies, contact the American Association of Naturopathic Physicians, 866-538-2267, *www. naturopathic.org*. Pregnant and breast-feeding women should avoid many natural remedies.

your doctor to measure your DHEA level by using a saliva test to confirm that you are deficient. This hormone should not be taken by people who have a hormone-sensitive cancer, such as breast or prostate cancer.

Also helpful: The herbs *astragalus* and *ginseng* are natural energy boosters. Drink a cup of astragalus or ginseng tea daily.

GLAUCOMA

This condition is caused by increased pressure within the eyeball. Regular eye exams should include a check for glaucoma. If it is detected, you may need prescription eye drops and should be under an ophthalmologist's care.

Natural approach: When glaucoma is detected early, dietary supplements can help reduce eye pressure. I recommend to my patients a combination dietary supplement of *methylsulfonylmethane* (MSM) (1,000 mg daily) and vitamin C for its anti-inflammatory effect. I also recommend two other dietary supplements—*alpha lipoic acid* (50 mg daily), which provides protection against free radicals that can exacerbate eye pressure...and *L-arginine* (1,500 mg, twice daily), which increases circulation.

Also helpful: The herbs *grape seed extract* (200 mg daily) and *green tea extract* (200 mg daily), both of which help prevent eye damage.

HEARTBURN

This fiery pain behind the breastbone is caused by stomach acid backing up into the esophagus. There are drugs that shut down stomach acid production, but a natural approach aims to improve digestion.

Natural approach: The probiotic *acidophilus* (one to three capsules before each meal) adds "friendly" bacteria that fight heartburn by aiding digestion...and the hydrochloric acid supplement *betaine* (150 mg once daily, with a meal) increases stomach acid levels in people who have a deficiency. Both supplements help the body break down protein and other food elements.

Also helpful: Aloe vera juice (one tablespoon, twice daily with meals) heals the intestinal lining, which helps prevent heartburn.

If heartburn develops, chew one to three papaya tablets or eat fresh papaya for quick relief.

HEMORRHOIDS

These inflamed veins in the rectum can be painful and often bleed.

Keep bowel movements regular to prevent straining on the toilet, which worsens hemorrhoids. Get at least 25 grams (g) of fiber in your daily diet. In addition to eating plenty of fruits and vegetables, add unprocessed wheat bran to soups, stews and salads...or take a fiber tablet. Be sure to drink eight to 10 glasses of water daily—otherwise, fiber can be constipating.

Natural approach: Vitamin C (500 to 1,000 mg daily) helps strengthen capillaries, including those in the rectum. Acidophilus (one to three capsules before each meal) aids bowel regularity.

Also helpful: Apply vitamin E oil or cream to hemorrhoids to ease any discomfort and promote healing.

PSORIASIS

The scaling, itchiness and inflammation of psoriasis are tormenting, but dietary supplements bring substantial relief for many people.

Natural approach: Fish oil capsules (500 mg, twice daily) and *selenium* (100 to 200 micrograms [mcg] daily) have been shown to reduce symptoms of psoriasis. Natural mixed carotenoids (5,000 to 10,000 international units [IU] daily) which convert to vitamin A in the body, if it is needed, and vitamin D (400 to 800 IU daily) promote healthy skin and protect against infection. Allow 30 days for this program to take effect.

Also helpful: Aloe vera gel, applied twice daily, soothes affected skin and relieves itching.

TINNITUS

This incessant ringing or buzzing in the ears is often worse at night and frequently interferes with sleep.

Natural approach: Calcium (500 mg daily) and magnesium (200 mg daily) help promote sleep when taken at bedtime...coenzyme Q10 (60 mg, twice daily) and any multivitamin-mineral complex that is rich in antioxidants protects against cell breakdown that can worsen this condition.

Also helpful: The herb *ginkgo biloba* (60 mg, three times daily) reduces tinnitus by improving circulation to the inner ear.

Chewing Gum...Drinking Water...and More Natural Ways to Relieve Heartburn

Elaine Magee, MPH, RD, nutrition expert for the WebMD Weight Loss Clinic, and author of numerous books on nutrition and healthy cooking, including *Tell Me What to Eat If I Have Acid Reflux.* New Page. *www. recipedoctor.com.*

Millions of Americans experience *gastroesophageal reflux disease* (GERD), the chronic backsplash of acid into the esophagus, more commonly known as heartburn. Acid reflux can injure the lining of the esophagus and lead to complications, including a condition called Barrett's esophagus, which may lead to cancer.

Symptoms of GERD include a burning sensation behind the breastbone, hoarseness, cough, asthma, belching and bloating. Medication can soothe symptoms, but it doesn't cure reflux. *Here's what to do to prevent the condition in the first place...*

FOODS TO AVOID

It's essential to limit foods that promote stomach acid, but keep in mind that what bothers one person may not bother another and that a cup of coffee may be fine in the morning but risky in the afternoon. *Most common offenders...*

- **Fried or fatty foods**
- **Chocolate**
- **Peppermint and spearmint**
- **Garlic and onions**
- **Coffee and nonherbal tea,** caffeinated and decaffeinated
- **Carbonated beverages**
- **Tomatoes and citrus fruits**
- **Hot peppers and chili powder**

OTHER TRICKS

- **Chew gum for one hour after a meal.** A study from the Veterans Affairs Medical Center in New Mexico found that this reduced the amount of time that acid was in contact with the esophagus.

- **Suck on lozenges.** This stimulates the production of saliva, which bathes the esophageal lining. Some people find that eating sweet pickles also increases saliva.

●**Drink water regularly** to dilute stomach acid and wash it from the esophagus. But limit your water intake close to bedtime.

●**Reduce fat content.** Steam, bake or broil instead of frying. Replace whole milk with 1% or skim.

●**Use caution when consuming alcohol.** Small amounts—one drink a day or less—may aid digestion, speeding up the movement of acidic stomach contents into the intestines. Too much alcohol has the opposite effect—and some people report a particular problem with red wine.

●**Keep portions small.** A full stomach is more likely to cause heartburn.

●**Eat dinner early.** Don't have anything to eat within three hours of bedtime, so there will be nothing to splash up into the esophagus when you lie down.

●**Lose weight.** Extra pounds put pressure on stomach contents and push acid up toward the esophagus.

●**Raise the head of your bed** by at least six inches—you can put wood blocks under the top two legs of your bed—or you can try a wedge-shaped pillow.

●**Sleep on your left side.** Doctors at Philadelphia's Graduate Hospital found that people who sleep on their left sides experience GERD less frequently than those who sleep on their right sides or backs.

Warning: See your doctor if you have heartburn more than twice a week.

You Can Think Away Irritable Bowel Syndrome

Jeffrey M. Lackner, PsyD, director, behavioral medicine clinic and assistant professor of medicine, University at Buffalo School of Medicine, Buffalo, NY.

Magnus Simren, MD, PhD, associate professor and consultant, Göteborg University, Göteborg, Sweden.

Emeran Mayer, MD, professor of medicine and physiology, University of California at Los Angeles.

Digestive Disease Week meeting, Los Angeles.

Short courses of cognitive therapy or hypnosis can alleviate the symptoms of *irritable bowel syndrome* (IBS) for the estimated 15% of adult Americans who have this disorder, according to several recent studies.

THE FIRST STUDY

In one study, Jeffrey M. Lackner, director of the behavioral medicine clinic and assistant professor of medicine at the University at Buffalo School of Medicine, assigned 59 patients to either a 10-week course of cognitive therapy, a four-week course, or a wait list.

Both the short and long cognitive therapy sessions included the same information, but the short course had a self-study workbook developed specifically for the study.

The therapy instructed IBS patients on how to undo some of their stressful habits, such as negative thinking patterns and poor coping skills, both of which can create anxiety and exacerbate IBS symptoms. "These people spend a lot of time in their head, engaging in worrisome thinking," Lackner says.

The study participants were encouraged to be more flexible in problem-solving and to learn skills, such as relaxation, that would help them take control of their symptoms. Muscle-relaxation training was also included in the therapy.

In total, 74% of the people who had the long course of therapy said their symptoms improved moderately to substantially, and 73% of the short-course patients reported the same improvements.

"Whether the patients went to 10 sessions or four, they achieved clinically significant improvements in symptom relief and quality of life and were satisfied [with the program]," Lackner says.

MORE STUDIES

In two other studies, hypnotherapy helped reduce the symptoms and improve the quality of life for people who have IBS, reports Dr. Magnus Simren, an associate professor and consultant at Göteborg University in Sweden.

One hypnotherapy trial involved 87 IBS patients; another looked at 48.

In each study, approximately one-half of the participants received 12 weekly "gut-directed" hypnotherapy sessions, in which the therapist helped the patients visualize a fully functioning gastrointestinal (GI) tract.

The other half of the participants were assigned to a control group that did not receive hypnotherapy.

Simren evaluated the patients at the start of the study, immediately after treatment, six months after treatment and 12 months after treatment, asking them to complete questionnaires that asked about their quality of life, anxiety, depression and GI symptoms.

There's a very important role for these kinds of mind–body approaches.

Emeran Mayer, MD

"The hypnotherapy groups improved significantly regarding GI symptoms," he says. "The control groups did not." Of the patients receiving hypnotherapy, 52% improved significantly, compared with just 32% of the control group.

Improvements lasted or even increased at 12 months, and were most marked for abdominal pain, bloating and distension. Anxiety and depression improved at one year in the smaller study of 48 patients, but not in the study of 87 patients. The reason for that disparity is unclear, Simren says.

HOW IT WORKS

Although experts are not sure just how cognitive therapy and hypnosis ease IBS symptoms, Lackner's and Simren's results are in line with other studies that have come to similar conclusions.

Dr. Emeran Mayer, a professor of medicine and physiology at the University of California at Los Angeles, believes that hypnotherapy works because it alters the way the brain reacts to stress, reducing levels of body arousal. "There's a very important role for these kinds of [mind–body] approaches," he says.

Simren says that patients who are eager for relief from IBS symptoms—which can include abdominal pain, cramps, bloating, food intolerances, constipation or diarrhea—don't really care how hypnotherapy works, just that it does. "I tell them, 'This is how you can get control of your symptoms,' and most are satisfied with that explanation," he says.

In addition, this type of therapy doesn't necessarily need to be ongoing, especially once patients learn the new skills.

Simren and Lackner suggest that IBS patients choose a therapist who has experience with this type of treatment. "It's very important that the therapist does have an interest in bodily symptoms, not just the mind," Simren says.

info To learn more about IBS, visit the American Gastroenterological Association at *www.gastro.org.* Click on "Digestive Conditions" under the heading "Patient Center."

Herbs that Have Proven Power to Heal

Mark Blumenthal, founder and executive director of the American Botanical Council (ABC), *www.herbalgram. org*, and senior editor of both the English translation of *The Complete German Commission E Monographs—Therapeutic Guide to Herbal Medicines* (Integrative Medicine Communications) and of *The ABC Clinical Guide to Herbs* (ABC).

It was headline news when *The New England Journal of Medicine* published a study that cast doubt on the effectiveness of echinacea. The message to the countless consumers spending more than $300 million annually on the purported cold-fighting herb? *Save your money.*

Researchers at the University of Virginia School of Medicine had found echinacea to be no more effective than a placebo at combating cold and flu symptoms.

But don't clear out your herbal medicine chest just yet.

What went largely unreported was that study participants received only 900 milligrams (mg) of echinacea daily—less than one-third of the dose recommended by the World Health Organization for combating upper-respiratory infections. That's akin to expecting one-third of a dose of aspirin to relieve a headache.

What's the other side of the story? Dozens of clinical studies point to echinacea's effectiveness, including a Canadian trial in which volunteers who took echinacea at the onset of colds experienced 23% milder and shorter symptoms, including sore throat, stuffy nose, chills and headache, than those who were taking a placebo

—a benefit that researchers link to a marked increase in circulating white blood cells and other cells of the immune system.

More work is needed to identify the optimal echinacea species (supplements are commonly derived from *E. purpurea*, *E. pallida* or *E. augustifolia*) and the most potent plant parts (roots, stems, leaves or flowers).

The best results have been achieved by taking 3,000 mg daily of an echinacea product that combines one of the above-mentioned species and parts at the first sign of a cold or flu and continuing this regimen until symptoms resolve.

Caution: If you're allergic to ragweed, avoid echinacea supplements that have been derived from stems, leaves or flowers—they may contain pollen and trigger a reaction. Use an echinacea root supplement.

Following are five other herbs that have scientific evidence on their side…

GARLIC

What it does: Helps prevent and possibly reverse arterial plaque buildup (atherosclerosis), a major cause of heart attack and stroke…reduces the risk of stomach and colorectal cancers…and acts as a blood thinner to reduce the risk of blood clots.

Scientific evidence: In a German study, 152 patients who had advanced atherosclerosis and took 900 mg of garlic powder daily for four years experienced a 3% decrease in existing arterial plaques in their *carotid* (neck) as well as their *femoral* (thigh) arteries.

Patients who took a placebo experienced more than a 15% *increase* in arterial plaques.

Potential side effects: Bad breath and indigestion. Because garlic has a blood-thinning effect, it should not be used if you take aspirin regularly or an anticoagulant drug, such as *warfarin* (Coumadin).

To minimize bleeding risk, ask your doctor about discontinuing garlic supplements at least one week before undergoing elective surgery.

Typical dose: One clove of fresh, minced garlic daily or 200 to 300 mg of standardized garlic powder, taken in pill or tablet form, three times daily.

GINKGO

What it does: Improves memory and concentration in people who have early-stage senile dementia or Alzheimer's disease, as well as in healthy adults, by increasing blood flow to the brain. May also relieve tinnitus (ringing in the ears), vertigo and altitude sickness, as well as vascular problems, such as *intermittent claudication*, a painful condition in the calf that is caused by decreased circulation to the legs.

Scientific evidence: An overwhelming majority of ginkgo trials have shown positive results. At least 33 randomized, controlled trials have shown that this herb enhances mental functioning or slows cognitive deterioration in older patients who have dementia. In addition, 13 other controlled studies have shown that ginkgo boosts memory and cognitive performance in healthy adults.

Potential side effects: Stomach upset, headache, rash and/or dizziness. Like garlic, ginkgo should not be taken with aspirin or a prescription blood thinner such as warfarin. The herb was previously believed to increase the effects of *monoamine oxidase inhibitor* (MAOI) antidepressants, such as *phenelzine* (Nardil), but this has been refuted.

Typical dose: 120 mg daily. Nearly all positive ginkgo trials have used one of three formulations that are produced in Germany and sold in health-food stores in the US under the brand names Ginkoba by Pharmaton Natural Health Products…Ginkgold by Nature's Way…and Ginkai by Abkit Inc.

MILK THISTLE

What it does: Because of its strong antioxidant activity, milk thistle detoxifies the liver and may help regenerate liver cells. It may be appropriate for patients who have alcohol-related liver damage or infectious or drug-induced hepatitis, as well as anyone who is regularly exposed to industrial pollutants.

Scientific evidence: At least 19 out of 21 clinical studies (a total of 2,200 people out of 2,400) have shown that milk thistle protects the liver against invasive toxins and possibly even stimulates the generation of new liver cells.

Potential side effect: Loose stools.

Typical dose: Take 140 mg of milk thistle three times daily.

SAW PALMETTO

What it does: Relieves symptoms of *benign prostatic hyperplasia* (BPH), a noncancerous swelling of the prostate gland, which causes frequent and/or weak urination and is common in men older than age 50.

Scientific evidence: In nearly two dozen clinical trials, saw palmetto has proven almost equal to prescription drugs, such as *finasteride* (Proscar) and *terazosin* (Hytrin), for relieving the symptoms of BPH. Unlike prescription prostate medications, which can cause side effects, including diminished libido, saw palmetto causes only minor adverse effects. Saw palmetto also does not inhibit the production of *prostate specific antigen* (PSA), a protein that, if elevated, may be an early warning for prostate cancer. Conventional BPH drugs suppress PSA, complicating prostate cancer screening.

Potential side effects: Stomach upset or nausea if taken on an empty stomach.

Typical dose: 320 mg daily. It requires four to six weeks to take effect.

VALERIAN

What it does: The root combats insomnia and acts as a mild sedative to relieve anxiety or restlessness.

Scientific evidence: All of the nearly 30 clinical studies to date have shown the herb to be effective against insomnia and anxiety. In a recent German trial, taking 600 mg of valerian root extract daily proved as effective as the prescription tranquilizer *oxazepam* (Serax) for improving sleep quality, but with fewer side effects. Unlike prescription sleep aids, valerian is not habit-forming, won't leave you feeling groggy the next morning and doesn't diminish alertness, reaction time or concentration.

Potential side effects: None known. It is best to avoid combining valerian with conventional sedatives, such as *diazepam* (Valium), since the herb may increase the drug's sedating effects.

Typical dose: 2 to 3 grams (g) of the dried, crushed root, infused as a tea…or 400 to 800 mg in supplement form, one-half hour before bed.

Unlock the Healing Power of Spices

David Winston, registered herbalist (RH), professional member of the American Herbalist Guild, and coauthor of *Herbal Therapy and Supplements: A Scientific and Traditional Approach.* Lippincott.

Traditional medicine has recognized the medicinal benefits of spices for thousands of years.

Now: A growing body of scientific evidence supports the use of spices to prevent—and even help treat—a variety of diseases, including arthritis, diabetes, cancer and Alzheimer's.* *Following are the new findings…*

CAYENNE PEPPER

What it does: Lowers cholesterol…helps prevent atherosclerosis…and reduces allergic responses. Cayenne's benefits can be attributed to the antioxidants, flavonoids and carotenoids it contains, all of which have anti-inflammatory effects and enhance circulation. An extract from cayenne pepper, called *capsaicin*, can be used in a topical cream to treat the pain from arthritis, shingles, bursitis, low-back ache and *neuropathy* (nerve pain). Capsaicin depletes nerve endings of *substance P*, a neurotransmitter that facilitates nerve transmission of pain.

Scientific evidence: A four-week study published in *The Journal of Rheumatology* found that patients who had osteoarthritis of the hands who applied capsaicin cream four times a day experienced reduced pain and tenderness.

Typical dose: Cayenne is available as a supplement in capsules and tincture. Take one capsule of cayenne pepper up to three times a day…or add three to eight drops of cayenne tincture to 4 ounces of water and drink two to four times a day. Apply topical cream containing capsaicin to painful areas as directed on the label. You can also season your food with powdered cayenne pepper or hot sauce.

Possible side effects: Cayenne pepper can cause gastric upset. If you take *warfarin* (Coumadin), do not use cayenne pepper supplements.

*Check with your doctor before using spices for medicinal purposes. They can interact with prescription medication.

Do not let topical capsaicin come in contact with your eyes or other mucus membranes—it can cause pain and burning.

CINNAMON

What it does: Helps prevent heart disease and type 2 diabetes.

Due to its antioxidant properties, cinnamon helps people who have *metabolic syndrome* (a cluster of factors, including excessive abdominal fat, high blood sugar and elevated blood pressure, that increase the risk of cardiovascular disease and type 2 diabetes) use the hormone insulin more efficiently.

Scientific evidence: A US Department of Agriculture (USDA) clinical study found that consuming capsules containing 1, 3 or 6 grams (g) of cinnamon daily (approximately ¼, ¾ or 1¼ teaspoons, respectively) for 40 days lowered blood levels of glucose and triglycerides (fats in the blood) by approximately 25% in adults who had type 2 diabetes. It also reduced LDL ("bad") cholesterol by up to 27%.

Typical dose: Use ½ to 1 teaspoon of powdered cinnamon daily on cereal or toast or mix into yogurt…take one capsule twice a day…or add 20 to 40 drops of tincture to 1 ounce of water and drink three times daily.

For tea, mix ¼ to ½ teaspoon of powdered cinnamon with 8 ounces of boiling water. Steep for 10 to 15 minutes, covered. Drink one 4-ounce cup up to three times a day.

Possible side effects: Because cinnamon can affect blood glucose levels, people who have diabetes should carefully monitor their blood sugar and ask their doctors if their medication needs to be adjusted.

GINGER

What it does: Reduces the pain and swelling caused by rheumatoid arthritis and osteo-arthritis…helps prevent the nausea and vomiting associated with motion sickness or pregnancy…enhances digestion and circulation…and eases intestinal gas.

Scientific evidence: Two clinical studies found that ginger relieved pain and/or swelling in 75% of arthritis patients.

Typical dose: Take one to two capsules with meals two to three times daily…or add 10 to 30 drops of the tincture to 1 ounce of water and drink three to four times daily.

For tea, mix ¼ to ½ teaspoon of powdered ginger (or use a ginger tea bag) with 8 ounces of boiling water. Steep for 10 to 15 minutes, covered. Drink 4 ounces up to three times daily.

Possible side effects: Ginger can have a blood-thinning effect, so check with your doctor before using it if you take an anticoagulant, such as warfarin. Ginger may cause an upset stomach in people who take doses larger than those described above.

TURMERIC

What it does: Helps prevent atherosclerosis, some types of cancer and Alzheimer's disease…reduces the pain and stiffness of rheumatoid arthritis and osteoarthritis…eliminates indigestion…and eases the symptoms of inflammatory bowel disease and irritable bowel syndrome (IBS). The beneficial effects of turmeric (also found in curry) are due to its anti-inflammatory compounds known as *curcuminoids*, as well as the essential oils and carotenoids it contains.

Scientific evidence: In a double-blind, placebo-controlled study, 116 people who had indigestion took either a 500-milligram (mg) capsule of curcumin (the substance that gives turmeric its yellow color) or a placebo four times a day. Nearly 90% of those taking curcumin experienced full or partial relief after seven days.

Typical dose: Take 250 to 500 mg of curcumin (standardized to 80% to 90% curcumin) three times daily…or add 40 to 60 drops of the tincture to 1 ounce of water and drink three to four times daily.

For tea, mix ½ teaspoon of powdered turmeric with 8 ounces of boiling water. Steep for 10 to 15 minutes, covered. Drink 4 ounces up to four times a day.

Possible side effects: Turmeric stimulates liver function, so it should be avoided by anyone who has gallstones or any other bile-duct obstruction. Preliminary studies show that curcumin may lessen the effectiveness of chemotherapy drugs, such as *doxorubicin* (Rubex) and *cyclophosphamide* (Cytoxan). If you are undergoing chemotherapy, talk to your doctor before taking curcumin.

■ ■ ■ ■

Curry Fights Skin Cancer

In a lab study of human cells, *curcumin* (the compound that makes curry yellow) was shown to interfere with the development of melanoma cells.

Past studies have shown that people who eat curry in abundance have lower rates of lung, colon, prostate and breast cancers.

Theory: Curcumin curbs inflammation, a risk factor for cancer.

Self-defense: Eat one-half tablespoon of curry every day.

Bharat B. Aggarwal, PhD, professor of cancer medicine, M.D. Anderson Cancer Center, University of Texas, Houston.

Natural Painkillers

Thomas Kruzel, ND, naturopathic physician, Scottsdale Natural Medicine and Healing Clinic, Scottsdale, AZ. He is associate professor of medicine, the National College of Naturopathic Medicine, Portland, OR, and past president of the American Association of Naturopathic Physicians.

If you have osteoarthritis or rheumatoid arthritis, the removal of *rofecoxib* (Vioxx) from the market because of reports linking it to heart attack and stroke took away one of your pain-relief options. You need a reliable painkiller—but does it have to be at the expense of your health? Absolutely not.

There are good alternatives. For centuries, herbs and other natural remedies have helped people cope with pain—without the unpleasant side effects and long-term health risks of many modern medications.

Natural painkillers, available at health-food stores, relieve arthritis pain, back pain and inflammation. Some deaden unpleasant sensations at the nerve itself. Others relax muscles or stimulate the release of *endorphins,* the brain's natural painkillers. Some painkillers strengthen affected joints. In some cases, they can take a bit longer to work than drugs, but they often provide all the pain relief you need.

HEALING HERBS

The best include…*

●**Arnica,** a homeopathic preparation that uses an ultra-diluted amount of the herb to stimulate pain relief. It is particularly effective at alleviating the soreness and stiffness of osteoarthritis and rheumatoid arthritis.

Typical dose: Follow label directions. Taken orally, in a 6X dilution, use three to four times a day…or in the stronger 30C dilution, once or twice daily. Arnica can be applied topically (as a cream or tincture) over the painful joint and covered with a heating pad.

●**Black cohosh,** a perennial herb native to North America. Although it is often used to curb menopausal symptoms, black cohosh is particularly effective for heavy, dull, aching rheumatoid arthritis and muscular pains.

Typical dose: 60 drops (approximately a standard teaspoon) of the tincture in 6 ounces of water three times a day. If you find that the herb causes mild stomach upset, take it with food.

●**Capsaicin,** the active ingredient of cayenne pepper. It is an effective topical painkiller.

Typical dose: Apply the cream two to three times daily.

●**Hops,** an herb that has a sedative effect. It can ease the nerve pain of rheumatoid arthritis.

Typical dose: One 300- or 500-milligram (mg) capsule two to three times daily…or 120 drops (approximately two teaspoons) of the liquid in 6 ounces of water three to four times daily.

●**Valerian,** a perennial plant native to North America and Europe. Better known as a sleep aid, valerian also relaxes extremely painful muscle spasms that can accompany arthritis.

Typical dose: One 300- or 500-mg capsule two to three times daily. If pain disrupts sleep, take one of the doses at bedtime.

NATURAL ANTI-INFLAMMATORIES

Inflammation triggers the pain of rheumatoid arthritis and flare-ups of osteoarthritis.

●**Protease enzymes,** derived from plants, are often taken to aid digestion, but they are also potent anti-inflammatories.

*Consult your physician before taking any of these herbs, especially if you are pregnant, nursing, have liver or kidney disease or are taking prescription medications.

Typical dose: Two 350-mg capsules three times a day between meals and two more capsules at bedtime.

•**Turmeric,** a popular spice (it is a major ingredient in curry powder), and *curcumin,* one of its key constituents, fight inflammation.

Typical dose: 500 mg three times daily.

FOOD FOR YOUR JOINTS

Natural arthritis care not only fights today's pain—but also aims to reduce tomorrow's aches by strengthening joints. One way of doing this is good nutrition. Consume an assortment of vegetables and fruits, especially green, leafy vegetables and antioxidant sources, such as carrots, broccoli, blueberries and cherries. Include cold-water fish, such as salmon, mackerel and halibut, at least three times a week.

Caution: Some people who have rheumatoid arthritis find that vegetables and fruits of the nightshade family (tomatoes, eggplant, green peppers, potatoes, etc.) worsen their symptoms.

If you have rheumatoid arthritis: Eliminate these foods from your diet for four to six weeks. Then reintroduce them one at a time to see if they worsen symptoms.

The following supplements are key for anyone who has arthritis...

•**Vitamin C** is a critical nutrient for the development of new joint tissue.

Typical dose: 2,000 to 5,000 mg daily in two divided doses at breakfast and dinner. Lower the dose if you develop diarrhea.

•**Minerals** are essential for strong bones and healthy joints.

Typical doses: Calcium (1,000 mg a day)... magnesium (500 mg a day)...and a multimineral supplement that contains manganese, zinc and boron.

•**Essential fatty acids** help control the natural chemicals that cause inflammation.

Typical dose: 1,000 mg of fish oil daily.

•**Glucosamine sulfate,** derived from crab, lobster or shrimp shells, and *chondroitin sulfate,* usually derived from shark cartilage, can be taken separately or together to supply the nutritional building blocks that are needed for new cartilage.

Typical dose: 1,500 mg daily, which often can be reduced to 500 mg when symptoms improve.

Important: It can take six to eight weeks for glucosamine and chondroitin to take full effect.

AT-HOME PHYSICAL THERAPY

In addition to taking natural painkillers, try these therapies...

•**Hot/cold therapy.** Alternately applying heat and cold increases and decreases blood flow to the joints, flushing out lactic acid, which irritates nerve endings.

What to do: First apply a heating pad on top of a moistened towel (place the heating pad in a waterproof bag for safety) to the painful joint for 10 minutes. Then, for two minutes, use a towel that has been moistened with cold water and chilled in the refrigerator. Repeat three or four times daily for acute pain.

•**Exercise.** Physical activity increases blood flow, which reduces pain in the long-term and helps improve the mobility of arthritic joints. But arthritis pain and concerns about joint injury can make people reluctant to exercise.

Solution: Do stretching exercises, yoga or tai chi in a warm room or warm pool—the warmth relaxes the muscles and eases pain. Exercising in a pool also reduces the impact on the joints.

MIND OVER PAIN

Stress-reduction techniques reduce the pain caused by arthritis and allow natural remedies to work more effectively.

•**Visualization** is particularly helpful.

What to do: Sit quietly in a place where you will not be disturbed, and play whatever music you find most relaxing. Close your eyes and imagine what your pain looks like, then visualize a scenario in which the pain becomes weaker and weaker.

Example: You might see the pain as a hot, red spot. Visualize it fading, cooling and gradually turning into a soft and soothing shade of blue. For best results, repeat this exercise daily for at least 10 minutes.

4 Herbs More Potent Than Viagra

Ray Sahelian, MD, board-certified family physician and nutritional consultant in private practice, Marina del Rey, CA. He is author of *Natural Sex Boosters* (Square One) and *Mind-Boosting Secrets* (Bottom Line).

The drug *sildenafil* (Viagra), introduced in 1998, revolutionized the treatment of sexual dysfunction. However, it and related drugs, such as *vardenafil* (Levitra) and *tadalafil* (Cialis), have significant limitations.

Although these impotence medications work well to promote blood flow to the penis, they have little or no effect on libido or sexual sensation in men—or in women.

These drugs also have potentially serious side effects, such as vision problems, and some doctors believe that they may be dangerous for men who have certain cardiac conditions, such as irregular heart rhythms or a history of heart attack or heart failure.

However, sex-boosting herbs have been used successfully for hundreds of years in Brazil, China, India and parts of Africa.

The following supplements,* which can be purchased at most health-food stores, can improve virtually every aspect of sexual performance, including increasing desire, creating stronger erections in men, and improving genital blood flow in men and women.

Start by choosing one herb that seems to best fit your needs. After one to two weeks, you can combine it with another supplement to enhance the effect. Or simply use a formula that combines these herbs.

Important: When combining herbs, cut the recommended dose of each in half to avoid potential side effects, such as restlessness.

HORNY GOAT WEED

This herb increases energy and libido in both men and women...and may produce firmer erections in men.

Horny goat weed reportedly got its name when a Chinese herder noticed that his goats

*Check with your doctor before taking any of these products.

became much more sexually active after eating the plant.

The herb is thought to influence levels of *dopamine* and other neurotransmitters that affect libido and mood. It also contains *flavonoids*, plant chemicals that dilate blood vessels and promote erections.

Scientific evidence: A study conducted in Beijing found that horny goat weed enhanced sexual activity in patients receiving dialysis for renal failure.

Typical dose: 500 to 2,000 milligrams (mg) daily. Start with 500 mg and increase, if needed. Side effects include restlessness and insomnia.

MUIRA PUAMA

This herb increases libido...orgasm intensity ...and skin and genital sensitivity in men as well as women.

The bark and roots of this Amazon tree, sometimes known as "potency wood," increase sexual desire and sexual fantasies in men and women, and also facilitate a woman's ability to have an orgasm.

Muira puama appears to work by promoting blood flow to the genitals.

Scientific evidence: A clinical study conducted at the Institute of Sexology in Paris found that taking muira puama for two weeks improved libido in 62% of the 262 men in the trial.

Typical dose: 500 to 1,000 mg in capsule form for three consecutive days each week.

Important: Muira puama should be taken in the morning—it can cause insomnia if it is taken in the afternoon or at night. It also may cause restlessness in some people during the daytime.

TRIBULUS

This herb increases energy and libido in both sexes...and improves erections in men.

This common roadside weed contains *proto-dioscin*, a chemical compound that is thought to increase the production of the sex hormone testosterone in both men and women.

It also dilates blood vessels in the penis, promoting firmer erections.

Scientific evidence: An animal study that was conducted at National University Hospital in Singapore showed that rats that were given tribulus for eight weeks had firmer erections.

Typical dose: 500 to 1,000 mg daily. Take tribulus for one week, then stop for one week, and so on. This minimizes the risk of side effects, such as restlessness and increased body temperature.

ASHWAGANDHA

This herb boosts mood and sexual desire and function in men and women.

It can improve sex drive in both sexes by acting as a relaxant, and it also helps men maintain an erection.

Ashwagandha produces a calming effect by mimicking the action of *gamma-aminobutyric acid* (GABA), a neurotransmitter in the brain that promotes relaxation.

It also boosts the production of nitric oxide, a substance that enhances penile erection and vaginal sensitivity by increasing the engorgement of the genital organs through blood vessel dilation.

Scientific evidence: A laboratory study conducted at the University of Texas Health Science Center found that ashwagandha inhibits the number of nerve cells that fire in the brain, much like the neurotransmitter GABA, resulting in an antianxiety and mood-enhancing effect.

Typical dose: 300 to 500 mg one to two times every day.

Important: For better absorption, take ashwagandha on an empty stomach.

Caution: Ashwagandha may cause drowsiness in some individuals. Do not drive after taking this herb.

■ ■ ■ ■

'Youthful' Scent

Women who wear a grapefruit scent appear to men to be approximately six years younger than they actually are.

Scents tested that had no effect: Broccoli, banana, spearmint leaves and lavender.

Alan Hirsch, MD, director, The Smell & Taste Treatment and Research Foundation, Chicago.

Saw Palmetto Won't Ease Enlarged Prostate

Stephen Bent, MD, assistant professor of medicine, University of California, San Francisco.

Ronald A. Morton, MD, professor of surgery, and chief, division of urology, Robert Wood Johnson Medical School, University of Medicine & Dentistry of New Jersey, and director, urologic oncology, Cancer Institute of New Jersey, both in New Brunswick.

Council for Responsible Nutrition.

The New England Journal of Medicine.

Millions of older American men use saw palmetto to treat an enlarged prostate, clinically known as *benign prostatic hyperplasia* (BPH), but a new study concludes that this herbal supplement is ineffective.

Several smaller studies had suggested that the extract might be of limited benefit, but this controlled, blinded study found that, "over a 12-month period, saw palmetto was no better than placebo in changing symptoms for this condition," according to lead researcher Dr. Stephen Bent, an assistant professor of medicine at the University of California, San Francisco.

THE STUDY

In the trial, researchers tracked the symptoms of 225 men over the age of 49 who had moderate to severe BPH. Half of the men took 160 milligrams (mg) of saw palmetto twice daily, while the other half took a placebo.

After one year, the researchers found no difference between the two groups in terms of symptoms, urine flow rates, prostate size, quality of life or blood levels of *prostate-specific antigen* (PSA), a marker for an enlarged prostate.

"Obviously, for anyone who holds saw palmetto in high regard, these results are a little bit disappointing," says Dr. Ronald A. Morton, director of urologic oncology at the Cancer Institute of New Jersey.

RESEARCH AMBIGUOUS

Bent notes that the research on the efficacy of saw palmetto for BPH has been ambiguous, with some studies suggesting a benefit and others finding it to be of no help at all.

"Those studies were of short duration, however, or they didn't use what is now the standard measure of symptoms," Bent says. Also, these prior studies were not always *blinded*, meaning the participants might have known if they were taking a placebo, which could bias the results.

Bent's team sought to address many of these issues, taking special care to ensure proper blinding and using a larger group of patients so the results would be statistically significant.

This research is "the most thorough and well-controlled study of the effect of saw palmetto on men with BPH that's ever been done," according to Morton.

---

*Obviously, for anyone who holds
saw palmetto in high regard,
these results are a little bit disappointing.*

Ronald A. Morton, MD

The researchers also went to great lengths to choose a top-notch product—in this case, a brand of saw palmetto capsules marketed in the United States by Rexall-Sundown Co. "We had an external advisory committee from the National Center for Complementary and Alternative Medicine—experts in the field—who evaluated a number of different extracts," Bent says. "They felt this was the best one."

In a statement, Andrew Shao, vice president of the Council for Responsible Nutrition, a supplements industry trade group, calls the findings "puzzling, given that more than 20 studies have shown promising findings for saw palmetto in alleviating symptoms commonly associated with prostate problems."

Morton agrees. "There are millions and millions of men out there who take saw palmetto. And if you review the literature on saw palmetto, it's really all over the map," he says

Shao admits that this study was well-designed, but speculates that the negative findings could be due to the study's focus on patients who had moderate to severe BPH. According to Shao, the bulk of the positive literature on saw palmetto involved men who had milder symptoms.

"The exclusion of those patients with mild symptoms may have reduced [the study's] ability to detect the benefits we've seen in other trials," he says.

WHAT TO DO

Because there's no evidence that saw palmetto poses any long-term safety risk, "if people are taking this and feel like they are getting some benefit, I think it's worth continuing," Bent advises.

Morton agrees that saw palmetto is probably safe, but he questions whether too many men plagued by BPH are using this ineffective remedy in lieu of conventional drugs whose efficacy is supported by clinical research.

"There are two medications that we commonly use for men with BPH," says Morton. "One includes drugs called *alpha blockers*, and the other group is *5-alpha-reductase inhibitors*. Alpha blockers cause a relaxation of the prostate that makes it easier for a man to urinate. And 5-alpha-reductase inhibitors shrink the prostate."

Either of these medications may be more effective than over-the-counter saw palmetto, he says.

info For more information on benign prostatic hyperplasia, visit the National Kidney and Urologic Diseases Information Clearinghouse at *http://kidney.niddk.nih.gov*. Click on "Kidney and Urologic Diseases," and scroll down to "BPH Benign Prostatic Hyperplasia."

Music Keeps Heartbeat Humming

Peter Sleight, MD, department of cardiovascular medicine, University of Oxford, Oxford, England.
Vincent Marchello, MD, vice president, medical affairs, Metropolitan Jewish Health System, and assistant professor of clinical medicine, Mount Sinai School of Medicine, both in New York City.
Heart.

New research has found that slow music produces a relaxing effect, and that musical pauses modulate heart rhythms and circulation patterns. The greatest benefits were seen in people who have musical training.

THE STUDY

Dr. Peter Sleight, of the department of cardiovascular medicine at the University of Oxford in England, and his team measured the physiologic responses of 12 musicians and 12 nonmusicians while they were listening to six different types of music. The music selections consisted of *raga* (Indian classical music), Beethoven's Ninth Symphony (slow classical), Red Hot Chili Peppers (funk), Vivaldi (fast classical), techno and Anton Webern (slow, dodecaphonic music).

Each participant listened to different sequences of music for two minutes, followed by the same selection for four minutes. Also included was a two-minute pause.

This is the first study to show that breathing can be easily and subconsciously entrained using music.

Peter Sleight, MD

Music that had fast tempos and simple rhythmic structures resulted in increased ventilation, blood pressure and heart rate, the researchers found. When the music was paused, heart rate, blood pressure and ventilation decreased, sometimes to levels that were even lower than the starting rate. This occurred regardless of the type of music, but the effect was stronger among the musicians, who are trained to measure their breathing with the music.

Slow music caused declines in heart rate, with the largest decline seen when the participants listened to raga music.

Overall, a person's musical preference had less of an impact on heart rate, blood pressure and ventilation than the music's pace, according to the researchers.

"Calm music with a slow tempo can entrain respiration to produce slower breathing," says Sleight. "This is the first study to show that breathing can be easily [and subconsciously] entrained using music."

Slower breathing has been linked to lower blood pressure and it may help the lungs work more efficiently.

MUSIC ENHANCES THERAPY

"Stress has its impact on cardiovascular disease. Music can not only reduce stress, but it can [also] enhance the therapy that one gets," says Dr. Vincent Marchello, vice president of medical affairs for the Metropolitan Jewish Health System and assistant professor of clinical medicine

at Mount Sinai School of Medicine, both in New York City.

Music already plays a therapeutic role for many of Marchello's patients. His staff has successfully used music to calm the behavior of agitated Alzheimer's patients. And in the post-surgery cardiac rehab ward, Marchello says, "Music can improve rehab therapy sessions and can make the sessions more efficient and shorten the time needed to get better."

Playing music that the patient likes may also have a positive impact on the therapy, Marchello notes. "Music is one thing we do to motivate patients. It has to be what they prefer."

Earlier research has shown that rhythmic poetry, such as Homer's *The Odyssey*, that is read aloud can synchronize the body's heart and respiration rates. Similar positive effects have been linked to the Catholic rosary prayers and to a yoga mantra.

Music has also been shown to have other beneficial properties, including improving athletic performance and enhancing motor function in people who have neurological impairments.

Up until now, however, there had been no comprehensive comparisons of how different types of music and the way they are presented might affect autonomic, cardiovascular and respiratory functioning.

info Learn more about music's effect on health at the Texas Center for Music & Medicine at *www.unt.edu/tcmm*.

■ ■ ■ ■

Breathing Device Lowers Blood Pressure

Approved by the US Food and Drug Administration (FDA), Resperate guides people through deep-breathing exercises. As breathing slows, muscles surrounding the small blood vessels relax, so blood flows more freely and blood pressure drops.

The device includes a sensor belt to monitor breathing, a handheld computer unit and headphones. Musical tones delivered through the headphones indicate when to inhale and exhale. Resperate should be used for 15 minutes at least three times a week.

Results after eight weeks: People who used Resperate for an average of 23 minutes per week had a 15-point decrease in blood pressure. The effect was greater in elderly people and people who had stage 2 hypertension. Most people who used the device also took blood pressure medication.

Resperate may be covered by insurance.

info For more information, call 877-988-9388, or visit the Web site, *www.resperate.com.*

William Elliott, MD, PhD, professor of preventive medicine, internal medicine and pharmacology, Rush University Medical College, Chicago.

Acupuncture Can Be as Effective as Botox

Mary Elizabeth Wakefield, licensed acupuncturist, New York City.
Shellie Goldstein, licensed acupuncturist, New York City and East Hampton, NY.
Laurie A. Casas, MD, associate professor of surgery, Feinberg School of Medicine, Northwestern University, Chicago, and spokeswoman, American Society for Aesthetic Plastic Surgery.

Facial acupuncture is gaining popularity, especially among Baby Boomers who want to diminish signs of aging.

There are other forces driving demand, too, including consumers who are tired or wary of repeated Botox injections. So, business-savvy acupuncturists are marketing their alternative approach as a holistic solution.

THE PROCEDURE

In facial acupuncture, the practitioner inserts small needles into "pressure points" in the face. According to supporters, this boosts blood flow to the area, producing tighter muscles and a more youthful appearance.

No one seems to know how many licensed acupuncturists in the United States offer such facial rejuvenation, but Mary Elizabeth Wakefield, a New York City acupuncturist, says she has taught more than 1,000 of her colleagues the technique.

Shellie Goldstein, an acupuncturist who practices in New York City and East Hampton, New York, has trademarked the name of her technique, Acufacial, which, she says, is good for the "marionette lines" around the sides of the mouth that appear when you smile, the nose-to-lip wrinkles called nasolabial lines and the frown lines between the eyebrows, as well as other areas.

Facial acupuncture "is as effective as Botox for fine lines, almost as effective with deeper wrinkles—and without paralyzing the muscles," Goldstein says.

DIFFERENCES IN COST AND TIME

Facial acupuncture tends to cost more and demand more time than Botox. Typical New York–area fees for facial acupuncture range from $140 to $200 per session, with 10 to 20 weekly sessions recommended, followed by monthly maintenance sessions. With that fee schedule, a typical first-year bill would be $2,800 or more, and $4,400 for two years. If you follow that schedule, Goldstein says, you can expect the effects to last for two years.

Acupuncture is as effective as Botox for fine lines— and without paralyzing the muscles.

Shellie Goldstein

For Botox injections, the average physician's fee is $376 (it may be higher in metropolitan areas), according to the American Society of Plastic Surgeons, and the procedure is repeated every three months.

SCIENTIFIC TESTS ARE NEEDED

Cosmetic surgeons don't dismiss the idea that facial acupuncture is effective, but for now published scientific evidence is lacking, they say.

Dr. Laurie A. Casas, a cosmetic surgeon, an associate professor of surgery at Northwestern University's Feinberg School of Medicine and a spokeswoman for the American Society for Aesthetic Plastic Surgery, says, "I never, ever dismiss any modality that has been around that many thousands of years." But, she adds, "I think it is critical that this group of very fine practitioners do some studies and then show us" that it works.

While some studies have been published suggesting that facial acupuncture reduces lines and wrinkles, Casas says that what is needed is a good scientific study—one in which acupuncture is performed on one side of the face and Botox or no procedure on the other side. Then, photo documentation could show the effects of each.

info To find an acupuncturist, visit the National Certification Commission for Acupuncture and Oriental Medicine Web site at *www. nccaom.org.*

■ ■ ■ ■

Super Sunburn Soothers

To ease the sting of a sunburn, apply cool raw slices of cucumber, apple or potato to skin. Or use aloe vera, either in commercial gel form or squeezed fresh from a plant. Never apply vitamin E—it may cause dermatitis. Soothe burned eyelids using tea bags that have been soaked in cool water. To make a compress for inflamed skin, soak a cloth in apple cider vinegar, witch hazel or a mixture of one part skim milk to four parts water and wring halfway. Apply for five to 10 minutes.

Caution: If blisters develop, do not treat the sunburn yourself—see a doctor.

Neal Schultz, MD, dermatologist, 1130 Park Ave., New York City 10128.

Sweet! All-Natural Cures For Bad Breath

Jamison Starbuck, ND, a naturopathic physician in family practice, a lecturer at the University of Montana, Missoula, and past president of the American Association of Naturopathic Physicians. She is a contributing editor to *The Alternative Advisor: The Complete Guide to Natural Therapies and Alternative Treatments.* Time Life.

Few doctors note the scent of a patient's breath during physical exams, but I'm a firm believer in this practice. *Halitosis* (bad breath) can provide several useful diagnostic clues. Although most people associate bad breath with poor oral hygiene, the more common cause is infection—such as a cold, tonsillitis or allergic congestion. Diets that are high in sugar and/or fat also lead to bad breath because

these foods trigger indigestion, which results in the undigested food becoming putrified.

Breath odor is due, in part, to what is happening in our lungs.

Example: For at least 24 hours after we eat garlic, our lungs excrete *methyl mercaptan*, the compound that causes garlic's odor. Brushing your teeth or gargling will temporarily mask the scent in your mouth, but it doesn't change the odor that's exhaled from your lungs.

If you think you have halitosis, ask your spouse or a close friend to smell your breath. *If the report is bad, consider these suggestions for the following common causes...*

●**Allergies or colds.** In addition to whatever treatment you choose for your allergy or cold, gargle with a solution combining saline and essential oils of eucalyptus and thyme. The essential oils not only clear away mucus and freshen breath, but they also act as an antiseptic to kill germs. My favorite gargling solution is Alka-Thyme, which is available at health-food stores or can be purchased from Heritage Products, 800-862-2923, *www.caycecures.com.* For best results, gargle for 60 seconds twice a day until your cold or allergy symptoms are gone.

●**Tonsillitis.** If you have enlarged tonsils, add fenugreek tea to your daily regimen. Fenugreek reduces swelling and inflammation in the tonsils and lymphatic system, eventually eliminating bad breath. Use 1 teaspoon of fenugreek seeds per cup of water. Gently simmer for 10 minutes, then strain and drink 16 ounces each day. If your tonsils remain enlarged for more than one week, see your doctor. You may have a bacterial infection.

●**Indigestion.** Coffee not only leaves a bitter residue in the mouth, but also interferes with digestion. Both of these problems lead to bad breath. That's why I prefer peppermint, spearmint or chamomile tea. These herbs freshen the mouth, enhance digestion and reduce gas.

If you're consuming a lot of sugar and/or fat, cut back on both. Substitute fresh fruit for sweets, eat vegetables and green salads, and drink eight glasses of water daily to improve your breath. Culinary herbs can also help. Carry dill, fennel or anise seeds with you instead of breath mints. Chew one-half teaspoon of one of the seeds.

The volatile oils in these seeds aid digestion and improve breath without the sugars and chemicals found in breath mints.

If these suggestions don't help, see your doctor. You may have a dental infection or a health problem, such as diabetes or liver or kidney failure, that natural bad breath remedies simply can't cure.

■ ■ ■ ■

Freshen Your Breath With a Cup of Tea

You can freshen your breath by drinking a cup of tea. *Polyphenols* found in green and black tea inhibit the growth of odor-causing bacteria. Drinking one to two cups of tea every day can help keep your breath fresh.

Christine D. Wu, PhD, professor of periodontics and associate dean for research, University of Illinois at Chicago College of Dentistry.

■ ■ ■ ■

Two Great Hiccup Stoppers

Pour a tall glass of water. While holding your breath and pinching your nostrils, take small sips until you feel like you are drowning. Stop, inhale deeply and breathe normally.

Alternative: Ice the nerve fibers responsible for hiccups.

Find your Adam's apple—for women, this is approximately two inches below the chin. Move your finger around your neck to just above the middle of your *clavicle*, the protruding bone at the base of the neck. Apply ice cubes to each side of the neck at those points until the hiccuping stops.

See your doctor if your hiccups last more than 48 hours.

John T. Walbaum, author of *The Know-It-All's Guide to Life*. Career.

11

Nutrition, Diet & Fitness

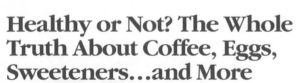

Healthy or Not? The Whole Truth About Coffee, Eggs, Sweeteners…and More

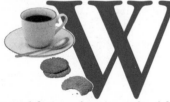

We're bombarded by conflicting information about foods and health, and the result is confusion. Is milk good for our bones or bad for our hearts? Is fish a source of healthful fats or dangerous toxins? Are artificial sweeteners smart low-calorie alternatives to sugar or dangerous chemicals?

Here is a closer look at the controversies about common foods…

FISH

Fish is a wonderful source of protein, vitamins, minerals and *omega-3 fatty acids*. However, the nutritional benefits of omega-3 fatty acids fall short of their hype. Some scientists claim that they are great for the heart as well as for improving children's ability to learn, but all we can say for sure is that omega-3s may be beneficial.

Also, because of water pollution and some fish-farming techniques, fish can contain *methylmercury* and *polychlorinated biphenyls* (PCBs). High amounts of these chemicals can cause children to experience muscle weakness, fatigue, headaches and severe developmental problems.

Bottom line: Eat fish if you enjoy it, but remember certain caveats…

• **Limit your consumption of large predatory fish,** which are likely to contain the most methylmercury (shark, swordfish, king mackerel, albacore tuna and tilefish), to no more than twice per week. Do not eat the fish at all if you are or might become pregnant—and don't feed these fish to children.

• **Select wild fish over farm-raised.** Farm-raised fish—salmon, in particular—can have higher concentrations of PCBs than the same fish that have been raised in the wild.

• **Don't regularly eat fish that have been caught in freshwater** without first checking

Marion Nestle, PhD, MPH, professor of nutrition, food studies and public health, New York University, New York City, and author of *What to Eat*. North Point.

222

with state health or wildlife officials. Unless you know that the water the fish came from is safe, assume that it's not. Consuming a few fish every year from a local lake or stream should be fine, but the health risks climb as you eat more.

COFFEE

It's full of caffeine, a mild "upper" and millions of people drink it by the quart every day—surely coffee must be bad for us.

In fact, there's little evidence that there's anything in coffee that's harmful to our health—and it may even be good for us. Coffee contains antioxidants believed to promote good health.

Bottom line: You can enjoy coffee without guilt, but don't put in too much sugar, milk or cream. A 12-ounce caffè latte breve at Starbucks has 420 calories and 23 grams (g) of saturated fat—more fat than you should consume in an entire day. If you become nervous or shaky when you drink coffee, you may be sensitive to caffeine. Reduce your intake or switch to decaf.

EGGS

Eggs are widely considered unhealthy because they are high in cholesterol—higher than any other food. But when eaten in limited quantities, eggs are good for you. They're relatively low in calories and are a good source of protein.

Some producers feed the hens flaxseed and fish oil to boost the eggs' omega-3 content—but these "omega-3 eggs" cost more, and it's not clear that they are actually any better for you.

Note: There's no difference between a brown egg and a white egg except the color of the shell.

Bottom line: The American Heart Association recommends no more than one egg per day from all sources. If your doctor has warned you to watch your cholesterol, cut down on eggs or eat egg whites, which have no cholesterol.

MARGARINE

Margarines do have significantly less saturated fat and cholesterol than butter, so a *non-hydrogenated* (no trans fats) margarine is a healthy alternative. It certainly is cheaper than butter. But if you are not eating much of either, this decision isn't going to have a major effect on your health. Personally, I prefer butter. I just don't eat much of it. If you like margarine, you can choose from vegan or organic margarines, omega-3 margarines and "light" low-calorie/low-fat margarines—but these cost significantly more than standard margarines, and the difference they make to your health will be small, at best.

Bottom line: If you like margarine, choose one with no trans fats.

ARTIFICIAL SWEETENERS

The US Food and Drug Administration (FDA) has approved artificial sweeteners because there is no compelling evidence that they cause harm at current levels of intake. But I am not a fan of them. I can't believe any food that has that kind of chemical taste can be good for you. Their single virtue is the absence of calories, but there is not much evidence that their use has helped people lose weight. Perhaps people who use them compensate by eating more calories from other sources. Or perhaps artificial sweeteners reinforce our preference for sweets. Personally, I prefer sugar—just not much of it.

Bottom line: If you are trying to lose weight, it is best to eat less, move around more and avoid junk foods.

MILK

For decades, dairy trade associations and lobbying groups have told Americans that drinking milk strengthens bones. Now they claim that dairy helps us lose weight. As in many aspects of nutrition, the evidence linking dairy foods to health conditions is complicated and contradictory. Dairy foods may have lots of calcium and other nutrients, but they are high in saturated fat (the bad kind) and calories.

Bottom line: If you want to avoid the fat and saturated fat, choose nonfat options. If you don't like or can't tolerate milk, you can get the nutrients it contains from other foods. Consuming dairy foods is not the key to bone health. The best advice for bone health—and for almost any other health condition—is to eat a diet containing plenty of fruits, vegetables and whole grains, don't smoke cigarettes, be active and don't drink alcohol to excess.

These good habits mean more to your health than the effects of any one food.

■ ■ ■ ■

Strong Onions Improve Health

Anew study has found that strong-flavored red and yellow onions and shallots tend to have the most *flavonoids*—antioxidants that help reduce the risk of heart disease, diabetes and some forms of cancer.

Rui Hai Liu, MD, PhD, associate professor of food science, Cornell University, Ithaca, NY.

The Miracle Food Every Man Should Eat...and Most Women, Too

Mark Messina, PhD, associate professor of nutrition, Loma Linda University, Loma Linda, CA, and former program director, diet and cancer branch, National Cancer Institute. He is an coauthor of The Simple Soybean and Your Health. Avery.

Soy is one of the few foods that the US Food and Drug Administration (FDA) allows to have a health claim on the label. The claim states that diets that are low in saturated fat and cholesterol and that include 25 grams (g) of soy protein per day may reduce a person's risk of heart disease.

Evidence suggests that soy may be helpful for a range of other diseases, including osteoporosis and some kinds of cancer. However, other studies suggest that it may increase the risk of breast cancer. *Here's what you need to know...*

SOY BENEFITS FOR YOU

Preliminary research suggests that soy may be helpful for the following conditions...

●**Cardiovascular disease.** The Japanese consume an average of 11 g of soy protein per day per person—and the rate of heart disease in Japan is among the lowest in the world. (Americans consume an average of 2 g of soy per day.) *How soy helps...*

●Soy protein lowers LDL ("bad") cholesterol by 4% to 5%—more when it is used as a substitute for red meat or other dietary sources of saturated fat. Soy protein may increase the activity of *cellular receptors*, which "trap" LDL and take it out of circulation.

●Soy is rich in *isoflavones*, a class of chemical compounds that act like weaker versions of the hormone estrogen. Isoflavones, known as *phytoestrogens*, enhance the ability of arteries to relax and/or dilate, improving blood flow. This is true for men and women.

●Soy lowers blood pressure by as much as 15 points, according to some studies. Other studies, however, have shown more modest or no effects.

●Soy has *linolenic acid*, which may reduce heart disease mortality by 20%.

●**Prostate cancer.** Japanese men have significantly less incidence of prostate cancer than American men, possibly due to soy. A study of cancer patients found that levels of *prostate-specific antigen* (PSA), an indicator of prostate cancer, leveled off in men who were given soy isoflavones for six months. Isoflavones are believed to inhibit the enzymes that fuel the growth of tumors.

Most men will develop prostate cancer at some point in their lives. This cancer grows slowly, so it may never cause related health problems—but prostate cancer still is the second-leading cause of cancer deaths among men (lung cancer is the first). I advise every man to eat soy.

●**Menopausal discomfort.** The phytoestrogens in soy are metabolized in the body into *equol*, an estrogen-like compound. Soy seems to be most effective for women who experience five or more hot flashes a day—it can reduce hot-flash frequency by up to 40%. Some menopausal women who eat soy also notice an improvement in vaginal dryness.

●**Diabetic renal disease.** One of the most serious complications of diabetes is kidney disease, which can lead to kidney failure. Substituting soy for animal protein lowers the *glomerular filtration rate*, a measure of kidney stress, and may slow kidney damage.

STUDIES NEEDED

Soy may be helpful for the following conditions, but research so far is inconclusive...

●**Osteoporosis.** Soy has been promoted for bone strength on the mistaken premise that Asian women have less incidence of osteoporosis than American women. Not true. While their rate of hip fractures is lower than in the US, the Japanese have twice the rate of vertebral fractures. The difference in hip fractures is probably due to a difference in anatomy, which makes the hip less likely to break on impact.

Other evidence suggests that isoflavones do promote bone strength. The US Department of Agriculture (USDA) and the National Institutes of Health (NIH) are currently allotting significant resources—approximately $10 million—for studies to determine whether isoflavones play a role in bone health.

●**Breast cancer.** Asian studies indicate that women who eat soy foods three or more times weekly have a reduced risk of breast cancer.

However, some researchers believe that soy may raise the risk of breast cancer. Most breast tumors are stimulated by estrogen. A diet high in isoflavones, which mimic some of estrogen's effects, could stimulate tumor growth in women who have these estrogen-positive tumors.

Animal studies conducted at the University of Illinois found that isoflavones increased tumor growth—yet similar studies at Harvard University showed the opposite. No one knows if soy isoflavones have any effect on breast cancer in humans. A recent two-year study of premenopausal women found that soy had no effect on breast tissue density, an indicator of cancer risk.

MORE ON SOY

Some people don't eat soy because they're just not familiar with it. The soybean is a member of the *legume* (pea) family. It forms clusters of three to five pods, each with two to four beans. Tofu, miso, tempeh and other foods made from soy contain isoflavones. Some soy products, such as soy sauce and soy oil, contain soy but are not good sources of isoflavones.

■ ■ ■ ■

Thai Tofu Kebabs

This recipe, from the Soyfoods Association of North America (*www.soyfoods.org*), is a great way to incorporate soy into your diet.

⅓ cup fresh lime juice (about 2 limes)
1 Tbsp soy sauce
1 garlic clove, chopped
2 Tbsp chopped Thai or Italian basil

½ tsp hot red pepper flakes
¼ tsp freshly ground black pepper
¼ cup olive oil
1 pound firm or extra firm tofu in one block
4-inch piece of cucumber, peeled
1 medium red onion, halved vertically and cut into half-inch crescents
8 cherry tomatoes

To make the marinade, combine the lime juice, soy sauce, garlic, basil, red pepper flakes, black pepper and olive oil in a resealable plastic bag. Cut the pressed tofu into 12 cubes. Add the tofu to the bag. Marinate in the refrigerator for at least four hours and up to 24 hours.

Soak four 10-inch bamboo skewers in water for 15 to 30 minutes. Preheat a grill to medium-high or a broiler.

Halve the cucumber lengthwise. Scoop out the seeds using a teaspoon. Cut each piece into 1-inch crescents.

To assemble, slip a cucumber piece almost to the bottom of a skewer. Add a tofu chunk. Slip on two or three onion crescents, followed by a tomato. Repeat.

Grill or broil kebabs for two minutes. Brush them with some marinade. Cook another minute. Turn and cook two to three minutes, until the tofu is hot and the vegetables lightly charred, brushing them with marinade halfway through. Serves four.

■ ■ ■ ■

Changing Your Goals

Federal recommendations suggest that Americans eat nine servings of fruit and vegetables a day—up from five servings. Consider the recommendations a goal—not a requirement. The biggest dietary health improvement comes to people who increase their intake of fruit and vegetables from one serving a day to two. Everything above that brings a smaller benefit. The same applies to the new exercise guidelines, which call for 60 minutes of exercise most days to avoid gaining weight. Consider that a goal—the old recommendation of 30 minutes still brings substantial health benefits.

Consensus of nutrition researchers, reported in *The New York Times.*

The Deadliest Fats Ever Made

Mary Enig, PhD, fellow, American College of Nutrition, and president, Maryland Nutritionists Association. She is author of *Know Your Fats* (Bethesda Press) and *Eat Fat, Lose Fat* (Penguin).

The US government recently mandated that trans fatty acids be listed on the nutrition facts label of every food. However, that's not enough to ensure that you're not getting these in your diet.

To learn about trans fatty acids—and how to avoid them—we spoke to Mary Enig, a biochemist and one of the first experts to warn people about the dangers of trans fatty acids.

THE MAKING OF TRANS FATTY ACIDS

Trans fatty acids, also known as trans fats, are solid fats that are produced artificially by a process known as *partial hydrogenation*.

Background: In the 1980s, many restaurants and food manufacturers switched to using vegetable oils, such as soybean, corn and canola, when the lard, butter and beef fat that were typically used for cooking were found to be high in saturated fat, which increases the risk for obesity and heart disease.

Because these vegetable oils are not stable when heated, manufacturers began using partial hydrogenation to make the oil more solid.

This process extends the shelf life of the oil and of the products made with it. The process also provides the texture, or "mouth-feel," of butter.

The hydrogenation process: A vegetable oil is first refined using chemical solvents and is then mixed with a metal catalyst, such as nickel oxide. The vegetable oil is then subjected to hydrogen gas in a high-pressure, high-temperature reactor. After that, deodorizing agents and bleaches are added.

This hydrogenation process not only creates a cheaper, cleaner-smelling, longer-lasting alternative to lard, butter and beef fat, it also changes the molecular configuration of the oil, resulting in a substance that bears no nutritional resemblance to the healthful vegetable oil from which it was derived.

Partially hydrogenated vegetable oil has become the primary fat used in food manufacturing in the US.

DANGERS OF TRANS FATS

Trans fats make the coronary arteries more rigid and contribute to the formation of blood clots, which can lead to heart attack or stroke. Trans fats also reduce HDL ("good") cholesterol levels and increase LDL ("bad") cholesterol.

According to a study by Dr. Walter Willett, chairman of the department of nutrition at the Harvard School of Public Health, approximately 30,000 premature heart disease deaths each year can be attributed to the consumption of trans fats.

According to Harvard University's landmark Nurses' Health Study, the consumption of just 2 to 3 grams (g) of trans fats daily—the amount typically found in three to six cookies—increases the risk of coronary heart disease by 21%.

Other studies have linked trans fat consumption to diabetes and obesity.

FOODS HIGH IN TRANS FATS

Approximately 40% of the food in supermarkets contains trans fats. This harmful substance is found in 95% of cookies, 80% of frozen breakfast foods, 75% of snacks and chips, 70% of cake mixes and almost 50% of all cereals. And these foods contain plenty of it.

Examples: Products that have the most trans fats include vegetable shortening, doughnuts, stick margarine, french fries (trans fats account for approximately 40% of the total fat content)…and many cookies and crackers (35% to 50% of fat content is from trans fats).

Eating establishments are exempt from the new trans fat labeling laws, but fast-food restaurants are among the worst offenders.

Example: A typical apple Danish from a doughnut shop contains approximately 2.7 g of trans fats…two vegetable spring rolls from a Chinese restaurant contain 1.7 g…five chicken nuggets and a large order of french fries from a fast-food restaurant contain nearly 4 g and 7 g, respectively…a piece of baked apple pie can contain 4.5 g.

READ LABELS CAREFULLY

In 2002, the American Heart Association's Scientific Conference on Dietary Fats said, "The optimal diet for reducing the risk for chronic disease is one in which trans fatty acids from manufactured fats are virtually eliminated."

Translation: There is no safe level of trans fats. To eliminate them from your diet, you must carefully read labels and the nutritional charts provided by some fast-food restaurants.

Caution: The US Food and Drug Administration (FDA) labeling laws allow a manufacturer to say "0 trans fats" if a product contains 0.5 g or less per serving. (For more information on why this is allowed on food labels and why it can be dangerously unhealthy, as those grams add up quickly, read the following article.)

SAFE FOODS

All fresh fruits and vegetables, fresh meat, poultry and fish, eggs, milk, cheese and yogurt are free of trans fats. Canned fish also is free of trans fats.

But watch out for processed cheeses, for example, the kind in many "snack packs"—they may contain trans fats.

Important: Trans fats are not formed when you cook—or even fry—at home with vegetable oil. They are created in frying oil only when the oil is reused after cooking a food that contains trans fats—a common practice in fast-food restaurants.

Trans Fat on Food Labels: Now You See It, Now You Don't

Barbara Schneeman, PhD, director, Office of Nutritional Products, Labeling and Dietary Supplements, US Food and Drug Administration.
Samantha Heller, MS, RD, senior clinical nutritionist, New York University Medical Center, New York City.

The latest US Food and Drug Administration (FDA) rules allow manufacturers to list "0 trans fats" on the labels of foods that have less than 0.5 grams (g) of trans fats per serving.

Because official serving sizes are often unrealistically small, it would be easy to consume several servings a day of products that have less than 0.5 g of trans fat, resulting in a significant intake during the course of a week.

Example: Benecol, a soft-spread substitute for margarine or butter, is advertised as promoting heart health by lowering cholesterol. It does this—but it also contains "less than" 0.5 g of trans fats per tablespoon.

This means that if you used one tablespoon four times a day, which is the amount recommended to lower cholesterol, you could consume nearly 14 g of trans fats in a week, just from Benecol spread alone.

Many companies are replacing trans fats with saturated fats. Just because something has zero trans fats doesn't mean people can eat as much as they want.

Samantha Heller, MS, RD

That's important because trans fats, like saturated fats, can raise the risk of heart disease by increasing levels of LDL ("bad") cholesterol.

Currently, the FDA estimates that Americans consume an average 5.8 g of trans fats per day.

EXPLANATION

Barbara Schneeman, director of the FDA's Office of Nutritional Products, Labeling and Dietary Supplements, says the reason the FDA is allowing foods containing less than 0.5 g of trans fats to be rounded down to 0 is that current detection methods for trans fats are not very reliable for amounts less than 0.5 g.

However, nutritionist Samantha Heller, from New York University Medical Center, takes a different view. "I don't understand why that's acceptable. It will add up over time." she says.

LOOK FOR 'HYDROGENATED'

To protect yourself from unknowingly consuming too many trans fats, Heller suggests,

"If you see a food with 0 trans fat, check the ingredient list. Look for the words, 'partially hydrogenated.' If you see partially hydrogenated, that means the product contains some trans fats."

The FDA adds that products that have shortening or hydrogenated oils in their ingredient lists also contain some trans fats, and if they appear at the beginning of the ingredient list, the product contains more trans fats than if they are further down on the list.

However, both Heller and Schneeman emphasize that trans fats are only part of the picture. "You can't look at trans fat alone. Some manufacturers might have eliminated trans fat by using products that are high in saturated fat," says Schneeman.

"What we encourage consumers to do to help lower their cardiovascular risk is to look at trans fat, saturated fat and cholesterol levels. A product can have 0 grams of trans fat, but what is the amount of saturated fat?" Schneeman adds.

"Be careful," says Heller. "Many companies are replacing trans fats with saturated fats. Just because something has zero trans fats doesn't mean people can eat as much as they want."

■■■■

What Are Trans Fats?

Trans fats are created when liquid oils are transformed into solids through a process called *hydrogenation.*

Trans fats are prevalent in many processed foods because they add to a product's shelf life and increase flavor stability.

Most of the foods that contain trans fats should be eaten in moderation anyway—even if they didn't contain trans fats.

Trans fats are often found in deep-fried restaurant foods, as well as in doughnuts, cookies, cakes and muffins.

info To learn more about trans fats, visit the US Food and Drug Administration Web site at *www.fda.gov/oc/initiatives/transfat.* Click on "What Every Consumer Should Know About Trans Fatty Acids."

Beware of These Dangerous Food–Drug Combinations

Earl Mindell, RPh, PhD, emeritus professor of nutrition, Pacific Western University, Los Angeles, and a director of the corporate board, Illinois College of Physicians and Surgeons. He is author of *Natural Remedies for 150 Ailments* (Basic Health) and *Bottom Line's Prescription Alternatives* (Bottom Line).

Some foods can interact with drugs in potentially dangerous ways. Foods, like drugs, are complex mixtures of chemical compounds. When some drugs and foods are taken simultaneously, the combination may increase or decrease blood levels of the drug in the body or speed or slow the drug's absorption into the bloodstream.

Example: Thiazide diuretics, one class of drugs used to treat high blood pressure and other conditions, cause the body to excrete potassium and magnesium. Taking them and eating salty foods can increase mineral loss and result in deficiencies.

That's why it's important to always ask your doctor or pharmacist if certain foods should be avoided when taking a medication. Drug instruction sheets provide minimal information. They are usually limited to whether to take medications with food (to protect the stomach) or on an empty stomach (to speed absorption).

MAIN OFFENDERS

●**Broccoli, cabbage and other leafy greens.** These foods are high in vitamin K, which can promote blood clotting and counteract the effects of blood thinners such as *warfarin* (Coumadin).

It's fine to eat small amounts—say, two or three weekly servings—of vitamin K–rich foods when taking an anticoagulant, but ask your doctor about eating more than that.

●**Grapefruit.** Both the juice and the whole fruit block liver enzymes that break down and clear drugs from the body. Eating grapefruit when you're on certain medications is like taking a higher dose, which can result in excessive levels of the drug in the blood.

Don't combine grapefruit with the statin drugs *lovastatin* (Mevacor) or *simvastatin* (Zocor)…

calcium channel blockers, such as *amlodipine* (Norvasc) and *diltiazem* (Cardizem)…benzo-diazepine tranquilizers (such as Valium)…or the antihistamine *loratadine* (Claritin). Wait one to two hours after taking any of these drugs before having grapefruit or grapefruit juice.

•**Bran muffins, whole-grain cereals and other high-fiber foods.** Fiber slows the absorption of *penicillin, ampicillin* and other antibiotics. In some cases, it binds to drugs in the intestine and prevents most of the active ingredient from entering the blood.

Warning: Fiber can also block the absorption of the heart drug *digoxin* (Lanoxin). Don't consume high-fiber foods or fiber supplements within two hours of taking this drug.

•**Dairy.** The calcium in dairy foods reduces the absorption of the antibiotic *tetracycline*. If you are taking tetracycline for an infection, take it one hour before or two hours after eating dairy foods or taking a calcium supplement.

•**Tyramine-rich foods.** Many cheeses (such as American, cheddar, blue and Parmesan), cured meats (such as salami, bacon and pepperoni), liver, red wine and beer contain *tyramine*. It's a chemical compound that can cause a potentially fatal rise in blood pressure in people who take older-generation antidepressants called *monoamine oxidase inhibitors* (MAOIs).

People who take MAOIs, such as *phenelzine* (Nardil) and *procarbazine* (Matulane), should never eat foods that contain tyramine. Ask your doctor or pharmacist for a complete list of foods that contain it.

•**Soft drinks.** The carbonation, sugar and phosphoric acid in soft drinks can greatly speed absorption and raise blood levels of *ketoconazole* (Nizoral), an oral drug taken for fungal infections. Avoid regular and diet sodas while taking this drug.

•**Rhubarb.** This vegetable contains natural chemicals that increase blood pressure and can reduce the effects of antihypertensive drugs such as *hydrochlorothiazide.*

Ask your doctor about: Eating five medium stalks of celery daily when taking antihypertensive drugs. Celery lowers blood pressure and can make the treatment more effective.

Organic Food Drives Pesticides Out of Your Body in Just Days

Chensheng Lu, PhD, assistant professor of environmental and occupational health, Emory University, Atlanta.

Nathan M. Graber, MD, fellow in pediatric environmental health, Mount Sinai School of Medicine, New York City.

American Association for the Advancement of Science meeting, St. Louis.

If you want to banish pesticides from your child's diet, research suggests that organic food will do the trick for two common pesticides. Researchers found that pesticide levels in children's bodies dropped to zero after just a few days of eating organic produce and grains.

"After they switch back to a conventional diet, the levels go up," says Chensheng Lu, coauthor of the study and an assistant professor of environmental and occupational health at Emory University in Atlanta.

THE STUDY

Lu says the impetus for the study was a previous research project that examined pesticide levels in 110 children and found only one child whose body was pesticide-free—a child who regularly ate organic food.

Parents should not feed their children less nutritious foods out of fear of pesticides.

Nathan M. Graber, MD

For the current study, funded by the US Environment Protection Agency (EPA), researchers recruited 23 children, ages three to 11, from Seattle-area schools. Researchers monitored levels of two organophosphorus pesticides—*malathion* and *chlorpyrifos*—in the children's urine during a 15-day period in which they alternated between their regular diets and diets featuring organic fruits, vegetables and grain products.

According to Lu, these pesticides are banned in residential areas, but are still used by growers.

The researchers found that the pesticide levels in the children dropped immediately when they started eating organic foods. The staying power of the pesticides was "relatively short," Lu says.

HEALTH RISKS NOT CLEAR

Lu acknowledges that the health risks of the pesticides in question are not entirely clear. "Whether [these results are] important in terms of health effects remains to be seen," he says, noting that scientists do not know exactly how the pesticides affect the body over time.

There is evidence that they're dangerous, says Dr. Nathan M. Graber, a fellow in pediatric environmental health at Mount Sinai School of Medicine. "We know that, at high doses, these pesticides can cause serious symptoms because they are toxic to the nervous system," he says, adding that there's "sound scientific reasoning" suggesting that low doses can hurt the developing brain.

What should parents do? Kids should be eating lots of fresh fruits and vegetables, regardless of whether they are organically grown, because the benefits greatly outweigh the risk, Graber says. "Parents should not feed their children less nutritious foods out of fear of pesticides."

Foods that are especially vulnerable to pesticide residue include strawberries, nectarines, peaches, apples, pears and cherries, Lu says. Bananas and oranges are not as vulnerable because you do not eat the part of the fruit that has been exposed to pesticides, he adds.

■ ■ ■ ■

Beware of Contaminated Fruits and Vegetables

Fruits and vegetables contaminated with bacteria such as *salmonella* and *E. coli* now cause more illness than raw chicken or eggs. The contamination comes from the use of manure as a fertilizer or from cross-contamination in home and restaurant kitchens.

Precaution: Wash fruits and vegetables under running water, use separate cutting boards for raw meat, poultry, fish and produce, and thoroughly wash countertops on which unwashed produce had been placed.

Caroline Smith DeWaal, food safety director, Center for Science in the Public Interest.

■ ■ ■ ■

Sprout Safety

Raw and undercooked sprouts can be as risky as undercooked beef and eggs. They may carry E. coli and salmonella, which can be especially dangerous for children, seniors and those who have weakened immune systems. The US Food and Drug Administration (FDA) is developing stricter safety standards for sprouts.

Michael Doyle, PhD, professor of food microbiology, and director, Center for Food Safety, University of Georgia, Griffin.

Myth: Willpower Is the Key to Weight Loss

James M. Rippe, MD, associate professor of medicine, Tufts University School of Medicine, Boston, and founder and director, Rippe Lifestyle Institute, a health research organization, Shrewsbury, MA. *www.rippehealth.com.* He is coauthor, with the editors at Weight Watchers, of *Weight Watchers Weight Loss That Lasts.* Wiley.

Most misconceptions about losing weight are based on a kernel of truth. These myths have complicated explanations that make them sound true. People who don't separate the myths from the facts are almost certain to have difficulties losing pounds and keeping them off.

Weight-loss expert and cardiologist Dr. James M. Rippe teamed up with Weight Watchers more than 10 years ago to rigorously study the group's techniques. Along the way, he has exposed some of the most common diet myths. *Here are his latest findings...*

Myth 1: **Most diets fail.** A 1950's study reported that approximately 95% of diets fail. This, and similar findings in 1992 from the National Institutes of Health, gives the impression that it is almost impossible to lose weight and keep it off. This destructive myth discourages many people from even trying to lose weight.

Reality: New information from two large databases—the Weight Watchers survey and the National Weight Control Registry Program—indicate that success rates are much higher than previously thought. On average, people who make a concerted effort to lose weight manage to keep off approximately 75% of the pounds for two years. After five years, most have kept off at least 50%.

Success rates are higher than they used to be because of advances in weight-loss methods. We now know that there are four key components—wise food choices, regular exercise, positive lifestyle changes (such as setting short- and long-term goals) and emotional support. People who incorporate all of these elements tend to be successful at losing weight and keeping it off.

Myth 2: **Willpower is the key to weight loss.** Many people assume that they haven't lost weight in the past because they lack the necessary mental toughness.

Reality: They often choose diets that are too difficult to maintain—no one has that kind of willpower. *Instead...*

•**Practice flexible restraint.** Put a moderate level of control on your eating. Studies have shown that people who exert high dietary restraint—counting every calorie, eating certain foods at specific times, etc.—are less successful than those who take a more balanced approach. The idea is to make sensible daily changes and avoid all-or-nothing thinking.

Example: Someone who eats too much at a party should make up for it not by fasting the next day, but simply by eating a little less.

•**Have nutritious food available.** Dieters often fail because of poor planning. Stock your refrigerator and pantry with sensible choices. Don't keep cookies, ice cream, potato chips or other unhealthy temptations in the house.

Myth 3: **You can lose weight through exercise alone.** Regular exercise is very important for weight loss—but it is almost impossible to lose weight through exercise alone.

Reality: It takes a lot of exercise to burn off enough calories to lose weight. To lose one pound of fat through exercise alone, a person needs to burn 3,500 calories more than what he/she is currently burning. For a sedentary, 170-pound person to lose one pound a week without dietary changes, he would have to walk at least five miles a day. It takes approximately one hour on a treadmill to burn off the calories from one

medium-sized bagel—and that's without butter or cream cheese.

The best way to lose is to combine physical activity with a reduction in calories.

Bonus: Exercise builds muscle, and muscle burns up to 70 times more calories than fat during normal metabolism. People who are physically active maintain a higher metabolism even during times of rest, which results in faster and easier weight loss.

People who are sedentary may have a drop in metabolism of 15% to 20% between the ages of 30 and 50. Those who stay active—particularly through muscle-building strength training—don't experience this decline and are less likely to gain weight than those who don't exercise.

Myth 4: **Calories don't matter.** Over the years, fad diets have identified particular foods or types of food as a leading cause of weight gain. In the 1990s, it was fat. Today, carbohydrates are the problem. There have also been claims that grapefruit, celery and other foods cause the body to burn additional calories. What each of these concepts has in common is the idea that calories are somehow less important than other factors in losing weight.

Reality: Cutting calories is the key to losing weight. It doesn't matter whether the calories come from fat, protein or carbohydrates. Shave 3,500 calories weekly by giving up desserts, for example, and taking smaller portions at meals.

Popular diets such as Atkins and South Beach are appealing because they're based on a fantastic promise—that you can lose weight quickly without much effort. But there's no evidence that restricting carbohydrates to the levels called for in these diets is any more effective than traditional dieting. It may even be counterproductive because few people are willing to stay on these diets very long.

Myth 5: **Weight-loss supplements are safe.** Health-food stores sell dozens of products that purport to safely increase metabolism and speed weight loss.

Reality: Some supplements are stimulants that increase heart rate, blood pressure and metabolism in addition to suppressing appetite. They may aid in weight loss temporarily, but they can cause severe side effects, including anxiety and insomnia.

Some of these products, such as those containing *ephedra* or *phenylpropanolamine*, have been banned because of the potential dangers.

■ ■ ■ ■

Laughter Burns Calories

Laughing out loud for 10 to 15 minutes uses up to 50 calories. People who laugh this much every day could lose more than four pounds in one year.

Maciej S. Buchowski, PhD, professor of family and community medicine, Vanderbilt University Medical Center, Nashville.

■ ■ ■ ■

After-Dinner Snacks Can Aid Weight Loss

If you are a "night snacker" or someone for whom after-dinner snacking significantly contributes to a weight problem, eating a low-calorie snack approximately 90 minutes after dinner may help curtail eating and overall daily caloric intake—as well as promote weight loss.

Good choice: A serving of low-calorie ready-to-eat cereal with fat-free milk.

Jillon S. Vander Wal, PhD, assistant professor, College of Nursing, Center for Health Research, Wayne State University, Detroit.

Dr. Leo Galland's Lose Weight Forever Diet

Leo Galland, MD, director, Foundation for Integrated Medicine, New York City. He has held faculty positions at Rockefeller University and Albert Einstein College of Medicine, both in New York City, and at the State University of New York, Stony Brook. He is author of *The Fat Resistance Diet* (Broadway) and *The Four Pillars of Healing* (Random House).

Weight loss isn't only—or even mainly —about calories. Surprisingly, we gain weight when natural weight-control mechanisms are disrupted by low-grade inflammation that is caused by poor diet and environmental toxins.

When people gain weight, the extra fatty tissue produces *leptin*, a hormone that suppresses appetite and speeds metabolism. In theory, this should cause people to lose the extra weight.

Instead, inflammation in fat tissue and blood vessels stimulates the production of chemicals that disable leptin's ability to suppress appetite and speed metabolism. This is called *leptin resistance.*

To combat leptin resistance, I have developed a fat-resistance diet based on cutting-edge research at premier institutions such as Harvard, Johns Hopkins and Rockefeller universities. Eating the proper foods can eliminate chronic inflammation and reprogram the body's weight-loss mechanisms.

ANTI-INFLAMMATORY FOODS

The focus of the diet isn't calorie control. The idea is to eat foods that supply anti-inflammatory nutrients. A major problem of most weight-loss diets is the use of artificial sweeteners and fat substitutes to reduce calories. Substituting these products for real foods deprives your body of key anti-inflammatory nutrients. *Main principles…*

•**Eat fish at least three times weekly.** The omega-3 fatty acids in fish have powerful anti-inflammatory properties. Fish that are rich in omega-3s and relatively low in mercury include anchovies, conch, herring (fresh or pickled, not creamed), mackerel (Atlantic only), sablefish, salmon (fresh, canned or smoked, wild or farmed), sardines (Atlantic), sturgeon and tuna (fresh or canned bluefin—not albacore).

•**Balance essential fatty acids.** The optimal ratio of omega-6 fatty acids to omega-3s is approximately 4:1. The ratio in the average American diet is closer to 20:1. A relative excess of omega-6 fats in tissues causes cells to produce excessive levels of pro-inflammatory chemicals called *prostanoids.* The best approach is to decrease the omega-6s and increase the omega-3s in your diet.

Foods high in omega-3s: Fish, flaxseed, walnuts and beans—navy, kidney and soy.

Foods high in omega-6s: Red meat, chicken, milk, eggs and most vegetable oils, including corn, sunflower and safflower.

●**Cut back on unhealthy fats.** Saturated fat—primarily found in beef, pork, lamb, dairy products and poultry skin—should be limited to no more than 10% of total calories. Don't eat any trans fat—this means avoiding any foods made with hydrogenated or partially hydrogenated vegetable oil. These include most commercial baked goods and some fast foods. Both saturated fat and trans fat greatly increase levels of inflammatory chemicals.

●**Get 25 grams (g) of fiber daily.** A high-fiber diet helps control appetite and reduce inflammation. A study by the Centers for Disease Control and Prevention (CDC) found that people who consume the most fiber have lower levels of *C-reactive protein* (CRP), a measure of inflammatory chemicals in the body. All plant foods contain some fiber. Among the best sources are beans, whole grains and vegetables.

●**Eat colorful fruits and vegetables.** Get at least nine servings daily. Produce that has deep colors and intense flavors is high in *flavonoids* and *carotenoids*, chemical compounds that have anti-inflammatory effects.

Important: Have at least one serving of blueberries, cherries or pomegranates daily. These contain *anthocyanins*, which are among the most potent anti-inflammatory agents.

●**Choose crucifers and alliums.** Crucifers are strong-flavored vegetables, including broccoli, cauliflower, cabbage and kale. Alliums include onions and garlic. Both classes of vegetables reduce chronic inflammation and lower the risk of cancer, particularly breast cancer. Eat at least one serving of each daily.

●**Use only egg whites or unbroken egg yolks.** The cholesterol in yolks has relatively little effect on cholesterol in the blood—but if the yolk is broken, the cholesterol is oxidized and produces inflammatory by-products. Poached or boiled whole eggs are fine. Avoid scrambled eggs and whole-egg omelettes.

●**Favor herbs and spices that are potent anti-inflammatories.** These include basil, cardamom, cilantro, cinnamon, clove, ginger, parsley and turmeric. Use them every day. Avoid chiles, cayenne pepper and jalapeños, which can trigger inflammation.

THREE STAGES

The diet progresses in phases…

Stage 1: Eat as much as you want of arugula, bell peppers, broccoli, cabbage, carrots, leeks, onions, romaine lettuce, scallions, shiitake mushrooms, spinach and tomatoes—as well as blueberries, cherries, grapefruit and pomegranates.

Eating three 4-ounce servings of high-protein foods every day helps suppress appetite and maintain muscle mass. Choose fish, egg whites, poultry and plain, fat-free yogurt. Meat lovers can eat red meat twice a week but should marinate beef using cherry or pomegranate concentrate (this reduces the inflammatory chemical compounds that are produced during cooking). You can have 1 or 2 tablespoons each day of nuts or seeds (especially flaxseed, walnuts and almonds). During this stage, get 25 g of fiber, primarily from vegetables.

Avoid grains—even whole grains—because they tend to raise insulin levels, thus increasing leptin resistance.

Most people stay in this stage for two weeks and lose six to 10 pounds.

Stage 2: This is the long-term weight-loss part of the diet. Stay on this until you reach your goal weight. You can expect to lose one to two pounds per week.

In addition to the Stage 1 foods, add some whole grains, such as oats and brown rice, and beans, lentils and other legumes (approximately 2 to 3 cups a week of each).

Stage 3: This is the lifelong maintenance phase. Increase the variety by adding potatoes, pasta and whole-grain breads.

■ ■ ■ ■

The Obesity Epidemic

The obesity epidemic could shorten US life expectancies by up to five years, reversing a 150-year trend. The prevalence and severity of obesity will continue to increase, and people in ever-younger age groups will experience the consequences of being overweight—heart disease, stroke, cancer, kidney failure, diabetes, etc. An estimated 30% of American children are overweight.

S. Jay Olshansky, PhD, professor of epidemiology and biostatistics, University of Illinois at Chicago.

Researcher Astounded as Yoga Melts Off Pounds

Alan R. Kristal, DrPH, associate head, Cancer Prevention Research Program, Fred Hutchinson Cancer Research Center, and professor of epidemiology, University of Washington, Seattle.

Janine Blackman, MD, PhD, assistant professor of family medicine and medical director, Center for Integrative Medicine, University of Maryland, Baltimore.

Alternative Therapies in Health and Medicine.

The ancient practice of yoga may do more than just improve strength and flexibility—it could also help people shed extra pounds in middle age, according to the first study to examine yoga's impact on weight loss.

Investigators report that overweight 45- to 55-year-olds who regularly practiced yoga lost an average of five pounds during the course of a decade. At the same time, normal-weight yoga practitioners gained three fewer pounds than people who did not practice yoga during this same 10-year period.

THE STUDY

To examine the relationship between weight loss and yoga, researchers at the Fred Hutchinson Cancer Research Center in Seattle surveyed 15,500 healthy men and women ages 53 to 57. The participants were queried on their weight history and physical activity since they were 45 years old.

Only 132 of the people surveyed said they practiced yoga regularly for at least four years. However, overweight yoga practitioners lost approximately five pounds, on average, during a 10-year period, while those who did not practice yoga gained an average of 13.5 pounds. People who were at a normal weight and regularly practiced yoga gained three fewer pounds during this period than those who didn't practice yoga (9.5 pounds compared with 12.6 pounds).

REACTION

"I was very surprised with the results. Considering that people gain approximately a pound a year during this time [of their lives], this is pretty substantial," says lead researcher Alan R. Kristal, associate head of the Cancer Prevention Research Program at the Hutchinson Center and a professor of epidemiology at the University of Washington. "Even the best dietary and behavioral approaches to weight loss are not all that effective. Now, with yoga, we have one more tool that may help with weight loss," he says.

Kristal says he isn't certain how yoga helps promote weight loss and maintenance, particularly because only vigorous yoga would burn enough energy to meet the American College of Sports Medicine's guidelines for weight management. However, he speculates that yoga could be indirectly beneficial by encouraging healthier eating and exercise habits. For example, yoga teaches body awareness and encourages physical discipline, so it may help a person know when they're full and promote a general sense of well-being, he says.

Dr. Janine Blackman, medical director of the University of Maryland's Center for Integrative Medicine, has another theory—the "mindful" nature of yoga creates a healthier response to stress, lowering stress hormones and preventing stress-driven eating.

"Middle age is a full time in life," Blackman says. "A better response to this stress can lower cortisol and other stress hormones, which helps physiologically. If cortisol is elevated, you're more likely to have insulin resistance, which is central to obesity."

STUDY LIMITATIONS

Both Blackman and Kristal agree that more research is needed because of this study's limitations. People in this study did not report the type of yoga they practiced—that's important, since the physical intensity of specific yoga techniques varies. The survey was also self-reported, relying on people's memories and assuming that they were honest. Kristal hopes a future observational study will help fill in these gaps and that, eventually, a large, randomized trial will be conducted.

In the meantime, Blackman, who recommends gentle yoga to her patients, says she will continue to do so. "Gentle yoga is a great way to ease into an active life, especially since overweight people are already less likely to exercise because it hurts," she says.

info For more information on yoga and other natural healing techniques, visit the National Center for Complementary and Alternative Medicine Web site at *http://nccam.nih.gov.*

■ ■ ■ ■

Chitosan Not Effective for Weight Loss

Marketers say that chitosan, which is made from shellfish, has fat-burning properties. However, in order to lose 1 kilogram (approximately 2.2 pounds) of body fat, you would have to take almost 10 capsules of chitosan a day for 25 months.

Judith S. Stern, ScD, professor of nutrition, University of California, Davis.

Diet Drug Works Best With Healthy Eating And Exercise

Thomas Wadden, MD, director, Weight and Eating Disorders Program, University of Pennsylvania School of Medicine, Philadelphia.

Susan Yanovski, MD, director, Obesity and Eating Disorders Program, US National Institute of Diabetes & Digestive & Kidney Diseases.

The New England Journal of Medicine.
Annals of Behavioral Medicine.

Three recent studies examined the effects of diet pills, lifestyle changes and daily weight monitoring to try to determine what works best in the fight against obesity.

STUDY #1:
MERIDIA PLUS LIFESTYLE CHANGES

The first study found that the weight-loss drug *sibutramine* (Meridia) is most effective when users also eat right and exercise.

In a one-year trial, researchers gave 224 obese adults 15 milligrams (mg) of Meridia every day. They randomly assigned some people to also receive counseling to teach them how to keep food records, shop for healthy foods and how to stay away from all-you-can-eat buffets and fast-food restaurants.

Lead researcher Dr. Thomas Wadden, director of the Weight and Eating Disorders Program at the University of Pennsylvania School of Medicine, says these changes, along with a healthy diet and physical activity, "help you modify the external environment," while drugs such as Meridia "help modify the internal environment," working on brain chemicals to lower appetite and help patients feel fuller, sooner.

The combination seems to work. According to the researchers, people taking Meridia who also changed their lifestyles lost an average of 26 pounds, more than twice as much as those who took the drug but made no lifestyle changes (11 pounds).

Most obesity experts say lifestyle changes, especially improved diet and exercise, are the real keys to losing weight. But many over-weight Americans still find it tough, according to Wadden.

"There's nothing worse than to be watching your calories and exercising, but the scale just doesn't budge," says Wadden. "You just feel like, 'My efforts are for naught.' That's when people tend to give up."

And that's when diet pills may come in handy, says Dr. Susan Yanovski, director of the Obesity and Eating Disorders Program at the US National Institute of Diabetes & Digestive & Kidney Diseases (NIDDK).

"All the weight-loss drugs have shown generally what I'd consider a modest weight loss compared with placebo, usually somewhere in the range of five to 15 pounds additional weight loss," says Yanovski.

Weight-loss pills "should not be used alone," Yanovski advises.

"Don't look for a quick fix from the drug store. Combining therapies seems to be much more effective than drug treatment alone," she says.

Study after study has shown that obesity can easily return when individuals stop exercising and eating right, or if they discontinue a weight-loss medication.

"We now realize that people may have to take weight-loss medications on a long-term basis," Wadden says, "just like they have to take other medications, such as those that control cholesterol or high blood pressure."

In the case of Meridia, that means long-term physician monitoring, because the drug can trigger a rise in pulse rate and blood pressure in approximately 10% of users, the researchers say.

Meridia is just one of two weight-loss drugs currently approved for use by the US Food and Drug Administration (FDA).

The other is *orlistat* (Xenical), and a third medication, *rimonabant* (Acomplia), showed promising results in a trial, and is currently undergoing FDA review.

The international study on rimonabant was led by Jean-Pierre Despres of Laval University in Sainte-Foy, Quebec, Canada, and involved more than 1,000 overweight or obese patients who had untreated high cholesterol The participants were placed on a low-calorie diet and given either daily rimonabant (at doses of 5 or 20 mg) or a placebo.

Don't look for a quick fix from the drug store. Combining therapies seems to be much more effective than drug treatment alone.

Susan Yanovski, MD

Rimonabant helped participants lose an average of approximately 15 pounds during one year. And the drug may have the added health benefit of lowering levels of dangerous blood fats known as triglycerides and boosting levels of HDL ("good") cholesterol.

"We know that rimonabant improves [cardiovascular] risk factors, but we don't know yet if that translates into a reduction in heart disease or death," Yanovski says.

"Rimonabant is a little bit different in that it acts not only on the brain but also on other tissues in the body, such as fat cells and those in the gastrointestinal tract," she says.

STUDY #3:
KEEPING TRACK

A third study found that people who get in the habit of weighing themselves every day are more successful at losing weight than those who do not monitor their weight daily.

The study looked at more than 3,000 obese or overweight individuals enrolled in weight-loss programs for two years.

Researchers at the University of Minnesota found that those who checked their weight daily lost more than those who didn't.

If people see that they have gained a few pounds, they may realize it's time to do something. It's probably easier to make that small correction than to make a larger one after they realize they have gained more than just a few pounds, says lead researcher Jennifer Linde.

All that monitoring and hard work could pay off, though—even minor weight loss can trigger major health benefits.

According to Wadden, "If people lost just 7% of their initial body weight—approximately 15 pounds through 150 minutes of exercise per week—they reduced their risk of developing type 2 diabetes by 58%. A little bit of weight loss goes a long way."

info Learn more about obesity at the Weight-control Information Network at *http://win. niddk.nih.gov/publications/understanding.htm.*

■ ■ ■ ■

When to Skip Your Workouts

Do you believe that you need to sweat out a cold or the flu at the gym?

If so, you're mistaken. Your body doesn't sweat out toxins during exercise, according to the War Memorial Hospital in West Virginia. Rather, your immune system works better when it's not stressed.

Moderate exercise can help boost your immune system, thereby decreasing the chance that you will catch a cold or the flu.

But a hard workout when you are already sick can impair your immune system for several hours, making your illness worse.

Once you're feeling better, give your body an extra few days to recover before you resume working out.

Allow three to four days of rest after a bad cold and at least a week after the flu.

When you return to your routine, practice the 50% rule—decrease your usual exercise time by half and go half-speed on the treadmill or exercise bike until you regain your strength and endurance.

■ ■ ■ ■

Everyday Exercise

Everyday and recreational activities can be rated by the degree of physical exertion required to complete them. You can achieve significant health benefits by accruing a total of 150 *cardiometabolic exercise* (CME) points per day. Use this chart to determine the CME points for various activities. The point values are based on a moderate level of exertion for 30 minutes, unless noted otherwise.

ACTIVITY	CME POINTS
Swim	230
Aerobics	200
Jogging (12-minute mile)	200
Mowing lawn (pushing hand mower)	200
Tennis (singles)	200
Golfing (carrying clubs)	165
Ballroom dancing	150
Gardening	150
Mowing lawn (pushing power mower)	145
Raking leaves	130
Yoga	130
Vacuuming	115
Bowling	100
Walking up stairs (10 minutes)	100
Washing car by hand	100
Cooking	60
Washing dishes	60
Laundering or ironing (15 minutes)	35
Walking down stairs (10 minutes)	30
Sexual activity (15 minutes)	25

Harvey B. Simon, MD, associate professor of medicine, Harvard Medical School, Boston, and author of *The No Sweat Exercise Plan*. McGraw-Hill.

Java Before the Gym? Think Again

American College of Cardiology news release.

Drinking coffee right before a workout may not be a good idea, according to the results of a recent study.

Researchers in Switzerland found that the amount of caffeine in just two cups of coffee limits the body's ability to increase blood flow to the heart during exercise.

THE STUDY

The study included 18 young, healthy people who were regular coffee drinkers. They did not drink any coffee for 36 hours prior to study testing. The researchers used high-tech *positron emission tomography* (PET) scans to measure the participants' heart blood flow before and after riding a stationary bike. Ten participants exercised in normal conditions and eight exercised in a room that simulated being at approximately 15,000 feet altitude.

Both groups repeated the testing procedure after taking a tablet containing 200 milligrams (mg) of caffeine—the amount in two cups of coffee.

The caffeine did not affect heart blood flow when the participants were inactive. However, after exercising, heart blood flow was slower when the study subjects had caffeine than when they did not.

Heart blood flow in the people who had caffeine was 22% lower in those who exercised in normal air pressure and 39% lower in those who exercised in the high-altitude room, the researchers report.

IMPLICATIONS

"Whenever we do physical exercise, myocardial blood flow has to increase in order to match the increased need for oxygen. We found that caffeine may adversely affect this mechanism," explains Dr. Philipp A. Kaufmann, of University Hospital Zurich and the Center for Integrative Human Physiology.

Researchers believe that caffeine may interfere with the normal signaling process that causes blood vessels to dilate in response to exercise.

"Although these findings seem not to have a clinical importance in healthy volunteers, they may raise safety questions in patients who have coronary artery disease, particularly before any physical exercise and at high-altitude exposure," the study authors say.

While some people regard caffeine as a stimulant, this study suggests it may not boost athletic performance. "It may be a stimulant at the cerebral level in terms of being more awake and alert, which may subjectively give the feeling of having better physical performance. But I now would not recommend that any athlete drink caffeine before sports," Kaufmann says.

info Iowa State University has more information about caffeine and athletes at *www.extension.iastate.edu/nutrition/supplements/caffeine.php.*

■ ■ ■ ■

'Talk Test' Means Better Exercise

Gauge your best level of exercise intensity with the *talk test*. If you can converse easily while exercising, you aren't working hard enough for maximum benefit. If you can't talk at all, then you are exercising too hard. When you just begin to have trouble speaking due to the intensity of the exercise, you are probably working at 80% to 90% of your maximum heart rate—the level for optimum benefit.

Carl Foster, PhD, professor of exercise science, University of Wisconsin–LaCrosse.

■ ■ ■ ■

When Muscles Are Sore, Stay Cool

To ease sore muscles, you should start by using cold therapy, and then move to heat, advise experts.

For relieving muscle pain caused by sprains and strains, the first step is to apply a cold compress for approximately 20 minutes every four to six hours for the first few days.

A cold pack, a plastic bag filled with ice or even a bag of frozen vegetables will serve the purpose. Wrap the cold compress in a towel or dry cloth to prevent frostbite when placing it on the skin. The cold should reduce the swelling and inflammation, as well as relieve pain.

After the pain and swelling have subsided, usually two to three days after injury, use heat therapy. The heat helps relax tight and sore muscles, and reduces pain. Apply heat to the injured muscle for 20 minutes up to three times a day using a hot water bottle, warm compress, heat lamp, warm bath or hot shower.

Heat is usually a better treatment than cold for chronic pain (i.e., arthritis pain) or for muscle relaxation.

info The National Institute of Arthritis and Musculoskeletal and Skin Diseases has more information about sprains and strains at *www.niams.nih.gov.* Click on "Health Information" and scroll down to "Sprains and Strains, Q & A."

Mayo Clinic news release.

■ ■ ■ ■

Muscle Myth

Muscles do not turn to fat when you stop working out. When people stop exercising, their muscles begin to shrink. This makes some people believe that muscle turns to fat. In reality, the ratio of fat to muscle simply changes.

Gerard P. Varlotta, DO, clinical associate professor, department of rehabilitation medicine, New York University Medical Center, New York City.

'Fast' Way to Increase Energy

Mark A. Stengler, ND, naturopathic physician, La Jolla Whole Health Clinic, La Jolla, CA, and associate clinical professor, the National College of Naturopathic Medicine, Portland, OR. He is author of numerous books on natural healing, including *The Natural Physician's Healing Therapies.* Bottom Line. *www.bottomlinesecrets.com.*

Fasting can be an effective way to detoxify the body and, subsequently, improve energy levels. It works by giving the organs and cells of the body a rest from some of the metabolic functions they perform every second of the day. This rest allows the body to expel toxins and cleanse the tissues.

During the first day of a fast, the body burns stored sugar, known as *glycogen*. The cells also begin to burn fat for fuel, while the brain continues to burn *glucose* (blood sugar).

During the second day of a fast, muscle tissue may be broken down into amino acids, which are then converted by the liver into glucose to feed the brain.

On the third day, the fasting body goes into *ketosis*. During this state, the liver converts stored fat into chemicals called *ketones*, which can be used by the brain and muscles, including the heart, to sustain energy levels.

Around the third day of the fast, most people lose their hunger pains and notice increased energy and a heightened sense of awareness and clarity of mind. People may lose up to two pounds per day during this stage.

There are many different types of fasts. A water-only fast (80 ounces of water daily for one to three days) is the most aggressive type and should be used only by people in good health.

Juice fasts (80 to 100 ounces of juice daily for two to five days) are also common and are especially useful for boosting energy. These fasts often include the fresh juice of carrots, lemons, apples, beets and celery. Wheatgrass juice, which helps detoxify the liver and kidneys, and other greens can also be added.

For a modified type of fast, you can eat homemade broths and soups (three to four bowls a day, containing carrots, celery, chicken broth, potatoes and spices)...or drink 30 to 40 ounces daily of detoxification meal-replacement drinks (containing rice or pea-protein, added vitamins and minerals, and detoxifying herbs, such as milk thistle and green tea extract), plus 32 ounces of water. Meal-replacement drinks are commonly available from natural health-care practitioners and at health-food stores.

People who have diabetes should avoid fasts. And, if you have a chronic health condition, you should fast only under the supervision of a medical professional.

People who do not react well to fasts often do better on the modified versions, such as those that use meal-replacement drinks.

If you have little experience in fasting, work with a nutrition-oriented doctor for guidance.

Up to 90% of Celiac Disease Cases Undiagnosed

Charles O. Elson, MD, professor of medicine, division of gastroenterology and hepatology, University of Alabama School of Medicine, Birmingham.

Celiac disease—a genetic disorder in which eating *gluten*, a protein found in wheat, barley and rye, causes damage to the small intestine—was long believed to be a relatively rare condition that emerged in childhood.

Now: Scientists at the Center for Celiac Research at the University of Maryland screened more than 13,000 blood donors throughout the US and discovered that the disorder afflicts approximately one in 133 Americans (a total of 3 million people).

Problem: Because its symptoms are so varied and unpredictable, as many as 90% of celiac sufferers remain undiagnosed.

WHAT IS CELIAC DISEASE?

When people who have celiac disease consume gluten, the protein spurs an abnormal immune response in their small intestines, which damages the intestinal lining and prevents the proper absorption of food. In children, this can result in a failure to grow.

In adults, it can cause a range of conditions including chronic diarrhea, bloating, flatulence, weight loss, abdominal or joint pain, fatigue, constipation, recurring miscarriage, infertility, tooth enamel defects, depression and/or anxiety.

Because celiac disease interferes with the absorption of iron, calcium and/or vitamin D, it can lead to iron-deficiency anemia or osteoporosis if it is left untreated. In rare cases, celiac disease can lead to intestinal cancers or lymphoma.

GETTING THE RIGHT DIAGNOSIS

Studies show that celiac disease patients endure, on average, 11 years of unexplained symptoms before being diagnosed. This is partly because many physicians don't think to look for celiac, especially if a patient does not have the classic symptoms—chronic diarrhea, abdominal bloating and weight loss.

However, most people who have celiac disease do not experience these symptoms, but instead have other gastrointestinal problems, such as constipation and abdominal pain.

Some celiac patients don't have gastrointestinal distress at all—they may experience frequent canker sores in the mouth or tingling in the hands and feet. A small percentage of patients develop a blistering, intensely itchy rash, called *dermatitis herpetiformis*, on their elbows, knees and buttocks. Many people who have celiac have no symptoms at all.

Bottom line: The only way to diagnose celiac disease is through a blood test and biopsy. The blood test detects certain antibodies that are produced when celiac patients consume gluten. If these antibodies are present, a biopsy is taken of the small intestine to check for damage to the lining. During this procedure, the doctor inserts an *endoscope*—a thin, flexible tube—through the mouth, esophagus and stomach, and into the small intestine to take a sample of intestinal tissue.

If both the blood test and the biopsy are positive, celiac disease is the presumed culprit. A gluten-free diet is prescribed—and if symptoms resolve within a few months of beginning the diet, the diagnosis is confirmed.

WHO SHOULD BE TESTED?

Screening for celiac disease is recommended for anyone who has unexplained, chronic gastrointestinal symptoms and one or more of the following celiac disease risk factors…

•**A first-degree relative (parent, child or sibling) who has celiac disease.** If an immediate family member has celiac disease, you have an 8% to 10% chance of developing it.

•**Type 1 diabetes,** rheumatoid arthritis, hypothyroidism or another autoimmune disorder.

•**Down's syndrome** (a chromosomal disorder resulting in mental retardation and physical abnormalities)…Turner syndrome (a rare genetic disorder in women, characterized by the absence of an X chromosome)…or Williams syndrome (a rare congenital disorder, characterized by mental and growth deficiencies).

•**Unexplained elevated liver enzymes.**

•**Unexplained iron-deficiency anemia.**

•**A first-degree relative who has osteoporosis or intestinal cancer.**

Important: If you suspect you may have celiac disease, do not eliminate gluten from your diet before consulting your physician. For your doctor to confirm a diagnosis of celiac, the blood test and biopsy of your small intestine must be done while foods containing gluten are still part of your diet.

LIVING WITH CELIAC DISEASE

If you're diagnosed with celiac disease, you can achieve complete remission of symptoms and restore intestinal health by adopting a gluten-free diet. This means eliminating all products containing wheat, rye or barley, which includes most breads, pastas, cereals and baked goods.

You'll also need to avoid unexpected sources of gluten, such as some marinades, gravies, soy sauce, cold cuts, frozen french fries, candy—even some lipsticks and postage stamps.

Important: You can't always tell by reading the label if a product contains gluten. Many common ingredients, including malt flavoring, caramel color, dextrin, hydrolyzed vegetable protein and modified food starch, may be derived from gluten-containing grains, so it is best to avoid all of them.

Because oats are typically processed in the same containers that the factories use to make wheat products, oats should also be avoided. Fortunately, some supermarkets offer specialty gluten-free foods.

Eating promises to get easier for celiac patients in the near future. In 2004, Congress enacted a bill requiring all foods containing wheat (plus seven other common allergens—milk, eggs, peanuts, tree nuts, fish, crustacean shellfish and soy) to clearly say so on the packaging. And by 2008, the US Food and Drug Administration (FDA) will establish guidelines that manufacturers must meet in order to label their products "gluten-free."

info For more information on celiac disease and advice on following a gluten-free diet, contact the Celiac Sprue Association, 877-272-4272, *http://csaceliacs.org*, or the Celiac Disease Foundation, which publishes a booklet, *Guidelines for a Gluten-Free Lifestyle*, available by calling 818-990-2354, or online at *www.celiac.org*.

■■■■

Surprising Cause of Illness

More than 2 million Americans may have a gluten intolerance, a condition that is also known as *celiac disease*. Most of them don't even know they have it. When such a person eats gluten—found in wheat, rye and barley—the small intestine becomes inflamed and nutrients are not absorbed properly. Classic symptoms include itchy skin rash, diarrhea, abdominal cramping and other intestinal problems.

But: Some celiac disease patients have anemia, headaches, hair loss, joint pain, liver inflammation and/or seizures. These people should be tested for a gluten intolerance.

Thomas Brunoski, MD, specialist in food and environmental allergies and nutritional medicine, Westport, CT.

Nutritional Deficiencies: Is Your Body Starving?

C. Leigh Broadhurst, PhD, research scientist, University of Maryland, College Park, and research geochemist, Agricultural Research Service, US Department of Agriculture.

Because of all the processed food now consumed in the US, getting the necessary nutrients from our diet has become increasingly difficult. Of course, we can turn to nutritional supplements, but research has consistently shown that fresh food—which has an abundance of healthful compounds that are believed to work synergistically—is usually our best source of valuable nutrients.

What most people don't realize: Choosing the right foods and food combinations allows you to consume these vital nutrients in a form that is most *bioavailable*, meaning the food components are efficiently digested, absorbed and assimilated.

What you must know to maximize the bioavailability of nutrients in your food…

•**Iron.** This mineral is critical for brain function and helps your immune system operate normally by increasing your resistance to stress and disease. Iron can help you avoid symptoms of fatigue, weakness and irritability.

Plant foods are rarely a good source of iron. For example, although spinach is a good source of magnesium, bone-building vitamin K and other important nutrients, the fiber and plant chemicals in the spinach leaf bind to iron, inhibiting the mineral's bioavailability.

Helpful: When shopping for meat, look for dark meat products, such as liver, beef or dark-meat turkey. They are the best sources of iron. Tofu and seafood (especially clams and shrimp) are also rich in iron.

•**Zinc.** This mineral is essential for a healthy immune system. It is highly bioavailable in red meat, though some zinc is also found in nuts (almonds and walnuts). Poultry is another good source of zinc.

Helpful: Consider adding oysters to your diet. They are one of the richest sources of zinc.

Caution: Raw oysters are often contaminated with bacteria.

•**Magnesium.** Up to 75% of Americans are deficient in this vital mineral, which is needed for heart health and strong bones as well as for blood sugar control.

Helpful: Vegetables are among the richest sources of magnesium. Eat raw or lightly steamed vegetables—highly processed or overcooked veggies lose their magnesium content. Whole grains are also much richer sources of magnesium than refined grains.

•**Calcium.** Many experts advocate the green, leafy vegetables for calcium, but these foods do not provide ample amounts of this mineral in a bioavailable form.

Sardines are an often-overlooked source of calcium, but they are not standard fare for many Americans.

Dairy foods remain the best regular source of calcium. Milk that has 1% or 2% fat is a good choice. Skim milk is not recommended because the bioavailability of fat-soluble vitamins, such as vitamin D, is diminished when you remove all the fat from milk.

Helpful: Avoid "fat-free half-and-half." This product provides no nutritional value—it is usually filled with corn syrup and other sugars to give it the creamy feel of real half-and-half.

•Selenium. The number-one source of this cancer-fighting mineral is the soil in which plants are grown. Soil in the Great Plains states contains adequate levels of selenium, so products from this area, such as whole-grain wheat, are generally good sources of selenium.

Helpful: If you are at an increased risk of cancer (due to family history, exposure to secondhand smoke or other carcinogens), consider taking a 50- to 200-microgram (mcg) selenium supplement.

Important: If you are currently undergoing treatment for cancer, talk to your doctor before taking selenium.

•Chromium. This mineral, shown in dozens of studies to help control levels of blood sugar, is poorly absorbed by the body. Unless you eat organ meats, such as liver, it is best consumed in supplement form.

Helpful: Everyone should consider taking a 200-mcg chromium supplement daily for general health. If you have diabetes, ask your doctor about taking 1,000 mcg of chromium daily.

•Carotenoids. More than 600 nutritious plant compounds known as *carotenoids* can be found in vegetables and fruits.

Examples: *Lycopene*, found in tomatoes, watermelon and pink grapefruit, may help prevent prostate cancer…*lutein* and *zeaxanthin*, found in dark green, leafy vegetables and corn, may help prevent and treat macular degeneration, the leading cause of vision loss in people older than age 65.

Helpful: Because carotenoids are fat-soluble nutrients (that is, they require some amount of dietary fat for optimal absorption), consume carotenoid-rich foods along with olive oil or other healthful fat sources. Low-fat salad dressings can be used, but avoid no-fat versions.

Also helpful: Steam or lightly simmer vegetables. Raw fruits and vegetables contain valuable enzymes, and cooking breaks the cell walls, thus increasing the bioavailability of many valuable nutrients.

Examples: To maximize the amount of cancer-fighting lycopene you get from tomatoes, make them into a sauce.

•Protein. On the bioavailability scale, meat, poultry, fish and eggs are among the best sources of protein. Although the protein found in lunch meats, such as ham and bologna, is bioavailable, these foods typically contain high levels of sodium and harmful fillers and preservatives known as *nitrates*.

Aim for 50 to 120 grams (g) of protein daily. One-half of a salmon fillet contains 42 g…one-half of a chicken breast contains 27 g…three ounces of top sirloin contains 25 g.

Helpful: To maximize the bioavailability of the nutrients that are found in beef, prepare it medium-rare.

For a convenient protein source that lasts for several days, roast a turkey breast or chicken in an oven cooking bag, slice it up and use it during the week.

As an alternative to meat, consider using whey protein powder—an excellent source of protein derived from milk.

Look for *cold filtered* and *ion exchanged* on the label, which indicates that the processing has removed *lactose* (milk sugar) and *casein* (a highly allergenic protein found in milk). This process breaks down the whey, making it more absorbable.

Next Nutrition as well as Jarrow each make excellent whey products. Only approximately 2% of the people who have dairy allergies are allergic to whey protein.

Whey protein powder can be easily added to a smoothie.

What to do: Mix one scoop of protein powder (typically 20 g of protein) with 8 ounces of water, milk or juice and ice in a blender. Add frozen blueberries or other fruit, if desired.

If you are allergic to whey protein, consider soy powder—the protein in soy powder is more easily utilized than that in other soy foods. Soy powder can also be used in smoothies.

Important: If you eat a vegan diet (no animal products of any kind), take a multivitamin as nutritional insurance. Plant-based diets do not contain adequate amounts of all nutrients.

■ ■ ■ ■

Are You Getting Too Much Iron?

Most Americans get enough iron from food, especially red meat, fortified grains and leafy vegetables.

Exceptions: People who have had blood loss from surgery or accidents…most pregnant or breast-feeding women…women who have heavy menstrual periods.

Caution: Even if you fall into one of these categories, don't take supplements that contain iron—including multivitamin/mineral supplements—until you have been tested for *hemochromatosis* (iron overload).

Reason: Excess iron exacerbates this hereditary condition and can lead to cirrhosis of the liver, heart failure, etc. A *serum ferritin* test can best measure the body's iron stores. In men, normal serum ferritin should be 20 to 300 milligrams per milliliter (mg/mL)…in women, 15 to 200 mg/mL.

Herbert Bonkovsky, MD, director, Liver-Biliary-Pancreative Center, University of Connecticut, Farmington, and chair of the scientific advisory board, Iron Disorders Institute.

These Supplements Won't Lower Heart Attack Risk— And They May Raise It

Joseph Loscalzo, MD, PhD, head of the department of medicine, Brigham and Women's Hospital, Boston.

Kaare Harald Bönaa, MD, PhD, primary investigator, NORVIT trial, professor of medicine and consultant cardiologist, Institute of Community Medicine, University of Tromsö, Norway.

Alice H. Lichtenstein, DSc, director, Cardiovascular Nutrition Lab and Stanley Gershoff Professor of Nutrition, US Department of Agriculture's Human Nutrition Research Center, Tufts University, Boston.

Council for Responsible Nutrition.

The New England Journal of Medicine.

Two new studies question the conventional wisdom that folic acid and B vitamin supplements cut cardiovascular risk. Healthcare practitioners have often prescribed these supplements in an attempt to reduce blood levels of *homocysteine*, a protein that has been linked to heart attack and stroke. However, the new research suggests that lowering homocysteine by supplementation has no effect on preventing heart attacks—and that these supplements may even trigger a slight rise in heart attack risk.

---

*B vitamins
do not prevent heart disease.*

Kaare Harald Bönaa, MD, PhD

"Combination vitamin therapies, which do lower homocysteine, have no effect on cardiovascular events, even though the homocysteine level is lowered," says Dr. Joseph Loscalzo, head of the department of medicine at Brigham and Women's Hospital in Boston.

THE FIRST STUDY

In the first study, called the Norwegian Vitamin (NORVIT) trial, Norwegian researchers randomly assigned 3,749 men and women who had had heart attacks to receive either folic acid along with vitamins B-6 and B-12, or a placebo.

During the three years of the trial, the researchers found that while homocysteine levels dropped an average of 27% among the people taking folic acid and vitamin B-12, this decline had no significant effect on whether they had or died from another heart attack. In fact, the people who were taking all three supplements actually had a slightly increased risk of having another heart attack, the researchers report.

"Doctors should not advise patients who have cardiovascular disease to take B vitamins in order to prevent heart disease or stroke," says lead author Dr. Kaare Harald Bönaa, a professor of medicine and consultant cardiologist at the Institute of Community Medicine at the University of Tromsö in Norway. "B vitamins do not prevent heart disease."

THE SECOND STUDY

In the Heart Outcomes Prevention Evaluation (HOPE) 2 study, researchers gave more than 5,500 patients who had diabetes or vascular disease supplements of folic acid and vitamins B-6 and B-12, or a placebo.

During the five years of the study, homocysteine levels dropped significantly among those receiving the supplements, but this did not translate into a significantly reduced risk of death from heart disease or heart attack.

There did, however, appear to be a slight reduction in the number of people who had a stroke among those taking the supplements, the researchers report.

Overall, the researchers say that, "combined daily administration of 2.5 milligrams [mg] of folic acid, 50 mg of vitamin B-6 and 1 mg of vitamin B-12 for five years had no beneficial effects on major vascular events in a high-risk population with vascular disease." They conclude, "Our results do not support the use of folic acid and B vitamin supplements as a preventive treatment."

STUDY LIMITATIONS

However, Anne Dickinson, a consultant and past president of the Council for Responsible Nutrition, a group that represents the supplements industry, says that because the two studies involved individuals who had a history of heart attack, heart disease, diabetes and other problems, the findings may not apply to relatively healthy Americans.

"These studies did not test whether B vitamins used by healthy people can help keep them healthy," Dickinson says. "Instead, they looked at whether B vitamins can treat or reverse heart disease in people who already have it. Vitamins should not be expected to perform like drugs—their greatest purpose is in prevention."

Alice H. Lichtenstein, director of the Cardiovascular Nutrition Lab at the US Department of Agriculture's (USDA) Human Nutrition Research Center at Tufts University, disagrees. She notes that even outwardly "healthy" Americans develop some level of atherosclerosis (hardening of the arteries) as they age, and therefore, the findings would probably apply to the average person, as well.

ANALYZING THE FINDINGS

Loscalzo believes that at the dosages used in the study, folic acid and B vitamins somehow counteract their beneficial effect of reducing homocysteine levels. "Some of those adverse effects may have to do with the complex metabolism of the vitamins," he speculates. "These vitamins are important for cell growth. It may be that the doses used might have stimulated the growth of cell and atherosclerotic plaque."

Vitamin therapy may not be the best way to lower homocysteine levels, he suggests. "These high doses of folic acid don't provide any benefit and shouldn't be used," Loscalzo says. Or perhaps lower doses are the key. "Lower doses are safe and may provide benefit, but we don't know that yet."

Lichtenstein agrees that high doses of vitamins may not be as beneficial as some experts had thought. "This is one of those cases where you see an association between a reduced risk of heart disease and levels of vitamins that would normally be consumed [through diet]. But when we go to considerably higher levels than people could consume from diet, we get disappointing results," she says.

■ ■ ■ ■

Deciphering Supplement Labels

Natural does not mean *safe*, and labels can often be misleading.

Smart: Check out the individual ingredients in the supplement, their effects and effectiveness. Use the US Department of Agriculture's (USDA) new Nutrition Information Web site, *www.nutrition.gov*. Consult your doctor before taking a new supplement. If a claim for a supplement sounds too good to be true, it probably is.

Fight Some Cancers with Vitamin D

Cedric F. Garland, DrPH, FACE, professor, department of family and preventive medicine, University of California, San Diego.

Lona Sandon, RD/LD, assistant professor of clinical nutrition, University of Texas Southwestern Medical Center, Dallas, and spokeswoman, American Dietetic Association.

American Journal of Public Health online.

You may be able to fend off colon, breast and ovarian cancer simply by getting enough vitamin D, a new analysis of previous research suggests.

THE NEW RESEARCH

Study coauthor Cedric F. Garland, a professor of medicine at the University of California, San Diego, and his colleagues examined 63 previous studies that looked at possible links between several types of cancer and a vitamin D deficiency. According to the researchers, the studies suggest that vitamin D can reduce the risk of colon, breast and ovarian cancers, among others, by as much as 50%.

The study authors found that people who are African-American, overweight, elderly or live in the Northeast are typically not getting enough vitamin D. They theorized on possible reasons for these results. The increased skin pigmentation of African-Americans reduces their ability to synthesize vitamin D. People who are overweight may also have a problem synthesizing vitamin D. As people age, they lose the ability to convert vitamin D into its usable form. And people who live in the Northeast may not get enough exposure to the sun, a source of vitamin D.

DEBATE CONTINUES

The debate over the value of vitamin D isn't over, however, says Lona Sandon, a spokeswoman for the American Dietetic Association.

The new research suggests a link between too little vitamin D and cancer, but doesn't *confirm* it, she says.

Why might vitamin D have a protective effect in the first place? "Vitamin D's main role is to keep the balance of calcium and phosphorous in the blood, which helps keep bones strong," Sandon says. "However, a lesser-known role is that it regulates cell growth and determines what a cell becomes. A vitamin D deficiency may allow cells to become cancerous rather than becoming healthy cells."

WHAT TO DO?

The experts are divided on dosage recommendations for vitamin D.

Garland urges everyone to consume 1,000 international units (IUs) a day of the active form of vitamin D (also known as vitamin D-3), which can be found in yogurt, cheese, orange juice, fatty fish and milk.

By contrast, Sandon says adults between the ages of 19 and 50 should get 200 IUs a day, equivalent to two glasses of fortified milk. People ages 50 to 70 should get 400 IUs, she says, while those 71 and older should get 700. But she acknowledges that "It is difficult to get this much vitamin D from food alone." She recommends that people take brief walks during lunch to get exposure to the sun, a source of vitamin D.

A supplement of the active form of vitamin D is another option, Sandon says.

info To learn more about vitamin D, visit the National Institutes of Health's Office of Dietary Supplements Web site at *www.ods.od. nih.gov/factsheets/vitamind.asp.*

▪ ▪ ▪ ▪

Are Cheap Vitamins as Potent as Expensive Ones?

Any brand of a single vitamin, such as vitamin C, is usually fine, but the potency varies among brands of multivitamins. Some less expensive brands, such as Wal-Mart's Spring Valley, are well-made, but some supermarket and drugstore brands may not be as reliable.

Name brands that are made by divisions of major pharmaceutical companies usually deliver what they claim.

Examples: Centrum and One-A-Day.

Tod Cooperman, MD, president of ConsumerLab.com, a consumer product watchdog organization, White Plains, NY.

▪ ▪ ▪ ▪

Vitamins May Fight Cravings

In a recent study, people who had taken multivitamins, B vitamins or chromium regularly for the past 10 years gained less weight than people who did not take them.

Possible reason: The body's craving for certain essential nutrients may cause hunger. Vitamin/mineral supplements may lessen hunger by supplying nutrients that would have been supplied by food.

Best: Take a multivitamin/mineral that provides chromium and the daily recommended intake of vitamins B-6 and B-12.

Emily White, PhD, epidemiologist, Fred Hutchinson Cancer Research Center, Seattle.

12

Pain Treatments

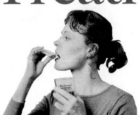

How Not to Get Addicted To Painkillers

Rush Limbaugh, radio personality, made headlines when he admitted that he was addicted to prescription painkillers. His announcement may have discouraged some people who have chronic pain from getting appropriate treatment, but Limbaugh is not typical.

Addiction is rare when prescription painkillers are used properly. The most powerful class of painkillers—opioids, such as *codeine, morphine* and *oxycodone* (Oxycontin)—are potentially addictive, but less than 1% of pain patients ever become addicted.

People who take these drugs can develop a drug tolerance and then require higher doses. If they stop taking the drug, they may experience withdrawal symptoms, such as heightened anxiety and pain, but they rarely exhibit the hallmark signs of addiction.

Warning signs of addiction…

- **Diminished ability to concentrate.**
- **Fixation on the drug.**
- **Watching the clock until the next dose.**
- **Hiding drug use** from your friends and family members.

To prevent addiction, first try to achieve pain relief through *nonsteroidal anti-inflammatory drugs* (NSAIDs), such as aspirin and ibuprofen. *If these aren't effective or if they cause stomach bleeding or other side effects…*

- **Ask your doctor about other non-opioid drugs** that help pain. Many antidepressants, including *amitriptyline* (Elavil), are effective at very low doses. The anticonvulsant *gabapentin* (Neurontin) works for nerve pain. These drugs are not addictive.

- **Try some pain-relief therapies, such as acupuncture and biofeedback.** Nondrug

Alan Rapoport, MD, neurologist, and founder and director, The New England Center for Headache, Stamford, CT, and clinical professor of neurology, Columbia University, New York City.

approaches often allow patients to take lower doses of painkillers or even discontinue them.

Helpful: Get treatment at a multidisciplinary center. Specialists at these centers are familiar with a wide variety of therapies. For information, contact the American Pain Foundation at 888-615-7246 or online at *www.painfoundation.org.*

If these approaches don't work, a pain specialist may recommend opioid drugs. *If you take an opioid…*

●**Limit use.** The risk of addiction tends to rise when a patient takes a prescription painkiller for one year or more.

●**Take a long-lasting drug.** Sustained-release opioids such as MS Contin can stay in the bloodstream for 12 hours and are less likely to cause addiction than shorter-acting drugs such as Percocet. Methadone is also long-lasting and a good choice for chronic pain.

●**Talk to your doctor immediately if you notice any addiction warning signs**—especially if you have a personal or family history of alcoholism or addiction.

■ ■ ■ ■

Combining Painkillers Can Be Dangerous

P atients who regularly take an over-the-counter (OTC) *nonsteroidal anti-inflammatory drug* (NSAID), such as *ibuprofen* (Advil), and aspirin in the same day have a two to three times higher risk of ulcers and gastrointestinal (GI) bleeding as those who take either alone.

Theory: Acidity in the GI tract reaches more harmful levels when the painkillers are combined.

If you must take multiple anti-inflammatory drugs: Ask your physician about adding a proton pump inhibitor (PPI), such as *lansoprazole* (Prevacid), to reduce stomach acid.

Joseph Biskupiak, PhD, research associate professor, department of pharmacotherapy, University of Utah, Salt Lake City.

Two-Thirds of High-Risk Patients Miss Key Meds

Neena S. Abraham, MD, assistant professor of medicine, Baylor College of Medicine, and physician investigator, Michael E. DeBakey Veterans Administration Medical Center, both in Houston.

Jeffrey Raskin, MD, chief of gastroenterology, Miller School of Medicine, University of Miami.

Gregory Haber, MD, director, division of gastroenterology and the Center for Advanced Therapeutic Endoscopy, Lenox Hill Hospital, New York City.

Gastroenterology.

F ewer than one-third of patients who are at high risk of gastrointestinal bleeding while taking *nonsteroidal anti-inflammatory drugs* (NSAIDs) are being prescribed medicines to prevent that bleeding, new research has found.

NSAIDs include over-the-counter (OTC) and prescription versions of aspirin, *ibuprofen* (Advil) and *naproxen* (Aleve).

Doctors have long recognized that long-term use of NSAIDs can increase the chance of gastrointestinal bleeding, so guidelines exist to identify patients at especially high risk.

However, many doctors are not giving these high-risk patients the medicines that can protect them against bleeding, says Dr. Neena S. Abraham, study author and an assistant professor of medicine at Baylor College of Medicine in Houston.

"While we know who's at high risk for upper gastrointestinal bleeding, somehow that knowledge is not being put into practice," she says.

THE STUDY

In their study, Abraham and her colleagues looked at more than 300,000 patients who were treated at 176 VA hospitals throughout the country. All were prescribed an NSAID for pain relief, and all were considered at high risk for upper gastrointestinal bleeding.

Among patients who had one or more risk factor, only approximately 27% were prescribed an NSAID prescription strategy aimed at reducing the risk of bleeding. Among patients who had at least two risk factors, close to 40% were prescribed a safer NSAID strategy, while approximately 42% of the patients who had three risk factors received this benefit.

THE DANGER

NSAIDs are the most commonly prescribed drugs in the United States, Abraham says, with millions of Americans using lower-dose OTC versions as well. They are used to treat pain from any number of ailments, including headache, arthritis, postoperative pain, muscle and backache and cancer pain.

> *This study really highlights some of the gaps between official society recommendations and clinical practice.*
>
> *Gregory Haber, MD*

Abraham adds that upper gastrointestinal bleeding, including ulcers that can perforate the stomach wall, occurs in approximately 4.5% of patients who take NSAIDs over the long term. Internal bleeding is especially dangerous for people older than age 65, since the risk of death linked to such bleeding is 30 times higher in this age group, Abraham says.

Other patients at high risk for bleeding include those who take a steroid and/or an anticoagulant in addition to an NSAID; patients who have a past history of upper gastrointestinal bleeding and patients who take NSAIDs in an amount exceeding the manufacturers' recommended dosage.

These risks are well-known, and numerous organizations, including the American College of Gastroenterology, the American College of Rheumatology and the VA Pharmacy Benefits Management Plan, have issued guidelines in the past several years to recommend preventive therapy for these patients, Abraham says. Guidelines are also being formulated to take into account recent research indicating that heart attack risk can increase among NSAID users.

RESULTS ARE SURPRISING

"I'm absolutely surprised by these findings," says Dr. Jeffrey Raskin, chief of gastroenterology at the University of Miami's Miller School of Medicine. "The risk factors for this have been identified since 1995, and I think we've educated so many people that it was surprising that physicians were not ordering additional therapy in this high-risk group."

Abraham says gastroenterologists, who treat NSAID-related side effects, are obviously aware of the importance of preventing bleeding, but doctors in other specialties as well as general practitioners may not be as mindful.

"It's a common health-care issue for us, but if you're in general practice with, say 100 patients, 10 of whom are on NSAIDs and only one of whom may have had bleeding, unless you've had an experience with it, you might not know," she says.

Other possible explanations for the study results may include disparities in prescription guidelines or financial constraints from insurers on ordering secondary medications, she says.

"This is an important study to publish and will provoke a lot of discussion, as it really highlights some of the gaps between official society recommendations and clinical practice," says Dr. Gregory Haber, director of the division of gastroenterology and the Center for Advanced Therapeutic Endoscopy at New York City's Lenox Hill Hospital.

info For more information on NSAIDs and how to avoid their dangerous side effects, visit the Mayo Clinic at *www.mayoclinic.com/health/pain-medications/PN00058*.

Best Pain Relievers for Headache, Arthritis, Backache and More

Jacob Teitelbaum, MD, director, The Annapolis Center for Effective CFS/Fibromyalgia Therapies, and author of *Pain Free 1-2-3!* (Deva) and *From Fatigued to Fantastic!* (Avery). *www.endfatigue.com*.

Most of us turn to *acetaminophen* (Tylenol) and *ibuprofen* (Advil, Motrin) for pain relief—but there can be more effective approaches, including combining conventional and natural pain relievers.

Caution: Check with your doctor before taking any new medication or supplement.

ARTHRITIS

There are two types of arthritis—*osteoarthritis*, in which cartilage between bones wears away… and *rheumatoid arthritis*, an autoimmune disease that inflames joints. For relief, people who have either type often take *nonsteroidal anti-inflammatory drugs* (NSAIDs), such as aspirin, *ibuprofen* and *naproxen* (Aleve, Naprosyn)—but 16,000 Americans die annually due to side effects from these drugs. And thousands more may have died from taking the recently recalled Vioxx and Bextra. *Instead, try…*

FOR OSTEOARTHRITIS

●**Glucosamine sulfate.** Take 1,500 milligrams (mg) of this supplement—made from *chitin*, which is derived from shellfish—along with 3 grams (g) a day of *methylsulfonylmethane* (MSM), a natural substance in the human body. These nutrients repair cartilage, reducing arthritis pain within six weeks. For maximum tissue repair, take these supplements for two to five months. For chronic arthritis, you may continue for up to a year.

●**Lidoderm.** Put a patch, available by prescription, on the joint. It contains the anesthetics Novocain and Lidocaine. Wear it for approximately 12 hours a day (one patch lasts that long) for two to six weeks. For a large area, some people may use as many as four patches (the package says three). Many patients experience a 30% to 50% decrease in pain within two weeks.

●**Willow bark and Boswellia.** These herbs work as well as Vioxx and Motrin. Take 240 mg of willow bark and 1,000 mg of Boswellia daily. It can take six weeks to work. For chronic arthritis, you may need to take these for up to a year to feel the full effect.

FOR RHEUMATOID ARTHRITIS

●**Fish oil.** Studies show that fish oil (one to two tablespoons a day for at least three months) can reduce inflammation and pain. Eskimo-3, available at health-food stores, and Nordic Naturals (800-662-2544, *www.nordicnaturals.com*) are two reputable brands. Keep taking the fish oil after the pain is gone as a preventive measure.

BACK PAIN

Back pain can occur for no apparent reason and at any point on the spine.

●**Lidoderm.** For low back pain, apply a Lidoderm patch in the morning and remove it in the evening. Expect relief in two to six weeks.

●**Colchicine.** Approximately 70% of all back pain can be eliminated without surgery, through six intravenous injections of the gout medicine *colchicine*. It enters the space between the discs of the vertebrae and reduces inflammation. Colchicine's main risk is a rare but severe allergic reaction (similar to that caused by penicillin).

CARPAL TUNNEL SYNDROME

When a nerve passing underneath a ligament through two bones in the wrist becomes swollen and pinched, it causes pain, numbness and tingling in the hand or forearm. *For relief…*

●**Vitamin B-6 and thyroid hormone.** Take 250 mg a day of B-6. Also, ask your doctor about a prescription for natural thyroid hormone. The combination of B-6 and thyroid hormone decreases swelling and usually clears up the problem in six to 12 weeks. You can remain on this treatment for six months to avoid a recurrence. During treatment, wear a wrist splint at night and, if possible, during the day.

HEADACHES

Tension headaches begin and end gradually. They can last for minutes or sometimes hours. The pain comes from tightened muscles across the forehead and/or at the base of the skull.

●**Tramadol hydrochloride** (Ultram) is often overlooked, but it is an effective prescription pain reliever. Take up to 100 mg as many as four times a day.

Migraines—severe headaches that may be preceded by lights flashing before your eyes and may be accompanied by nausea, vomiting, sweating and dizziness—can last for hours, even days. *Natural remedies are more effective than prescription drugs at preventing migraines…*

●**Butterbur,** from the butterbur plant, can prevent—and even eliminate—migraines. Take 50 mg three times a day for one month, then one 50-mg dose twice a day to prevent attacks. Take 100 mg every three hours to eliminate an acute migraine. Use only high-quality brands, such as Enzymatic Therapy (800-783-2286, *www.enzy.com*) and Integrative Therapeutics' Petadolex (800-931-1709, *www.integrativeinc.com*).

●**Sumatriptan** (Imitrex). When a migraine is developing, 75% of patients experience tenderness and pain around the eyes. Sumatriptan knocks out 93% of migraines if it is taken before the pain around the eyes occurs. When it is taken later, it helps in only 13% of cases. Therefore, if you have a migraine, it is best to take sumatriptan within the first five to 20 minutes.

●**Magnesium.** In the doctor's office or the hospital emergency room, intravenous magnesium can eliminate a migraine in five minutes.

IRRITABLE BOWEL SYNDROME

Irritable bowel syndrome (IBS), also known as spastic colon, is a digestive disorder characterized by bloating, abdominal cramps and diarrhea and/or constipation. *Consider...*

●**Peppermint oil.** For symptomatic relief, take one or two enteric-coated peppermint oil capsules three times a day. Peppermint oil decreases spasms of the bowel muscles. Effective brands include Enzymatic Therapy (800-783-2286, *www. enzy.com*) and Mentharil, available at most health-food stores.

●**Hyoscyamine** (Anaspaz, Levsin). Take this prescription antispasmodic as needed. It relaxes the muscular contractions of the stomach and intestines. Dosages range from 0.125 to 0.375 mg, taken 30 to 60 minutes before a meal.

SHINGLES

This itchy, blistering rash—called shingles or *herpes zoster*—is caused by the same virus that causes chicken pox. It strikes in middle or old age and usually afflicts one side of the upper body. The virus affects the nerves, so it can leave victims in chronic pain, a condition called *postherpetic neuralgia* (PHN). *Discuss these options with your doctor...*

●**Ketamine.** This prescription anesthetic can decrease shingles pain within days in 65% of the cases. Apply a gel containing 5% ketamine two to three times daily to the painful area.

●**Lidoderm.** Place a patch over the area of maximum pain.

●**Neurontin.** This prescription medication can also reduce pain. To avoid side effects, start by using 100 to 300 mg, one to four times a day.

●**Tricyclic antidepressant.** A prescription tricyclic such as *amitriptyline* (Elavil) can relieve nerve pain. To avoid side effects, use a low dose of 10 to 50 mg.

■ ■ ■ ■

What Is Mesotherapy?

Mesotherapy has been used in Europe for more than 50 years for relief from pain that is caused by injured muscles, as in some chronic back pain and in arthritis. It is a virtually painless technique that involves injecting natural compounds—i.e., anti-inflammatory herbs, such as *coumarin* or *arnica*, or medications, such as the bronchodilator *aminophylline* (Trophylline)—into the *mesoderm* (middle layer of the skin) using tiny needles approximately the size of an eyelash. Currently, mesotherapy is being used in the US primarily for cosmetic purposes—it improves blood flow and plumps up the mid-layer of the skin to help reduce wrinkles and cellulite. It also reduces inflammation and pain in the treatment of sports injuries, such as Achilles tendinitis and sprains. The number of injection sessions varies, but can reach 15 or more for cosmetic treatments. The cost ranges from $300 to $500 per session, and it is usually not covered by insurance.

Dan Hamner, MD, sports medicine physician and owner and founder, Peak Energy Program, New York City.

What's New in Arthritis? Diagnosis...Treatment... Living Well

John D. Clough, MD, rheumatologist, The Cleveland Clinic, and publisher, The Cleveland Clinic Press. He is author of Arthritis: A Cleveland Clinic Guide. *Cleveland Clinic.*

New developments in medications and improvements in surgery have brightened the outlook for people who have arthritis. While most forms of arthritis remain incurable, many can be made bearable or better.

Arthritis is an umbrella term for approximately 100 forms of joint ("arthr") inflammation ("itis") involving warmth, redness, tenderness, swelling, stiffness and pain ranging from annoying to disabling. To complicate matters, many conditions with similar symptoms—and requiring different treatment—can masquerade as arthritis.

Examples: Fibromyalgia (muscle pain)… osteoporosis (brittle bones)…side effects of cholesterol-lowering drugs with names ending in "statin"…polymyalgia rheumatica, involving pain and stiffness in the hips or shoulders—common after age 50 (especially in women) and highly treatable using *prednisone* (Deltasone) but a cause of blindness if untreated.

Surprises: A swollen knee, hip or pain in the spine may signal tuberculous arthritis from tuberculosis contracted years before. Mild, fleeting arthritis can result from rheumatic fever following strep throat.

Ideally, arthritis is identified in its early stages and treated aggressively before irreversible damage can occur. Lab tests narrow the possibilities, but for most forms of arthritis, no single test can confirm the diagnosis.

Best bet: See a rheumatologist—a physician specializing in diseases of the joints, muscles and bones. Later, an internist or a general practitioner given the diagnosis and treatment plan can oversee your care.

To find a rheumatologist, ask your doctor, local hospital, county medical association or a friend for recommendations…or search the American College of Rheumatology Web site, *www.rheumatology.org.* Look for board certification in both internal medicine and rheumatology.

THE BIG FIVE

Equipped with a diagnosis, learn about your form of arthritis. The majority (95%) of Americans who have arthritis have one of five types…

•**Osteoarthritis.** By far the most common form of arthritis in the US, osteoarthritis strikes more than half of people over age 65 and 80% of those over age 75.

What it is: Cartilage, which cushions the ends of the joint bones, disintegrates. The bones then rub together and can eventually wear out.

Most often affected: Neck, lower back… hips, knees…fingers, toes. Involvement in the

ankle and elsewhere is usually triggered by an injury or surgery.

Osteo patients tend to take a lot of *acetaminophen* (Tylenol) and *nonsteroidal anti-inflammatory drugs* (NSAIDs), including *ibuprofen* (Advil, Nuprin) and *naproxen* (Naprosyn, Aleve). In large amounts, these effective and seemingly innocuous over-the-counter drugs can be toxic, even deadly. Ask your doctor how much is safe for you.

Easier on the stomach: Cox-2 inhibitors, which are selective NSAIDs that block *prostaglandins*—hormones that cause inflammation of the joints. Cox-2 inhibitors—*rofecoxib* (Vioxx, withdrawn from the market in 2004), *celecoxib* (Celebrex) and *valdecoxib* (Bextra, withdrawn from the market in 2005)—were welcomed with open arms in the late 1990s until a few patients had heart attacks or strokes.

You may still take a Cox-2 inhibitor if your doctor advises and monitors you. Or you may be advised to return to ibuprofen or naproxen.

Glucosamine and chondroitin, sold without a prescription, are among the building blocks of cartilage. Some osteoarthritis sufferers say that these supplements help. With your doctor's approval, you can try them if you want.

When meds no longer quell osteoarthritis pain, a trade-in may be the answer. Hip and knee replacement surgery, performed for more than 30 years, has advanced dramatically. Shoulder replacement has long been a possibility, as has elbow replacement—although the latter is not usually as successful.

On the horizon: Wrist and ankle replacement. Meanwhile, many people who have osteoarthritis of the ankle are getting good results using ankle fusion, in which some ankle joints are fused together. The ankle contains so many joints that range of motion remains good.

•**Rheumatoid arthritis.** In rheumatoid arthritis, the immune system goes haywire, attacking joints throughout the body.

Results: Pain, deformity and disability.

The most exciting developments in the fight against rheumatoid arthritis and some other forms of arthritis are new drugs that fight inflammation. The remarkable *tumor necrosis factor* (TNF) inhibitors block a type of protein called a *cytokine* that triggers inflammation when present in large amounts.

TNF inhibitors are expensive but covered by Medicare Part B. They include *infliximab* (Remicade), approved for use in rheumatoid arthritis in 1999, and *adalimumab* (Humira), approved for use in advanced rheumatoid arthritis in 2002 and in psoriatic arthritis and early rheumatoid arthritis in 2005.

Remicade is given intravenously in a healthcare facility every six to eight weeks. Humira is self-injected every two weeks.

Another effective TNF inhibitor is *etanercept* (Enbrel), approved for use in rheumatoid arthritis in 1998 and in psoriatic arthritis in 2002. Etanercept requires an injection under the skin that can be given at home.

• **Gout.** Remember Jiggs, from the comic strip "Bringing Up Father," whose hassock-supported, bandaged foot radiated lightning bolts of pain? He had gout, a form of arthritis in which uric acid accumulates in the blood and crystallizes in a joint—often, but not always, the ball of the big toe—causing excruciating pain.

The best drug for lowering uric acid is *allopurinol* (Zyloprim). Anti-inflammatories such as *indomethacin* (Indocin) and, in chronic cases, drugs such as *probenecid* (Benemid, Probalan) that reduce the level of uric acid in the blood do wonders for gout.

Diet may help. Restrict foods containing high levels of purine, a heterocyclic aromatic organic compound that produces uric acid crystals. Limit alcohol...organ meats (liver, kidneys)...game fowl (duck, goose)...dried legumes (lentils, chickpeas)...and some seafood (scallops, sardines, shrimp, herring). For a free brochure called "Gout," with a list of food to avoid, contact the Arthritis Foundation, *www.arthritis.org*, 800-568-4045.

• **Seronegative spondyloarthropathies.** These half-dozen conditions involve the spine.

Among the most common: Ankylosing spondylitis, which causes back pain and stiffness, worst in the early morning...psoriatic arthritis, which approximately 20% of the people who have psoriasis develop and which responds well to TNF alpha inhibitors and to the cancer drug *rituximab* (Rituxan), a monoclonal antibody.

• **Systemic lupus erythematosus (SLE).** Arthritis is the primary symptom of lupus, a dysfunction of the autoimmune system.

Relief: Prednisone, a corticosteroid...*cyclophosphamide* (Cytoxan), a cancer drug...and several other medications. These allow many lupus patients to live fairly normal lives with minimal problems.

GET MOVING

Formerly, because it's painful to move, people who had arthritis sat still and got steadily worse. We now know that inactivity is a mistake. For most people who have arthritis, careful exercise is recommended to keep limbs limber.

Physical and occupational therapy have an important place in treating arthritis. Applying heat and practicing strengthening and range-of-motion exercises may help.

Because of the many faces of arthritis, therapy must be designed and supervised individually—and reviewed regularly—by trained professionals. What eases one person's pain may exacerbate another's.

Ask your doctor to recommend a physical therapist who can show you how to protect yourself from injury...a physiatrist, a physician specializing in physical treatments for muscular, skeletal and neurological problems...or an occupational therapist, who can explain how to protect your joints from stress during your usual activities. Swimming pools are superb exercise settings for many people with arthritis.

■ ■ ■ ■

Choosing Easy-to-Use Products

Consider these shopping suggestions from the Arthritis Foundation...

• **Avoid products that are difficult to grasp** or require twisting to open and close.

Example: Levers are better than knobs.

• **Seek out lightweight products,** especially cookware, cooking utensils and cleaning tools.

• **Buy products, such as shoulder bags, that are shaped so that they can be carried close to the body,** reducing pressure on arms, hands and back.

• **Choose products that have texture.**

Example: Drinking glasses that have bumpy exterior surfaces.

●**Simplicity counts.** Products that have intricate pieces are harder to use, clean and store.

Shanon Whetstone Mescher, certified health education specialist (CHES) and consultant, Arthritis Foundation.

Breakthrough Treatments For Rheumatoid Arthritis

Harry D. Fischer, MD, chief of the division of rheumatology, Beth Israel Medical Center, and associate professor of clinical medicine, Albert Einstein College of Medicine, both in New York City. He is coauthor, with Winnie Yu, of *What to Do When the Doctor Says It's Rheumatoid Arthritis.* Fair Winds.

Rheumatoid arthritis isn't just about achy joints. This condition can also affect other parts of the body.

In severe cases, rheumatoid arthritis can cause dangerous heart inflammation (*pericarditis*)… lung inflammation (*pleurisy*)…and sight-damaging eye inflammation (*scleritis*).

People who have rheumatoid arthritis should be treated early, not only to prevent permanent joint deformities but also to guard against the inflammation-related complications that are associated with the disorder. Most of the joint destruction caused by rheumatoid arthritis occurs in the first six to 12 months following diagnosis.

At one time, doctors mainly focused on relieving symptoms using pain medication.

Now: Drug therapies are aimed at curbing the progression of this debilitating disorder.

ARE YOU AT RISK?

Rheumatoid arthritis can occur at any age. Approximately 75% of patients are women, which suggests that hormones may play a role in the disease. Some researchers believe that a viral or bacterial infection may trigger the disorder in some patients. Smoking and stress are thought to contribute to rheumatoid arthritis—but not cause it.

Rheumatoid arthritis is characterized by joint stiffness and swelling, often in symmetrical patterns on both sides of the body. Fatigue and a low-grade fever may also occur.

NEW TREATMENTS

Rheumatoid arthritis almost always requires drug therapy. Drugs can significantly reduce pain in more than half of the patients and offer some relief to the others.

People who have rheumatoid arthritis should seek treatment from a rheumatologist (a medical doctor who specializes in the treatment of diseases that involve the joints, muscles and associated structures).*

Rheumatologists typically prescribe *nonsteroidal anti-inflammatory drugs* (NSAIDs), such as *ibuprofen* (Advil) and *naproxen* (Aleve), or the corticosteroid *prednisone*, to control the pain and inflammation of this condition.

A majority of rheumatoid arthritis patients are also prescribed a medication known as a *disease-modifying antirheumatic drug* (DMARD), which is designed to reduce pain and inflammation and slow the progression of the disease.

●**Nonbiological DMARDs** are synthetic medications that have been available for many years. These drugs reduce joint damage. *Nonbiological DMARDs include…*

●*Methotrexate* (Rheumatrex). This drug suppresses the immune system and minimizes joint destruction. Most patients who take methotrexate experience reduced pain and joint swelling within weeks. It is one of the best drugs for slowing the progression of rheumatoid arthritis.

Potential side effects include nausea, diarrhea and, in rare cases, liver scarring and/or inflammation. For this reason, periodic liver function tests are required.

●*Hydroxychloroquine* (Plaquenil). This antimalarial drug suppresses immune attacks on the joints. It is often combined with methotrexate to try to achieve better results. Potential side effects include nausea and decreased appetite and, in rare cases, *retinopathy*, a disorder of the retina that results in vision impairment. If you take this drug, you should have regular eye exams.

●*Sulfasalazine* (Azulfidine). This medication, often used for mild symptoms or in combination with other drugs for severe symptoms, can cause stomach upset, headache and, in some cases, a decrease in disease-fighting white blood cells.

*To find a rheumatologist in your area, contact the American College of Rheumatology (404-633-3777, *www. rheumatology.org*).

Important: In addition to liver function tests, people who take nonbiological DMARDs require regular blood tests to monitor changes in blood counts.

• **Biological DMARDs** resemble substances that are naturally present in the body. Most patients who take these newer, more specifically targeted drugs experience improvements in a short time—and some even report complete remission.

Three biologic agents are currently available that inhibit or block a cell protein known as *TNF-alpha*. TNF-alpha produces the inflammatory response.

• *Etanercept* (Enbrel). It is usually injected once or twice weekly.

• *Adalimumab* (Humira). It is given by injection once every two weeks, although it is sometimes given weekly.

• *Infliximab* (Remicade). This drug is taken in combination with methotrexate. It is given by intravenous (IV) infusion in a doctor's office, usually once every eight weeks. At times, it can be given as frequently as every four weeks.

These drugs may increase the risk of infection. They can also reactivate tuberculosis (TB) in patients who were previously exposed—even if they never had symptoms. A TB skin test is required prior to starting therapy.

Drawback: These drugs are extremely expensive, costing $13,000 to $30,000 annually, depending on the dose.

NEW DRUG CHOICES

Several new drugs do not have the long-term data of the DMARDs, but they are an option for patients who don't respond to DMARDs.

• **Abatacept** (Orencia). Approved by the US Food and Drug Administration (FDA) in December 2005, abatacept inhibits the activity of *T-cells*, immune cells that play a central role in joint inflammation. Abatacept may increase the risk of infection.

• **Rituximab** (Rituxan). Used for 10 years to treat lymphoma, this drug was recently approved to treat rheumatoid arthritis. It reduces *circulatory B-cells*, a type of white blood cell that has been shown to play a role in the development of rheumatoid arthritis. Rituximab is given by IV infusion once every few months. It may also increase infection risk.

■ ■ ■ ■

Types of Arthritis

Rheumatoid arthritis is caused when the immune system begins attacking the body itself, causing pain and inflammation in the joints.

It is one of the most serious and disabling types of arthritis, is most common among women and often begins when people are in their 30s and 40s.

By contrast, osteoarthritis is caused when the cartilage that covers the ends of bones in the joint deteriorates, producing pain and loss of movement as bone begins to rub against bone, according to the Arthritis Foundation.

Ouch! Arthritis Patients Missing Out on Aspirin Therapy

Lee Colglazier, MD, rheumatologist, Crestview Hills, KY.

Eric Ruderman, MD, associate professor of medicine, Feinberg School of Medicine, Northwestern University, Chicago.

People who have rheumatoid arthritis (RA) should take a low-dose aspirin once a day because they are more likely to develop heart disease. But new research suggests that many patients aren't getting this message, potentially putting them at risk.

Researchers found that just 18% of RA patients are using aspirin therapy, widely considered an effective and inexpensive way to prevent heart attacks. Meanwhile, a similar group of people who have other types of arthritis are significantly more likely to take aspirin every day—in fact, 25% of them do, the study found.

THE STUDY

The researchers surveyed 18,123 arthritis patients for three years. The majority—14,114—had the rheumatoid form.

Of the RA patients, only 18.4% took an aspirin every day to prevent heart disease, compared with 25.1% of the patients who had other forms of arthritis.

For reasons that are not entirely clear, people who have RA are twice as likely to develop heart disease, says study coauthor Dr. Lee Colglazier, a rheumatologist in Crestview Hills, Kentucky, who worked on the study as a rheumatology fellow at Wake Forest University School of Medicine in Winston-Salem, North Carolina. Some theories suggest that the inflammation triggered by RA contributes to cholesterol buildup and artery blockages.

SEARCHING FOR AN EXPLANATION

The reason for overlooking aspirin therapy is not clear, but it may have something to do with rheumatologists and primary-care doctors failing to consider a patient's overall health, says Dr. Eric Ruderman, an associate professor of medicine at Northwestern University's Feinberg School of Medicine. "Maybe we're not looking at the rest of the picture as much as we should," he says.

The findings are mystifying, especially because RA patients are hardly strangers at doctors' offices, Colglazier says. "Maybe they're seeing the doctor a lot, [and] a lot of acute things are going on, [so] doctors don't have time to say, 'Let's address prevention.' "

Ruderman agrees, adding that primary-care doctors might not realize the heart-risk urgency facing RA patients.

Perhaps "they don't view these patients with the same concern that they may view a diabetic or a patient who has significant hypertension or elevated cholesterol," he says.

■ ■ ■ ■

Rheumatoid Arthritis Symptoms

Rheumatoid arthritis is an inflammatory condition that affects an estimated 2 million Americans. It typically occurs in the hands and feet, resulting in swelling, pain and joint deformities. Rheumatoid arthritis is an *autoimmune disease* (a malfunction in the immune system that causes the body to attack cells), which affects the *synovium*, the thin membrane that surrounds the joints.

Faster Treatment for Rheumatoid Arthritis

Scott J. Zashin, MD, clinical assistant professor, division of rheumatology, University of Texas Southwestern Medical Center, Dallas, and author of *Arthritis Without Pain: The Miracle of TNF Blockers.* Sarah Allison.

Traditionally, doctors recommended that patients "go slowly" in treating rheumatoid arthritis—start by using *nonsteroidal anti-inflammatory drugs* (NSAIDs), such as *ibuprofen* (Advil, Motrin), followed by stronger drugs, as needed, through the years. But this approach doesn't always work. In the past, up to 20% of patients who had rheumatoid arthritis were disabled two years after diagnosis, and 50% were disabled 10 years after diagnosis.

Newer approach: Treatment using drugs called *tumor necrosis factor* (TNF) blockers. Rheumatoid arthritis patients have excessive amounts of the cell protein *TNF-alpha*, which mobilizes white blood cells to travel to affected joints and cause inflammation, pain, stiffness and, eventually, joint damage. TNF blockers bind to TNF-alpha, rendering it inactive and relieving symptoms—sometimes in less than two weeks—and slowing down joint deterioration and deformity.

WHO SHOULD TAKE TNF BLOCKERS?

A newly diagnosed patient is usually treated by an NSAID, possibly combined with short-term steroid therapy. If that isn't effective within a few weeks, he/she might be given an antirheumatic drug, such as *hydroxychloroquine* (Plaquenil), *methotrexate* (Rheumatrex) or *sulfasalazine* (Azulfidine). If adequate results still aren't achieved in 12 to 24 weeks, the next step may be a TNF blocker. The US Food and Drug Administration (FDA) has approved three TNF blockers to treat rheumatoid arthritis. They appear to be equally effective. Your doctor can help you decide which is best for you.

•**Etanercept** (Enbrel) is taken by self-injection, usually twice a week. It is not yet determined if a new once-a-week formula is as effective.

•**Adalimumab** (Humira) is also taken by self-injection, usually once every two weeks.

●**Infliximab** (Remicade) is given by intravenous infusion, usually in a doctor's office, once every six to eight weeks.

THE DOWNSIDE

TNF blockers are extremely expensive, costing at least $15,000 a year.

They are taken as long as the condition is active—often for life. The cost may be covered by insurance—check with your insurance company.

The drugs may cause itching, pain or swelling at the injection site. *More serious risks...*

●**Infection.** TNF blockers increase the risk of infection because they suppress the immune system. People who develop respiratory or other infections are often advised to discontinue the drugs until the infection is successfully treated. People who have insulin-dependent diabetes (type 1) have a high risk of infection and are not good candidates for TNF-blocker therapy.

Important: A tuberculosis (TB) skin test is required prior to starting a TNF blocker. TB can be activated in patients who have had any prior exposure, even if they never had symptoms of TB.

●**Cancer.** Some types of cancer, such as lymphoma, which affects the lymph system, have been associated with TNF blockers. However, recent studies suggest that chronic inflammation, rather than the treatment, is responsible for the higher cancer risk.

Beat Pain Now with Self-Hypnosis

Bruce N. Eimer, PhD, president, Alternative Behavior Associates (*www.hypnosisgroupcom*), and author of *Hypnotize Yourself Out of Pain Now!* New Harbinger.

More than 100 million Americans have intractable pain from arthritis, cancer, fibromyalgia, an accident or another source. If conventional measures, such as medication, surgery and physical therapy, haven't allayed it sufficiently, you can learn to relieve it yourself through the power of your mind.

Hypnosis is not about losing control or failing to "wake up." Hypnosis is not sleep. It is a long-established, well-respected form of therapy. Self-hypnosis uses many of the same techniques.

THE PUZZLE OF PAIN

Pain is a survival mechanism. It warns us that something is wrong. Self-hypnosis teaches the central nervous system to be less sensitive to pain signals. It prevents pain messages from flowing to the brain, changes the way the brain interprets them and switches on the part that restores relaxation. Your conscious mind tells your unconscious mind to lower the volume.

Self-hypnosis is safe and convenient, has no negative side effects and can accompany and boost other forms of therapy.

MY STORY

After 10 years of counseling patients who had chronic pain, a major car accident left me with neck, back, leg and bone pain. I also have scoliosis (a curved spine), which triggers muscle pain, and arthritis.

Using self-hypnosis techniques, I greatly reduced my pain. In addition, self-hypnosis helped me prepare emotionally and psychologically for back surgery, promoted positive expectations of a quick recovery and helped me brace for possible disappointment.

Caveat: Before trying self-hypnosis, see a medical professional to make sure that your problem isn't being caused by something physical that can be fixed.

EVALUATE YOUR PAIN

Reconnaissance to evaluate the enemy is the first step in conquering it. To assess the enemy —your pain—write down in a notebook identifying details that will change the pain from vague to specific, making it finite, approachable, reducible.

On a scale of 0 (no pain) to 10 (the worst pain imaginable), rate your pain's intensity right now... at its worst...at its best...at different times of day ...after taking medication...after various activities or treatments...and later, after self-hypnosis.

How do you react to pain? What makes it worse or better?

RELAXATION HELPERS

Also, to prepare for self-hypnosis, think about whether you tend to be most receptive to sights (how a beach looks), smells (ocean brine), sounds (seagull calls, waves breaking) or touch (warm sand under your feet).

To find out: Think of the activity you enjoy most (hiking, gardening, sex). What combination of senses (sight, sound, smell, touch, taste or a nontraditional sense, such as movement) does it primarily involve? You will use this information to relax yourself in self-hypnotism exercises.

RETREAT TO A SAFE PLACE

Everybody daydreams. When you daydream, you're in a hypnotic-like state. Self-hypnosis provides a way to take charge of your daydreams and find a mentally comfortable place where you are protected from pain.

After some practice, you will attain deep physical and mental relaxation—a natural antidote to stress and pain.

Benefit: You'll replenish and restore energy reserves drained by continual pain.

Bonus: Scientific evidence suggests that if you practice self-relaxation regularly, your immune system will become stronger and more effective at shielding you from pain and stress.

Helpful: Tell yourself what you want to happen, then think and imagine that it is happening.

Sit comfortably with your back, neck and head supported and your feet on the floor or a low stool. Close your eyes to block out distractions. Take three deep breaths to unwind. Then breathe normally.

Concentrate on relaxing your eyes, eyelids and surrounding muscles until they don't feel like opening. Tell yourself that deep relaxation is spreading through your body. Imagine that you are experiencing a pleasant floating sensation.

Open your eyes briefly. Close them again and repeat the entire procedure two more times.

Then deepen your relaxation by slowly counting backward to yourself from 20 to one. Tell yourself that you are becoming more and more deeply relaxed with each number. Pay attention to your breathing without trying to change it. Enjoy drifting into a pleasant daydream.

ACT ON THE PAIN

Using your senses, reshape the pain into something less disturbing. *Examples...*

●**Back pain.**

Assess: Stiff, tight and achy.

Retreat: Daydream that you're in a hot tub at a mountain spa.

Action: Imagine the bubbling waters softening the hardness, loosening the tightness, soothing the achiness.

●**Headache.**

Assess: Tightness in forehead, sharp stabbing around left eye.

Retreat: Daydream that you're sitting comfortably. On your head is a block of ice that has air holes for your eyes, nose and mouth.

Act: Feel the soothing coolness numbing the painful sensations...and the cool, smooth, insulating comfort surrounding your head.

EMERGE FROM YOUR DAYDREAM

After approximately five minutes, when you've had enough relaxation and are ready to rouse yourself, slowly count from one to three. At three, blink your eyes tightly, then open them and tell yourself that you're coming back feeling wide awake, alert and refreshed, sound in mind and body, and in control of your feelings.

Bonus: To use this exercise to fall asleep, do not count from one to three at the end. Instead, after your daydream, let yourself drift into a natural sleep state. When you wake up from your nap or night's sleep, you will feel refreshed, alert and rested.

Practice self-hypnosis at least twice a day in a safe place, preferably not when very hungry or full...and *never* while driving a car or operating machinery. After one week, you should find it easy to slip into a light trance-like state when it is appropriate to do so.

ASSESS YOUR PROGRESS

Refer to your initial assessment of the pain recorded in your notebook. Has the pain changed since you began self-hypnosis? Has its intensity lessened? Are its qualities softer? Are the sensations more tolerable?

If so, then self-hypnosis is working for you. If not, there are numerous other self-hypnosis methods to try.

A qualified hypnotherapist can provide a good start to learning self-hypnosis. Choose a licensed mental health professional, typically a clinical psychologist or social worker. Ask about his/her training, experience and credentials in using clinical hypnosis for pain management. Trust your gut feelings about the person as well.

Although effective self-hypnosis takes practice, success brings the reward of pain reduction. By identifying and routinely using coping methods that work best for you whenever you need them, you can ease your pain, enhance your well-being and improve your ability to function all day, every day.

 Visit the American Society of Clinical Hypnosis Web site at *www.asch.net.*

■ ■ ■ ■

Cough Away Pain—It Works!

Coughing reduces the pain of a needle being inserted into the skin for a local anesthetic, an intravenous (IV) line or when blood is drawn.

Reason: Coughing at the moment the needle is injected distracts a part of the brain that also perceives pain.

Important: Before trying this approach, ask the practitioner to observe whether you move your arm when you cough.

Taras I. Usichenko, MD, professor of anesthesiology, Ernst Moritz Arndt University, Greifswald, Germany.

Heal Your Pain... Help Your Health

Jennifer P. Schneider, MD, PhD, board certified in internal medicine, addiction medicine and pain management, and author of *Living with Chronic Pain.* Hatherleigh.

One in 10 Americans has moderate to severe chronic pain, most often due to osteoarthritis, back ailments or injury. Unfortunately, pain is often *undertreated.*

Pain control is not a *luxury*—it is a medical *necessity.* Chronic pain can cause muscle weakness due to inactivity, insomnia and fatigue. It can even "rewire" the nervous system, increas-

ing your sensitivity to pain signals and causing pain in areas that were previously pain-free.

PAIN INVENTORY

Your doctor's ability to prescribe the right treatment depends on knowing exactly where, when and how your body hurts. *Before your next appointment, create a personal pain inventory by answering the following questions...*

●**Where is the pain?** Is it shallow and near the surface of your skin or deep below the surface? Is it worse in any particular location or equally bad all over?

●**When do you feel pain?** Is it worse in the morning or at night? Does it hurt all the time or only when you move? Which movements cause pain? Is your pain affected by stress, changes in weather, exercise or sleep?

●**How bad is the pain?** Rate your pain on a scale of 0 to 10, where 0 represents no pain and 10 is the worst pain you've ever had. These ratings might change during the day—for example, you may wake up with level 3 pain, but progress to level 7 by the evening. Or you may have no pain most of the time, but level 8 pain when you perform specific movements, such as sitting down, standing up or walking.

●**What does the pain feel like?** Is it sharp, stabbing, dull, burning or throbbing?

●**How has the pain interfered with your life?** Does the pain interfere with your sleep? What activities or aspects of your life are limited by pain? Physicians use this information to determine how aggressively to treat the pain, so be honest and thorough in describing how your life has changed.

●**What relieves the pain?** What have you tried, and what has worked? Include all prescription and over-the-counter (OTC) medications, rest, ice packs, applied pressure, herbal remedies, etc.

WORKING WITH YOUR DOCTOR

Most primary-care physicians can diagnose and treat common causes of pain, such as back pain, headaches and osteoarthritis. Depending on your problem, your doctor may refer you to a neurologist, orthopedic surgeon, rheumatologist or other specialist. These doctors may determine that you need surgery or other procedures to treat the underlying cause of your pain.

People who are in pain tend to minimize movement because it hurts. But the less you move, the weaker your muscles become, which worsens the pain when you do try to move. To end this vicious cycle, engage in as much physical activity, such as walking, as you can.

Your doctor may need to try different drugs to see which works best for you. Often, a "cocktail" of medications, instead of just one type, provides the best pain relief. For each medication prescribed, ask the doctor how soon it will begin working and what side effects you can expect.

Example: Some pain relievers can cause constipation.

Make a follow-up appointment before leaving the office. You may need frequent visits while your medications are being adjusted. Once your pain is controlled, you will probably need to see your doctor less often. Prepare a new pain inventory before each visit.

MEDICATIONS TO CONSIDER

Following are some potent pain-fighting therapies, many of which are underused...

•**Anti-inflammatory drugs.** Because these medications both relieve pain and decrease inflammation, they are typically used to treat arthritis and other painful conditions that cause inflammation. The pain reliever *acetaminophen* (Tylenol) does *not* treat inflammation. First-generation *nonsteroidal anti-inflammatory drugs* (NSAIDs) include *ibuprofen* (Motrin, Advil) and *naproxen* (Naprosyn, Aleve). These medications can cause gastrointestinal bleeding and elevated blood pressure, so they may only be appropriate for some people for a limited amount of time. A second-generation NSAID, such as the prescription Cox-2 inhibitor *celecoxib* (Celebrex), is less likely to cause bleeding, but might increase the risk of heart attack and stroke. Your doctor should weigh the risks against the benefits before recommending treatment using anti-inflammatory medication.

•**Opioids.** These medications are typically used to treat moderate to severe pain. Opioids include *codeine, morphine, hydrocodone* (Vicodin), *fentanyl* patches (Duragesic), *oxycodone* (OxyContin), and *oxycodone combined with acetaminophen* (Percocet). These drugs have been so stigmatized by their illicit use that many doctors are afraid to use them to ease pain in patients for whom they would be appropriate.

When used as directed, opioids are no more dangerous than any other drugs and can be taken indefinitely, if needed. Although most patients who take opioid analgesics for more than approximately three weeks become physically dependent on them, few become addicted. Physical dependency means the body has become used to the drug, and when it is stopped, withdrawal symptoms, such as muscle pain, vomiting and diarrhea, can occur. This can be avoided if your doctor tapers the drugs slowly. Addiction occurs when there is a loss of control over the drug use, continued use of the drug despite negative consequences and a mental focus on getting and using more than the prescribed amount.

•**Topical analgesics.** Some types of pain, especially pain on the surface of the skin—such as from shingles or osteoarthritis joint pain—respond well to drugs that are absorbed through the skin.

Examples: The *lidocaine* (Lidoderm) patch and *capsaicin* (Zostrix) cream.

•**Antidepressants.** *Venlafaxine* (Effexor) and *duloxetine* (Cymbalta) have been shown to relieve the nerve pain that accompanies shingles and diabetic neuropathy.

•**Anticonvulsants.** Typically used to control seizures, *topiramate* (Topamax) eases migraines, and *gabapentin* (Neurontin) is helpful for people who have diabetic neuropathy or shingles pain.

If You Think You'll Feel Better, You Will

Jon-Kar Zubieta, MD, PhD, associate professor of psychiatry and radiology, University of Michigan Medical School, Ann Arbor.
Journal of Neuroscience.

Pain relief may be mind over matter. According to new research, just the belief that a pill will relieve pain can cause the release of *endorphins*, the brain's natural pain-fighting chemicals. This finding is the first direct evidence that endorphins play a role in the well-known *placebo effect.*

THE STUDY

Lead author Dr. Jon-Kar Zubieta, an associate professor of psychiatry and radiology at the University of Michigan Medical School, and his team induced pain by injecting a concentrated saltwater solution into the jaws of 14 healthy young male volunteers. The injections were given while the men underwent *positron emission tomography* (PET) scans of their brains.

During one scan, the men were told they would receive pain medication, but were given a placebo instead. The men were then asked to rate the intensity of their pain on a scale of 0 to 100. After the experiment, they provided more detailed pain ratings.

---

*If you receive a drug
and you believe it is active,
the drug itself might
not be doing very much.*

Jon-Kar Zubieta, MD, PhD

The researchers found that after giving the men the placebo, the amount of concentrated saltwater needed to maintain the pain increased, indicating that sensitivity to pain was reduced. Thinking they were getting a pain medicine actually allowed the participants to tolerate more pain, the researchers conclude.

"We looked at the response of pain control systems in the brain," Zubieta says. "We observed that a placebo that was believed to be a [medication] was able to enhance the release of these antipain opioids. In fact, in some areas of the brain, the release [of endorphins] was related to how much the participants believed the drug was going to be effective," Zubieta adds.

THE POWER OF PLACEBO

"When there is a belief that something may take place, this belief actually activates systems in your brain that are directly modifying experience," says Zubieta. "If you receive a drug and you believe it is active, the drug itself might not be doing very much."

Zubieta believes these findings show something about how humans function. "Understanding these mind–body connections are important," he says. "There are many treatments that are believed to be effective, when in reality they may not be more effective than placebo."

Harnessing the placebo effect may have some positive therapeutic applications, Zubieta says. "You want to enhance the placebo effect under some circumstances," he says. "And in some others, you want to reduce it—like when you do a clinical trial."

info The Creighton University Web site provides more information about the placebo effect at *http://altmed.creighton.edu/homeo pathy.* Click on "Placebo Effect."

■ ■ ■ ■

Quick Pain Relief Tricks

When you're in pain, it's hard to think of anything else. But redirecting your thoughts can be helpful. *Following are some other techniques to try...*

●**Instruct yourself to think and behave in a functional way.** *I will take a walk to increase the circulation of blood in my legs, bring oxygen to my tissues and lift my mood.*

●**Decatastrophize.** Reframe your pain as less terrible than it feels. *I've been here before. I'm in charge. I can handle it.*

●**Distort your perception of pain.** Use your imagination to transform how the pain feels. Shift your attention to sensations, thoughts or feelings that are easier to cope with. Let these new thoughts generate sensations that oppose the pain.

Example: When pain strikes, imagine that one of your hands is immersed in ice water. Concentrate on telling your hand to become totally numb. Then place your hand on the part of your body that hurts most. Imagine the numbness flowing into the part of your body that needs pain relief. If you can't reach that place, such as your back, put your hand on your stomach and let the cold flow through your body to your back.

●**Distract yourself.** Refuse to pay attention to the pain. Ignore it like an annoying car alarm. Shift your attention somewhere else. Tell yourself,

I will concentrate on the sensation of rubbing my fingers together...focus my attention on my breathing...squeeze my tension into a fist, then relax my hand and let the tension fly out.

Study the sensations as if they were separate from you. Tell yourself, "No pain lasts forever."

Bruce N. Eimer, PhD, president, Alternative Behavior Associates, and author of *Hypnotize Yourself Out of Pain Now!* New Harbinger.

Cognitive Therapy Eases Back Pain as Well As Physical Therapy

Rob Smeets, MD, consultant, rehabilitation medicine, Rehabilitation Centre Blixembosch, the Netherlands.

Scott Eathorne, MD, associate chairman of primary care and medical director of athletic medicine, Providence Hospital, Southfield, MI.

Musculoskeletal Disorders.

People who have chronic lower-back pain can benefit as much from cognitive behavioral therapy as they do from physical therapy, a new Dutch study suggests.

Study participants who had low-back pain reported improvements in function and reductions in pain whether they received 10 weeks of physical therapy or 10 weeks of cognitive therapy, according to researchers. Interestingly, those people who received a combination of cognitive and physical therapy did not do better than those on either treatment alone.

THE STUDY

The study looked at 212 people who had chronic low-back pain. The participants were randomly assigned to one of four groups—active physical therapy (APT), cognitive behavioral therapy (CBT), a combination of APT and CBT or no treatment at all.

Active physical therapy was designed to restore aerobic capability and to increase back muscle strength. Participants rode a bicycle and did back-strengthening exercises. Cognitive behavioral therapy helped the patients cope with their pain and taught them how to overcome their reluctance to undertake physical activity.

THE RESULTS

At the end of the 10-week study, both treatment groups had an improvement in their function and pain scores and a drop in their levels of complaints compared with the group that received no treatment. The combination group also improved, but only as much as either treatment group alone.

People who have chronic back pain tend to start avoiding things that may actually be helpful to them.

Scott Eathorne, MD

The study participants all completed numerous psychological and physical function questionnaires at the start and end of the study. One questionnaire that was used to gauge improvement was the Roland Disability Questionnaire, which asks 24 questions about the limitation on physical function due to back pain. The higher the score, the more disabled a person is by back pain. The average score on this questionnaire increased by almost three points for the group that received no treatment. However, scores went down an average of 2.25 points for the active physical therapy group, 2.65 points for the cognitive behavioral therapy group and 2.27 points for the combination group.

"People with disabling low-back pain should be [active], and this can either be achieved by physical training or cognitive behavioral training," says lead author, Dr. Rob Smeets, a consultant in rehabilitation medicine at the Rehabilitation Centre Blixembosch in the Netherlands.

"Physical training is slightly preferable for people with a relatively low level of disability at the start of treatment, but the cognitive behavioral treatment is preferred when people are moderately to severely disabled," he says.

THE BENEFITS OF CBT

Dr. Scott Eathorne, medical director of athletic medicine at Providence Hospital in Southfield, Michigan, says he wasn't surprised that cognitive behavioral therapy had such an effect.

"People who have chronic back pain tend to start avoiding things that may actually be helpful to them. But cognitive behavioral therapy can change how they think about themselves," he says. "CBT not only addresses the physical aspects of the pain, but it starts to look at how the patients think about their pain and how they behave."

Both Smeets and Eathorne say they were somewhat surprised that the combination therapy wasn't more effective than either treatment alone. Smeets says it could be that there is a limit to the amount of improvement that's possible. It also could be that the people in the combination treatment group didn't adhere as closely to the study protocol as the other treatment groups, or the combination group might have been too small to produce any statistical difference, he says.

Smeets and his colleagues are following the study participants to see if the results will be long lasting.

"A multidisciplinary approach to back pain management is really key," says Eathorne. "We need to design treatment approaches to take into account physical, emotional and behavioral aspects of back injuries."

Back pain is an extremely common condition, affecting four out of five Americans at some point in their lives, according to the National Institutes of Health (NIH).

info To learn more about back pain and treatment options, visit the National Institute of Arthritis and Musculoskeletal and Skin Diseases Web site at *www.niams.nih.gov.* Click on "Health Information" and look for "Back Pain."

■ ■ ■ ■

Low-Back Pain Relief

Low-back pain can be relieved by antidepressants. A recent review of published studies found that people who experienced chronic low-back pain who took the tricyclic antidepressant *nortriptyline* (Aventyl) had less pain and needed fewer painkillers than those taking a placebo.

Theory: The analgesic properties of these antidepressants, which inhibit the uptake of the neurotransmitter *norepinephrine,* help relieve back pain.

If you have chronic low-back pain: Talk to your doctor about adding an antidepressant to your painkiller regimen.

Thomas O. Staiger, MD, associate professor of medicine, University of Washington, Seattle.

■ ■ ■ ■

How to Sit to Save Your Back

Most of us spend more time sitting than in any other position. Sitting exerts 30% more pressure on the spine than standing. It's the main reason that back pain is the number-one cause of work-related disability in the US.

There are no good chairs. No matter how much money you spend on a chair or how ergonomically well-designed the chair is, sitting will still be hard on your back. *To protect your spine...*

●**Support your *lumbar* (lower) spine** by slipping a roll of paper towels between your back and the chair. To hold the paper towels in place, put string through the hole and tie the roll to the back of your chair, parallel to the floor. It's a lot cheaper than buying a fancy pillow or a chair that has an adjustable lumbar support— and you can remove the towels, as needed, to get the right level of support.

●**Shift your weight every few minutes.** Arch your back...lean forward...lean back... shift your weight from one buttock to the other. Movement prevents excessive strain on any one muscle or joint.

●**Get up and walk around** for 30 seconds at least once every 45 minutes.

Joseph Weisberg, PhD, founder and owner, North Shore Rehabilitation, Great Neck, NY, and coauthor of *3 Minutes to a Pain-Free Life.* Atria.

Yoga Eases Low-Grade Back Pain

Karen Sherman, PhD, MPH, epidemiologist and researcher, Group Health Cooperative, Seattle.
Andrew Sherman, MD, assistant professor and head of medical rehabilitation, the Spine Institute, Miller School of Medicine, University of Miami.
Annals of Internal Medicine.

A new study compared yoga, conventional therapeutic exercise and the information contained in a popular back pain book to determine which was the most effective in treating chronic low-back pain.

The results showed that people who participated in weekly yoga classes for 12 weeks experienced the greatest benefits.

THE STUDY

Karen Sherman, an epidemiologist and researcher at Group Health Cooperative in Seattle, and her colleagues chose 101 participants between 20 and 64 years of age who had chronic but not serious low-back pain.

The researchers separated the participants, mostly women in their 40s, into three groups. One group took classes in *viniyoga*, a therapeutic type of yoga that's relatively easy to learn and emphasizes safety.

The second group attended specially designed therapeutic exercise classes taught by a physical therapist and comprised of stretching and strength training. The third group was asked to read *The Back Pain Helpbook*.

For people who are looking to do something for themselves, you could clearly say that yoga is the best.

Karen Sherman, PhD, MPH

During the 26-week study, the participants were interviewed four times, including prior to the start the study and at the end, to assess their pain level, ability to do daily tasks and how much pain medication they took.

All three groups reported improved function. However, those who took the yoga class experienced the greatest gains—78% of the group improved by at least two points on the Roland Disability Scale, a standardized measure that assesses the limitation on physical function due to back pain.

Of the people who participated in the exercise class, 63% reported at least a two-point improvement, while 47% of those who read the book reported a similar benefit.

The yoga participants also reduced their use of pain medicine more than those in the other two groups. At the end of the 26 weeks, only 21% of the people in the yoga class were taking medication for their back pain; 58% had been doing so prior to the start of the study. The use of pain medication for the exercise group dropped to 50% from 57%, and those who read the book actually increased their use of pain medication—from 50% to 59%, according to the researchers.

"For people who are looking to do something for themselves, you could clearly say that yoga is the best," says Sherman.

WHY YOGA HELPS

Sherman says yoga may be effective in alleviating back pain because many people are unaware of how they move their bodies. The breathing component of yoga makes people more conscious of their bodies and of movements that might contribute to their back problems, she says.

Sherman says that this is the largest study to date that compares different therapies for chronic low-back pain. Larger studies may tease out the benefits of yoga compared with other forms of exercise.

She also emphasizes that it is important to choose the right yoga instructor if you are experiencing back pain.

A TAILORED APPROACH

Dr. Andrew Sherman, head of medical rehabilitation at the Spine Institute at the University of Miami's Miller School of Medicine, says that although this study shows that yoga is helpful in treating back pain, the best therapy is one that is tailored to each patient. Someone who is under stress and has tight muscles might be a good candidate for yoga, but another person who has very weak muscles might also benefit from other strength-building exercises, he says.

Because this study included only approximately 35 people in each group, a larger study is needed before yoga can be shown to be definitively better than other therapies, he says. "You can't throw other therapies under the bus based on 35 patients."

info For more information on back pain, visit the US National Library of Medicine's MedlinePlus Web site at *www.medlineplus.gov*. Click on "Health Topics."

Back Pain Relief Combo Is Effective

Consortium of Academic Health Centers for Integrative Medicine news release.

Used together, conventional and alternative treatments can help patients alleviate low-back pain better than using mainstream treatment alone, US research has shown.

THE STUDY

A study at Brigham and Women's Hospital looked at 19 patients who had low-back pain—six received conventional care and 13 received *integrated* care, which included acupuncture, chiropractic, internal medicine, massage therapy, neurology, nursing, nutritional counseling, occupational therapy, orthopedics, psychiatry/mind–body, physical therapy and rheumatologic.

Over the 12-week study period, the patients in the integrative care group had a significantly greater reduction in pain scores and a greater improvement in function than the conventional care group.

The promising results suggest that this combination approach to treating low-back pain warrants further evaluation, the study authors say.

info The National Center for Complementary and Alternative Medicine has more information about a variety of treatments at *http://nccam.nih.gov/health/whatiscam.*

■ ■ ■ ■

Devil's Claw Relieves Back Pain

Back pain can be relieved by using the herb *devil's claw.**

A recent meta-analysis of 12 previous studies found that a daily dose of 60 milligrams (mg) of *harpagosides*, which are in devil's claw, is as effective in treating low-back pain as a standard dose of the prescription drug Vioxx. Vioxx was pulled off the market because it was linked to heart problems.

Caution: Do not take devil's claw if you are taking blood thinners or have any clotting disorders.

Joel J. Gagnier, ND, postgraduate fellow, Institute of Medical Sciences, University of Toronto, Ontario, Canada.

*Check with your doctor before taking this product.

■ ■ ■ ■

Back Pain Treatment

Some doctors are now using machines designed to straighten and strengthen the back's *extensor* muscles—the muscles you use when you bend backward. By using this method, doctors hope to relieve pain and allow patients to avoid back surgery.

Reality: Any exercise that conditions key postural muscles—abdominals, hip flexors and back muscle extensors—can help relieve pain. These machines can help but contribute nothing special.

Best: Carefully prescribed, standardized exercises tailored for your individual back problem.

Norman Marcus, MD, medical director, Norman Marcus Pain Institute, 30 E. 40 St., New York City 10016.

Spot and Treat Shingles Quickly to Avoid Years of Pain

Leon Kircik, MD, medical director of Physicians Skin Care and Dermatologic Research, PLLC, Louisville, KY, and consulting physician at Jewish Hospital, Louisville, KY, and Staten Island University Hospital, New York City.

Shingles is a painful nerve ailment caused by the reactivation of the chicken pox virus in adulthood. One out of every five Americans will have shingles at some point in his/her life.

While the disease can occur at any age, it usually strikes after age 50 and is most common among people ages 65 to 80. Shingles rarely occurs more than once and typically lasts a week to 10 days. But if medication is not used promptly, that single episode can result in painful nerve damage that persists for years.

WHAT CAUSES SHINGLES?

To get shingles, you must have been exposed to the chicken pox virus earlier in your life.

After someone has chicken pox, typically as a child, the virus that caused it—a type of herpes virus called *varicella-zoster virus* (VZV) or *herpes zoster*—retreats to nerve cells along the spinal cord, where it remains for life.

When immunity to VZV declines, either due to age or because the immune system has been weakened by a disease (such as cancer or AIDS) or medication (such as chemotherapy), the virus can suddenly flare up again as shingles.

SYMPTOMS TO WATCH FOR

One of the unique aspects of shingles is that it occurs only on one side of the body, along the affected nerve. The first signs tend to be an unusual tingling, burning or itching sensation or an abnormal sensitivity along one arm, leg or cheek, sometimes accompanied by flu-like symptoms. This indicates that the virus has become active in the nerve root. Within a few days—the time it takes for the virus to reach the skin—a rash made up of painful, fluid-filled blisters develops in the area where the nerve sensations occurred.

Left untreated, the blisters usually dry up on their own in seven to 10 days. Prompt drug treatment can shorten the episode to three or four days. Once the rash clears up, however, 20% of shingles patients experience ongoing nerve pain in the affected area that can last for months or even years—a condition called *post-herpetic neuralgia*. In the most severe cases, even the slightest touch causes such excruciating pain that even normal activities become impossible.

Very important: The best way you can prevent post-herpetic neuralgia is to take antiviral medication within 72 hours of the first signs of tingling, burning or itching—before any blisters appear. (Just as when you have a herpes-related cold sore, medicine is used at the first sign of tingling, before the sore actually appears.) Once the virus has reached the skin—in 48 to 72 hours—it's too late for the medication to have any preventive effect.

Other dangers of shingles: Shingles sometimes affects a nerve supplying the face. When this happens, the virus can spread to the eye or ear, leading to blindness or deafness if it's not treated quickly. Until they've dried up, the blisters are contagious, and direct contact with them could spread chicken pox (not shingles) to someone who has never had chicken pox.

If you have fresh shingles blisters, be especially careful not to get near a child who hasn't had chicken pox or has not been vaccinated against it, anyone who has a compromised immune system or any pregnant women who haven't had chicken pox (the fetus could be at risk if she catches chicken pox).

DIAGNOSING AND TREATING SHINGLES

If you feel a strange sensation that you suspect may be shingles, your best bet is to see a dermatologist at once. Diagnosing the early signs of shingles, before the rash appears, can be difficult. The rash itself can also be misleading, because it may resemble herpes simplex or contact dermatitis. A trained dermatologist will be able to spot the symptoms of shingles immediately and confirm the diagnosis by a viral culture.

Once diagnosed, the shingles patient is immediately started on a seven- to 10-day course of the antiviral drug *acyclovir* (Zovirax)—taken five times a day—or *valacyclovir* (Valtrex) or *famciclovir* (Famvir), both of which are taken twice a day. As mentioned above, the earlier the antiviral drugs are given, the more effective they will be. To prevent long-term complications, they should be started no later than 72 hours after the first signs of shingles appear.

Additional treatments may include topical antibiotics, such as Bactroban ointment, to prevent infection, and topical steroids, such as hydrocortisone, to help dry up the blisters and reduce painful inflammation. The infected area must also be kept clean as an additional safeguard against secondary infections.

In severe cases, such as in people who have weak immune systems, shingles can cover the entire body or spread internally. In both of these cases, the patient may need to be hospitalized and given acyclovir intravenously. If the eye or ear becomes involved, then the patient will need to be referred to an eye or ear specialist for appropriate treatment. If the patient develops post-herpetic neuralgia, appropriate pain management will also be required.

■ ■ ■ ■

Ouch! Shingles Is on the Rise

As more children get immunized against chicken pox, more adults may get shingles.

Reason: The same virus causes both illnesses. Some scientists believe that exposure to children who have chicken pox helps adults develop immunity against shingles—so more vaccinated kids could mean a higher risk of shingles for adults.

Marietta Vazquez, MD, assistant professor of pediatrics, Yale University School of Medicine, New Haven, CT.

New Vaccine Blocks 50% of Shingles Cases

Jesse Goodman, MD, director, Center for Biologics Evaluation and Research, US Food and Drug Administration.

Norman Baylor, PhD, director, Office of Vaccines Research and Review, Center for Biologics Evaluation and Research, US Food and Drug Administration.

Donald H. Gilden, MD, professor and chairman, department of neurology, Health Sciences Center, University of Colorado, Denver.

Anne Louise Oaklander, MD, PhD, director, Nerve Injury Unit, Massachusetts General Hospital, and associate professor of neurology, Harvard Medical School, Boston.

The US Food and Drug Administration (FDA) has approved Zostavax, a new vaccine that can protect up to 50% of people age 60 and older from developing shingles.

Shingles is caused by the *varicella-zoster virus*, the same virus that causes chicken pox. After someone has had chicken pox, the virus lies dormant in nerve tissue. As people get older, the virus can reappear in the form of shingles—usually clusters of blisters that develop on one side of the body and that can cause severe pain that may last for weeks, months or years.

THE ONLY VACCINE

"This is the only vaccine that reduces the risk or reactivation of the varicella-zoster virus," says Dr. Jesse Goodman, director of the FDA's Center for Biologics Evaluation and Research.

The vaccine is not intended for people who currently have shingles. "The vaccine will not treat shingles. The whole idea of this vaccine is to prevent people from getting it," says Norman Baylor, director of the FDA's Office of Vaccines Research and Review at the Center for Biologics Evaluation and Research. "It is essentially boosting an older person's immunity against the virus, in order to prevent the virus from emerging and causing shingles," he adds.

The vaccine is not recommended for people whose immune systems are compromised, such as people who have HIV/AIDS or patients receiving immunosuppressant therapy, Baylor says.

REACTION

"I am absolutely delighted that it got approved," says Dr. Donald Gilden, professor and chairman of the department of neurology at the University of Colorado Health Sciences Center. "It has been tested for 10 years and shown to reduce the incidence of shingles by 50%."

Baylor believes this vaccine will have a significant impact on a growing and painful problem for the increasing elderly population. Gilden agrees. "It's not going to wipe out shingles," he says, "but it will reduce the incidence of shingles very effectively."

"This is a terrific advance, with major implications in preventing a serious, common, chronic pain condition," says Dr. Anne Louise Oaklander, director of the Nerve Injury Unit at Massachusetts General Hospital and an associate professor of neurology at Harvard Medical School.

Oaklander says the vaccine offers a great benefit and very little risk. "The benefits are potentially enormous," she says, "not only in lessening illness from shingles but in preventing post-herpetic neuralgia, a devastating pain condition that commonly develops in older shingles patients."

info The National Institute of Allergy and Infectious Diseases can provide more information about shingles at *www.niaid.nih.gov/ factsheets/shinglesfs.htm.*

13

Savvy Consumer

Best Ways to Avoid Deadly Hospital Errors

The hospital is one of the most dangerous places you'll ever go. Patients are exposed to bacteria and viruses…subjected to tests and procedures with high risks…and given drugs that should be closely monitored—but sometimes aren't.

Between 44,000 and 98,000 Americans die annually from hospital errors. Although hospital patients can't control everything that happens in the hospital, they can lower their risks more than they realize.

Example: Use only a hospital that's accredited by the Joint Commission on Accreditation of Healthcare Organizations. This type of accreditation means the hospital is evaluated every three years to ensure that it meets the best standards in cleanliness, infection control, drug administration guidelines, etc. More than 15,000 health-care facilities are accredited—but many others aren't. To check, go to *www.qualitycheck.org*, or call 630-792-5800. *Other ways to stay safe…*

PICK THE BEST HOSPITAL

Teaching hospitals affiliated with major medical universities tend to have the latest technology and best-trained staff. If you require major surgery (such as a transplant operation) or have a life-threatening condition (such as an aortic aneurysm or pancreatic cancer), a teaching hospital is your best option. Smaller hospitals are fine for patients with "routine" health problems, such as pneumonia or a broken leg.

Warning: In the summer months, teaching hospitals are largely staffed by new residents and interns. Their lack of experience can adversely affect patient care. If you can, avoid teaching hospitals during the first two weeks of July, when the new school year begins. *Other points to consider…*

Michael F. Roizen, MD, chief, division of anesthesiology, critical care medicine and pain management, The Cleveland Clinic. He is author of *RealAge* (Cliff Street) and coauthor, with Mehmet C. Oz, MD, of *You: The Smart Patient* (Free Press).

●**Is it a "magnet" hospital?** Medical centers with outstanding nursing programs earn this designation from the American Nurses Credentialing Center (800-284-2378, *www.nursecredentialing.org*). Patients in these hospitals benefit from improved care...less staff turnover...and high-quality physicians, who are more likely to work at a hospital with magnet status.

●**Are there full-time intensivists and hospitalists?** Intensivists are doctors who specialize in treating critically ill patients. Hospitalists are doctors who treat only hospital patients. Both types of specialists provide superior hospital care and don't maintain private practices "on the side."

●**How often does the hospital perform the procedure you're undergoing?** The best outcomes usually occur at hospitals where a given procedure is performed most often, on average.

Examples: A top-flight hospital will perform at least 500 open-heart procedures annually...100 carotid-artery grafts or surgeries...and 25 mastectomies.

CHOOSE THE BEST SURGEON

Only use a surgeon who is board certified in the specialty that is related to your operation —neurosurgery, cardiac surgery, etc. Look for the letters "FACS" (Fellow, American College of Surgeons) after his/her name. This means that the surgeon has been evaluated for competence and ethical standards.

Helpful: Call the hospital anesthesiology department, and ask one of the anesthesiologists which surgeon he would pick. (Anesthesiologists often are free between 3 pm and 5 pm.) They know all the surgeons and have no reason not to give a straight answer.

Once you have some recommendations, choose a surgeon who does only a few types of procedures. Research has shown that surgeons who specialize—in nerve-sparing prostate surgery, for example—have better results and fewer complications than the national average.

Caution: Don't shave your surgical site before surgery. You'll wind up with thousands of invisible nicks that increase the risk for infection. Let the operating room staff do it. They use special creams that prevent nicks.

Important: Ask the anesthesiologist to provide a blanket (if it won't get in the way) to keep you warm during surgery. Patients who maintain *normothermia* (normal body temperature) have a lower risk for infection and other complications.

PREVENT HOSPITAL INFECTIONS

Each year, an estimated 2 million hospital patients develop an infection. With the emergence of antibiotic-resistant bacteria, even a minor initial infection can be fatal.

We all know the importance of hand washing, so insist that visitors (including nurses and doctors) wash their hands before touching you. A quick rinse doesn't help. Studies show that you must wash vigorously with soap and warm water for at least 15 seconds to remove all bacteria. As an alternative, hand-sanitizing gel, which is now located outside many hospital rooms, may be used by visitors.

Other self-defense strategies...

●**Keep a bottle of hand-sanitizing gel at your bedside.** Use this hand cleanser yourself before eating.

●**Beware of the TV remote control.** One study found that remote controls in hospitals have three times more bacteria than doorknobs or nurse call buttons. To protect yourself, cover the TV remote with a new medical glove. You'll still be able to change the channels.

●**Ask about the stethoscope.** Doctors and nurses are supposed to clean their stethoscopes with alcohol between patients—but some get too busy and forget. Uncleaned stethoscopes have been linked to hospital infections.

DRUG PROTECTION

Drug mistakes—giving the wrong drug, a dangerous drug combination or the wrong dose— often occur in hospitals. Ask your primary-care doctor to supervise all of your health care, including drug prescriptions. If that isn't possible, ask one of the hospitalists to do it. Patients with one supervising doctor face fewer risks.

Each time you're given medication: Show your ID bracelet. To ensure that you're getting the right drug (medical test or procedure), ask the nurse to check your ID wrist bracelet.

Ask the nurse to tell you what each drug is and why you're taking it. Don't take a drug unless you're sure it's the one that you're supposed to be taking. If you're receiving a medical test or procedure, confirm that it's the correct one.

Finally, ask a family member or friend to help monitor your daily care. This is especially important if the patient is not able to do so.

Dial 911! US Emergency Care Needs Help

Frederick C. Blum, MD, president, American College of Emergency Physicians, and professor of emergency medicine, pediatrics and internal medicine, West Virginia University School of Medicine, Morgantown.

Stephen Epstein, MD, emergency physician, Beth Israel Deaconess Medical Center, and instructor, Harvard Medical School, both in Boston.

National Report Card on the State of Emergency Medicine.

Emergency care in the United States has been given a "C-" grade by the American College of Emergency Physicians on the first-ever *National Report Card on the State of Emergency Medicine.*

Their study found that the emergency care system is overcrowded, provides limited access to care, is hampered by soaring liability costs and has a limited ability to deal with public health or terrorist disasters.

A NATIONWIDE C- AVERAGE

Each state and the District of Columbia was graded on a scale of "A" through "F" based on the state's access to emergency care, quality and patient safety, public health and injury prevention and medical liability environment.

Not a single state achieved an overall A. California had the highest ranking, followed by Massachusetts, Connecticut and the District of Columbia—all of which received an overall grade of B. Arkansas, Idaho and Utah received the lowest ranking—a D.

LIABILITY AND COSTS ARE FACTORS

Dr. Frederick C. Blum, president of the American College of Emergency Physicians and also a professor of emergency medicine, pediatrics and internal medicine at West Virginia University School of Medicine, says that one of the main obstacles to providing quality emergency care is medical liability. In many places, the cost of mal-

practice insurance has forced doctors, particularly specialists, to give up their practice, he says. This trend is making it more difficult for emergency departments to get specialists to see patients in the emergency room. It also increases the burden on emergency departments, since patients who would have gone to a specialist may go to the emergency department instead, Blum explains.

In addition, many hospitals are closing their emergency departments because of financial considerations. "At a time when emergency-department visits are going through the roof, the number of emergency departments has declined because hospitals have found it's more economically attractive to close the emergency department than to keep it open and lose money," Blum says.

> *It's like musical chairs. The number of emergency departments is decreasing, while the number of patients is increasing. We are running out of chairs.*
>
> *Stephen Epstein, MD*

These problems all have a significant impact on the quality and safety of care being given, Blum says.

GOVERNMENT ACTION NEEDED

To solve some of these problems, Blum believes that both state and federal action is needed, particularly in the areas of liability reform, reimbursement for emergency department visits, disaster and terrorist preparedness and public health education and legislation.

"People tend to count on and take for granted emergency care," Blum says. "But there are a lot of problems that are facing the people who deliver that care."

Dr. Stephen Epstein, an emergency physician at Beth Israel Deaconess Medical Center in Boston, agrees. "It's like musical chairs," he says. "The number of emergency departments is decreasing, while the number of patients is increasing. We are running out of chairs."

A LARGER CRISIS

Epstein notes that the problem in emergency departments is only a symptom of a larger crisis. "Hospitals have to operate at near 100% capacity in order to survive," he says.

Because of this, many hospitals have closed off areas and have fewer beds available. "A number of us are afraid that if we had a flu pandemic, we would not have places to hospitalize people," Epstein says.

info The American College of Emergency Physicians can tell you more about the state of emergency medicine in the United States at *www.acep.org/webportal*.

■ ■ ■ ■

Keep These ER Aids in Your Wallet

Regularly update information that could be lifesaving in the emergency room. *Don't leave home without a...*

- **List of your drug allergies** (or the statement "no known drug allergies").
- **List of all current medications,** prescription and nonprescription (herbs, vitamins, antacids), including dose and reason.
- **Health insurance** and/or Medicare card.
- **Your baseline electrocardiogram (ECG)** —a miniature copy, laminated. Take your ECG readout to a copy place, reduce it to wallet size and cover it with self-stick clear plastic sheets, sold at stationery and office supply stores.

Why: Comparing a new ECG with an old one can increase the accuracy in the diagnosis of heart problems.

Joel Cohen, MD, medical director, MD RoomService/ DoctorCare, a house call practice, Scottsdale, AZ (www. mdroomservice.com), and author of ER: Enter at Your Own Risk—How to Avoid Dangers Inside Emergency Rooms. New Horizon.

Coping with Health-Care Conflicts

Abraham Verghese, MD, director, Center for Medical Humanities and Ethics, University of Texas Health Science Center at San Antonio. He is author of My Own Country: A Doctor's Story. Simon & Schuster.

Many hospital patients and their families don't realize that at every hospital, in addition to all the advanced drugs and technical procedures, there's also a group of people—doctors and others—who spend a great deal of time focusing on the personal, human and moral issues of medicine—an ethics committee. Members of this committee help work through the many troubling medical issues that can arise.

To find out more about the work of these committees and explore other doctor–patient ethical issues, we spoke with Abraham Verghese, MD, a preeminent figure in medical ethics and head of the University of Texas Health Science Center at San Antonio's humanities and ethics curriculum.

●**Who is on a hospital's medical ethics committee, and what can they do for patients and families?** Membership varies from place to place, but it's not only doctors. There also may be a lawyer, a chaplain, a nurse and a nonmedical professional from the community. Special training isn't required, but all of these participants will have expressed an interest in medical ethics and patients' rights. At most large hospitals, one member will carry a beeper, on a rotating basis, in case there's a need for an ethics consultation.

Sometimes hospital staffers themselves want to consult the ethics committee—for example, if a recommendation by the hospital's oncology team to aggressively treat an end-stage cancer patient doesn't sit well with the patient's primary care team. But often, family members disagree about treatment issues, which may trigger an ethics committee consultation.

●**What would a typical family scenario be?** Unexpected end-of-life decisions are the most common. The medical system is not equipped to make such judgments in acute emergencies. It will deliver the maximum care even if that's not what the patient would have wanted.

That's why planning ahead by creating advance directives, such as a living will or a durable power of attorney for health care, is so important. Many people say the idea of remaining on a breathing machine is repugnant to them. But, having said that, most people don't have the proper documentation in place to prevent that scenario.

Here's a typical dilemma: A patient has had a massive stroke and is now on a ventilator in the ICU. The patient's prognosis is grim. Most of the time, the family will agree to remove the ventilator and discontinue treatment, other than that which makes the patient comfortable. But oftentimes, one or more family members disagree. They think their mother is going to get better. Or maybe an adult child doesn't trust his father's second wife to make this kind of decision.

If there's any such conflict, especially in this type of critical situation, the ethics committee will be called in to hear all sides and then make a recommendation to the health-care team.

●**But ethics issues aren't only about dying or incompetent patients, are they?** You're right—and it's important for us as doctors to recognize our boundaries. For a long time, medicine tended to be very paternalistic. Doctors acted as though they alone knew what was in the best interest of their patients.

That era is gone. Today, it's an era of patient autonomy. For example, if you're a mentally competent adult and your belief system does not allow you to have a needed blood transfusion, you won't receive a transfusion.

●**How do you teach your medical students to handle such difficult ethical situations?** We put students in simulated scenarios, walk them through real case histories and let them wrestle through to a solution. Real personal exposure helps, too.

Example: We illustrate the concept of patient autonomy—the right to make one's own decisions—by telling them the story of Dax Cowart, who, at age 26 in 1973, was horribly burned and lost his sight and the use of his hands in a propane explosion in west Texas. On his way to the hospital and then many times over the course of many very painful treatments, he articulated clearly that he didn't, in fact, want treatment—he just wanted to be allowed to die.

In 1974, Dax became the subject of a landmark video, *Please Let Me Die*, in which he questions what it means to be an American if a citizen is unable to halt unwanted medical treatment. We show our students the video and, after the after the lights come on, Dax himself is standing there to discuss his experience.

One of the things students always ask is, "Aren't you glad that you came through all this, and didn't the physicians do the right thing?" And he tells them that they don't understand—even though he's married now and a lawyer, he still wishes that he'd been allowed to die. He should

have been the one to decide. A mentally competent patient should have the autonomy to make informed decisions about his medical care.

●**Many medical consumers are fed up with the impersonality of the health-care system. How do you advise med students and doctors in their everyday work?** It's true that the American public has become disenchanted with physicians' attitudes. It's a great paradox because, on the one hand, we've never had more technology and a greater ability to cure than we have today. Yet the popularity of healers who use spiritual and other non-scientific remedies is growing because they deal with aspects of healing that we doctors seem to ignore.

We need doctors who will sit with patients, touch them, talk with them. As a doctor, you can't always say that you have the answer, but you can say, "I'm really interested in what has happened to you. I'm going to get to the bottom of this. Whatever happens, I'm going to be there with you."

I remember once going to the home of an AIDS patient who was dying. I went out of ignorance, not knowing what else to do. There were no drugs in those days, but I suddenly realized, by the way the family came around me sitting at his bedside, that I was helping the patient and his family come to terms with his death.

That's a mysterious thing but, if you're a smart doctor, you don't fight it or be too self-conscious about it. You just let it happen. If you think about it, that's what the old horse-and-buggy doctors used to do. It just makes sense.

How to Be a Health Advocate

Charles B. Inlander, health-care consultant and president, People's Medical Society, a nonprofit consumer health advocacy group, Allentown, PA. He is author of more than 20 books, including *Take This Book to the Hospital with You: A Consumer Guide to Surviving Your Hospital Stay.* St. Martin's.

For more than 30 years, I have recommended that health-care consumers ask a friend or family member to accompany them on doctors' appointments. It makes sense. Having a family member or friend present is like having another set of ears to hear what the doctor is saying and a second voice to ask the questions that need to be asked.

Most doctors appreciate an advocate being present, especially if the patient is under great stress or is otherwise unable to comprehend all that's being discussed. Any patient who has a serious health problem or faces a major course of medical treatment would be wise to take someone along on doctors' appointments. When a person's health is at stake, it can be incredibly stressful, which means the patient is probably not operating at 100% of his/her mental capacity.

But just accompanying someone on a doctor's appointment is not enough. *Here's how to be a good advocate...*

●**Write questions in advance.** We've all heard this time and time again, but there really is no substitute for writing down the questions you want to ask the doctor. To use your time with the doctor most efficiently, go one step further. Divide the questions into two categories. First list the questions that apply directly to the patient, such as "What do you expect to find from this test?" or "Should the medication be taken in the morning or evening?" Then list the questions that involve the advocate or caregiver, such as "Will he need assistance at home after the surgery?"

●**Be sure the patient is included.** Once at the doctor's office, make sure the doctor speaks directly to the patient at all times. Too often, the doctor assumes that the patient won't understand what's being discussed and speaks to the advocate. But even if the patient doesn't understand, he still can hear and probably feels nervous. It's very reassuring when the doctor focuses on the patient. On the other hand, if the doctor ignores the advocate's questions, it may be helpful for the patient to say, *I've brought along my friend (daughter, neighbor, etc.), and I'd like her to be included in all discussions.* During the appointment, the advocate should take notes. If the doctor asks the patient a question, the advocate first should let the patient try to answer. If he cannot, then the advocate can respond, if appropriate. Before leaving, the advocate should verbally review what the doctor has said.

●**Don't forget the office staff.** The advocate should introduce himself to the receptionist and

any staffers who assist during the appointment. Be sure also to get the name of the doctor's primary nurse. Tell the receptionist and the doctor's nurse, if possible, that you are a friend or relative of the patient. Ask if it is okay if you call either of them directly if you have any follow-up questions or concerns. Ask for the best times to make such calls.

Most important, don't be shy. Remember that you are representing a person who is relying on you for help.

Many Hospitals Don't Require Board Certification For Pediatricians

Gary L. Freed, MD, director, general pediatrics, and director, Child Health Evaluation and Research Unit, University of Michigan, Ann Arbor.
Christine K. Cassel, MD, president, American Board of Internal Medicine.
The Journal of the American Medical Association.

New research shows that many hospitals and health plans do not require pediatricians to be board-certified, a finding that may have implications for patient safety and quality of care.

"You don't have to be board-certified to practice in most hospitals in America, and only around 40% of health plans require a general pediatrician to be certified at any time of association with the health plan," says study author Dr. Gary L. Freed, director of the Child Health Evaluation and Research Unit at the University of Michigan in Ann Arbor.

THE STUDY

In this study, 78% of 200 hospitals surveyed nationwide did not require general pediatricians to be board-certified when they first received hospital privileges. However, 70% did require pediatricians become board-certified at some point. Almost half (48%) of those that required board certification had a time frame within which certification was needed, but 42% did not.

Of the 193 US health plans the researchers surveyed, 90% did not require general pediatricians to be board-certified when they were initially credentialed by the plan. Although 41% of the health plans required the pediatricians be certified at some point, the majority (61%) had no time frame in which this should happen. Only 40% of health plans require subspecialists to become board-certified.

"It appears that many hospitals and many health plans are not using the tools that are available to them to help ensure that the public has the highest quality of care that can be provided," says Freed.

IMPLICATIONS

The study raises the question of whether certification translates into better patient care. "There have been few studies that have looked at differences in quality of care," Freed says. "It's an important area for future research. Just as there are no randomized trials of airline pilots who get recertified in the simulator and those who don't, it's likely that the public would want their pilots to have regular certification processes to make sure they stay sharp. One should expect nothing less from physicians."

The public wants their pilots to have regular certification processes to make sure they stay sharp. One should expect nothing less from physicians.

Gary L. Freed, MD

Dr. Christine K. Cassel, president of the American Board of Internal Medicine, says, "This is a time of tremendous change in health care. There's a whole lot going on around quality assessment, and making it more visible to the public. This is important. The public needs to understand how hospitals and health plans assure that physicians have met certain standards."

BACKGROUND

Until 1987, certification from the American Board of Pediatrics (ABP) was valid for the entire career of the doctor. Now, the ABP requires renewal of certification, through a stringent review process, every seven years. "Starting in 1987 for pediatrics, they began limited certificates, to be able to say that, in fact, medicine does change, and it's not a static endeavor, and you need to be sure that people keep up to date," Freed explains.

"The only national standard that reflects specialty training is board certification," Cassel says. "My presumption is that you're going to see hospitals and health plans looking much more carefully at board certification going forward. It's a strong indicator, and it's getting stronger."

info The American Board of Pediatrics can provide more information on the certification process at *www.abp.org.*

New Regulations Help Doctors Stay Up-to-Date

Robert Steinbrook, MD, national correspondent, *The New England Journal of Medicine.*
Troyen Brennan, MD, JD, MPH, Brigham and Women's Hospital, Boston.
F. Daniel Duffy, MD, executive vice president, American Board of Internal Medicine.
Richard J. Baron, MD, Greenhouse Internists, PC, Philadelphia.
The New England Journal of Medicine.

With medical information and practice changing at lightning speed, making sure your doctor keeps up with the latest breakthroughs could prove vital to the care you receive.

It's the job of professional certification boards to assess just how well physicians are keeping abreast of these changes. Now, those certification requirements are in the process of undergoing a major change.

10 YEARS AT A TIME

One of the biggest changes is that a doctor's board certification will not be set for life, but instead will be limited to no more than 10 years.

"The nature of board certification is changing," says Dr. Robert Steinbrook, a national correspondent for the *The New England Journal of Medicine.* "Historically, physicians were certified once. Now, physicians are expected, as part of a process of continuing education, to maintain their certification."

Each specialty will have its own ways to monitor and assess competence, but certification will be for only six to 10 years.

While the new 10-year rule will not apply to doctors certified before 1990, certifying boards are actively encouraging these doctors to participate in the new certification program.

---

*A smarter doctor who is
more aware of the recent changes
in health-care techniques is a better doctor.
And patients will get higher-quality care.*

Troyen Brennan, MD, JD, MPH

Dr. Troyen Brennan, from Brigham and Women's Hospital in Boston, believes this change is a good way for doctors to keep abreast of the latest developments in medical practice, which is changing faster than ever before. "It is a reason for people to demonstrate that they have kept up and know what the most recent information is," he says.

"A smarter doctor who is more aware of the recent changes in health-care techniques is a better doctor," Brennan says. "And patients will get higher-quality care."

BETTER PATIENT CARE

Dr. F. Daniel Duffy, executive vice president of the American Board of Internal Medicine, says the changes "move certification beyond an examination of knowledge and judgment to an evaluation of actual performance and practice."

Key to the new process is a team approach and systems that help achieve better care. "I learned a lot, and felt that I was a better doctor as a result of [the new certification process]," says Brennan. "The move toward required recertification is a way of ensuring that medical practice is good, and continues to be good."

Dr. Richard J. Baron, from Greenhouse Internists, PC, in Philadelphia, believes that revamping the certification process will lead to better patient care.

"Traditionally, we have thought about what we do as a one-patient-at-a-time approach. The new process is a way to look at the patients we take care of as a population of people, and enables us to get a sense of how we are doing taking care of the whole group," he explains. "It's a different way to look at excellence in medical care."

"The motivation behind the changes is excellent," Steinbrook says. "Whether all the goals will be achieved is hard to say. I think we will have to wait and see."

DOING THE RIGHT THING

Duffy admits that for many physicians the new process will be time-consuming. "We are not used to sitting down and systematically looking at our practices," he says. "Until we get accustomed to that and build that into our culture, it's going to seem like a burden and something we didn't choose to do.

"But when physicians do it, they realize—wow, the value of doing this is really terrific!" Duffy says. "And people really want to do the right thing."

Board-certified specialties include: Allergy and Immunology, Anesthesiology, Colon and Rectal Surgery, Dermatology, Emergency Medicine, Family Medicine, Internal Medicine, Medical Genetics, Neurological Surgery, Nuclear Medicine, Obstetrics and Gynecology, Ophthalmology, Orthopaedic Surgery, Otolaryngology, Pathology, Pediatrics, Physical Medicine and Rehabilitation, Plastic Surgery, Preventive Medicine, Psychiatry and Neurology, Radiology, Surgery, Thoracic Surgery and Urology.

info The American Board of Internal Medicine has more information on physician certification at *www.abim.org.*

Nearly Half of Americans Getting Substandard Health Care

Steven M. Asch, MD, Rand Health, and West Los Angeles Veterans Affairs Health Care System, and associate professor of medicine, University of California at Los Angeles.

Elizabeth A. McGlynn, PhD, associate director, Rand Health.

The New England Journal of Medicine.

All Americans are at risk of receiving substandard health care, regardless of gender, race, income or even insurance status. In fact, a recent study found that only 54.9% of the patients surveyed received the care that experts usually recommend for their condition.

"There's no question that disparities exist, but the big variations are not between groups, but between what people are getting and what people should be getting," says Dr. Steven M. Asch, study author and with Rand Health. "Everyone—men and women, rich and poor, insured and uninsured—is at risk. No matter who you are, it's almost a flip of the coin as to whether you get the care that experts want for you."

THE STUDY

The study, conducted by Rand Health, is the third in a series of studies on health-care quality in the United States.

Using both telephone interviews and reviews of patients' medical records, the researchers collected data on approximately 6,700 patients in 12 metropolitan areas who had received care for 30 acute and chronic conditions between 1996 and 2000. Health care was assessed using 439 quality indicators, which was validated by 36 specialists who are considered leaders in their field.

No matter who you are, it's almost a flip of the coin as to whether you get the care that experts want for you.

Steven M. Asch, MD

Two important notes: The researchers only looked at what happened during the visit, not at the patient's access to care or what happened after the patient left the office (for example, filling a prescription).

Among the study's findings...

●**Women received more recommended care than men** (56.6% vs. 52.3%).

●**Women were more likely than men to receive preventive care** (58% vs. 50%) and chronic care (58% vs. 55%). But women were less likely than men to receive needed acute care (52% vs. 58%).

●**Generally, quality of care declined as people got older.** People younger than age 31 received more recommended care than those older than 64 (57.5% vs. 52.1%).

●**African-Americans (57.6%) as well as Latin Americans (57.5%) got slightly more recommended care** than Caucasians (54.1%).

●**People who had incomes greater than $50,000 per year received more recommended care** than those who earned less than $15,000 (56.6% vs. 53.1%).

●**Insurance status had no effect on the quality of care received.**

EXPLANATION

Because medical information changes virtually every day, it may be complicated to adequately care for patients, the researchers speculate.

"Over the past five to 10 years, there's been an explosion of medical knowledge, and of the possibilities of what can be done for you," says Elizabeth A. McGlynn, senior author of the paper and an associate director of Rand Health.

TECHNOLOGY MAY HELP

The technology to cope with all of this information is available, it's just underused in health care, Asch says. "The system is not set up, [but] information technology can make a difference," he explains.

Asch notes that the Veterans Affairs system is already using upgraded information technology and "care has improved dramatically"—approximately two-thirds of veterans are now receiving the recommended care.

"We wouldn't tolerate this in almost any other sector of society," he continues. "We wouldn't tolerate it if a pilot had to memorize his pre-flight checklist before he flew cross-country. It's a complicated thing to give medical care, and to do it right you need assistance."

info Visit the Agency for Healthcare Quality and Research at *www.ahrq.gov* for more information on issues of medicine and quality.

Lifesaving Medical Tests Doctors Too Often Overlook

David Sandmire, MD, associate professor, department of biological sciences, University of New England, Biddeford, ME, and coauthor of *Medical Tests That Can Save Your Life: 21 Tests Your Doctor Won't Order...Unless You Know to Ask.* Rodale.

A 50-year-old man I knew went for an annual checkup. His doctor pronounced him in excellent health. Eight months later, the man had a major heart attack and died.

His death could have been prevented. If the doctor had talked to the patient at length, he would have discovered that one of his relatives had *hemochromatosis,* a dangerous condition in which the body retains too much iron, causing heart problems. A simple $35 blood test would have confirmed the condition—the patient could have been treated and would still be alive today.

Dozens of screening options can diagnose deadly diseases in the earliest stages, when treatment has the greatest chance of success—but doctors, pressured by increasing patient loads and hamstrung by what insurers will cover, don't always order them when they should.

KEY TESTS

The following conditions can be detected by simple tests. *These tests may not be covered by insurance—check with your insurer—but consider paying for them even if they're not...**

●**Diabetes.** Type 2 diabetes affects 17 million American adults and children, yet close to one-third don't know they have it because symptoms may not appear for a decade. Approximately 200,000 people die each year from the complications of type 2 diabetes. Hundreds of thousands more experience blindness, kidney failure and/or nervous system damage.

Test: A *fasting blood glucose* test is taken after you have not eaten for at least eight hours. If your results are above 110 milligrams per deciliter (mg/dL), you should have the more definitive *oral glucose tolerance* test. After you ingest a high-sugar drink, your blood glucose level is measured every hour for three hours. If your glucose level rises more than expected and doesn't return to normal by the third hour, you have diabetes.

Who should consider testing: Obese people who have a body mass index (BMI) of 30 and higher (to calculate BMI, go to *www.diabetes.org*)...African-Americans, Latinos and Native Americans older than age 45...anyone who has a close relative who is a type 2 diabetic.

Cost: Approximately $12 for a fasting blood glucose test...approximately $25 for an oral glucose tolerance test.

●**Coronary heart disease (CHD).** In CHD, the walls of the coronary arteries are narrowed

*Test costs vary based on facility and region.

or blocked by a buildup of fatty plaque. CHD is the single largest killer of men and women in the US. Elevated *C-reactive protein* (CRP) levels are a sign of inflammation and are a better predictor of heart disease in women than LDL ("bad") cholesterol levels. A standard blood test measures C-reactive protein in the blood.

Test: The new *high-sensitivity C-reactive protein* test measures levels more accurately than the old test. This is vital because studies now show that any reading higher than 1 milligram per liter (mg/L) puts you at above-average risk for CHD. (The older test wasn't able to detect a level that low.) Formerly, it was thought that only readings greater than 5 mg/L put you at risk.

Who should consider testing: Anyone who has high cholesterol or high blood pressure... people who have diabetes...people whose parents or siblings have or had CHD...smokers.

Cost: $25 to $50.

●**Hemochromatosis.** This disease causes the body to absorb too much iron, resulting in heart problems, arthritis and a decreased life expectancy. One in 10 Americans has the single mutated gene that causes secondary hemochromatosis, a milder form of the disease.

Test: A *percent transferrin saturation* blood test screens for an abnormal metabolism that signals a propensity to overaccumulate iron. If the test is positive, a genetic blood test for hereditary hemochromatosis should be performed.

Who should consider testing: Male Caucasians of Northern European descent, particularly of Celtic ancestry...individuals who have relatives that have had hemochromatosis.

Cost: $20 to $50 for percent transferrin saturation test...$125 to $165 for genetic testing.

●**Hepatitis C virus (HCV).** Approximately 4 million Americans are infected with HCV, but less than 30% are diagnosed because most of them have no symptoms. Left untreated, HCV can lead to cirrhosis and liver cancer.

Test: An *enzyme-linked immunosorbent assay* (ELISA) blood test can detect the presence of hepatitis C antibodies. If the test results are positive, you'll need to have an *HCV ribonucleic acid* (RNA) test to determine how recently you were exposed to the virus and how much of it is in your blood.

Who should consider testing: People who received blood transfusions or organ transplants prior to 1992 (when the blood supply was not screened for HCV)…health-care workers who get accidental needle sticks…intravenous drug users …those who have had multiple sex partners.

Cost: $70 to $100 for an ELISA test…approximately $100 for an HCV RNA test.

●**Pancreatic cancer.** The five-year survival rate of this deadly disease is just 4% because symptoms rarely appear until the tumor grows large enough to interfere with the function of nearby organs, such as the stomach, small intestine and liver. Early detection can raise the five-year survival rate to nearly 40%.

Test: *Endoscopic retrograde cholangiopancreatography* (ERCP) can detect abnormalities of the pancreas, including a precancerous condition known as *dysplasia*, approximately 90% of the time. A physician guides an endoscope down through your stomach and small intestine to inject a dye into the ducts in the pancreas. X-rays are taken and examined. If anything suspicious is seen, a biopsy is performed.

Who should consider testing: People who have *pancreatitis*, an inflammatory condition that occurs when digestive enzymes attack the pancreas itself instead of breaking down food in the small intestine. Symptoms include mild to severe abdominal pain, often accompanied by nausea, vomiting and fever. People who have an inherited defect in the BRCA2 gene also should be tested. This is found in approximately 1% of Ashkenazi Jews and in some women who have a family history of breast cancer.

Cost: $1,500 to $2,000.

YOUR RISK PROFILE

The more informed a doctor is about your health and risk factors, the more likely he/she is to order tests that could save your life. You can help your doctor by creating your own detailed risk profile. *Include…*

●**Personal medical history**—major diseases, injuries and operations you have had and any residual effects. Patients often forget childhood illnesses, so ask close relatives. Also, list allergies, including those to medications.

●**Genetic makeup**—your racial and ethnic background.

●**Extended family medical history**—diseases that family members have or have died from, such as type 2 diabetes, cancer and coronary artery disease. Also include family conditions such as obesity and depression.

●**Lifestyle.** Be honest with yourself and your doctor about smoking, alcohol consumption, diet and exercise. Ask family and friends for objective opinions.

■ ■ ■ ■

If You Think Your Doctor Is Making a Mistake…

S peak up. A new survey shows that patients usually don't say anything—which puts them at risk for medical errors. Patients were more likely to speak up about possible medication mistakes than about possible incorrect diagnoses or inappropriate treatments.

Helpful: Affirm your respect for the doctor's position and competence before suggesting that he/she may have made an error.

Joseph Grenny, president, VitalSmarts, a research and training firm, Provo, UT, and coauthor of *Crucial Conversations: Tools for Talking When Stakes Are High.* McGraw-Hill.

5 Questions Your Doctor Should Ask—But Won't

Leo Galland, MD, director, Foundation for Integrated Medicine, New York City. He has held faculty positions at Rockefeller University and Albert Einstein College of Medicine, both in New York City, and at the State University of New York, Stony Brook. He is author of *The Fat Resistance Diet* (Broadway) and *The Four Pillars of Healing* (Random House).

I n the US, the typical doctor's office visit lasts seven to 10 minutes. During that time, the doctor reviews your medical history, asks questions about your symptoms, performs an exam and orders tests, if necessary.

This approach can be effective for emergencies or acute illnesses, such as earaches, bronchitis or chest pain. It doesn't work as well for chronic diseases, such as diabetes, arthritis, asthma or fatigue.

Reason: Doctors don't ask the questions that reveal the key facts about a person's life that can significantly affect the development and progression of disease.

Example: One of my patients had severe rheumatoid arthritis. She failed to improve even with the latest, most powerful drugs. None of her doctors thought to ask about her diet, which was triggering the release of inflammatory chemicals that exacerbated her symptoms.

I ask my patients to complete a 20-page questionnaire before their initial visit. In many cases, their answers give important clues to an accurate diagnosis.

Even if your doctor doesn't ask the questions listed below, you should bring up these issues with him/her during your appointment.

Following are questions your doctor should ask—but may not…

●**Have you ever felt better after avoiding particular foods?** Up to 40% of Americans that are considered *healthy* report having an intolerance to one or more foods.

Why it matters: Millions of Americans react to wheat, dairy or other specific foods or food groups. Food intolerance is a frequent cause of diarrhea and other digestive problems. It also can cause fatigue and headache. Patients often suffer for years before being accurately diagnosed. The quality of a person's diet can have a significant impact on the risk of chronic or recurrent disease…energy levels, mood and body weight…recovery from infection…and the control of chronic disorders, such as diabetes and high blood pressure.

What you can do: If you have unexplained symptoms, such as headache or diarrhea, keep a food diary to record everything you eat and drink over a three-day period, including spices and condiments such as pepper and mustard. The most common culprits are milk products, wheat, corn, yeast, sugar, spices and artificial colors and flavors. Eliminate a suspected problem food from your diet for five to seven days. Do your symptoms improve when you avoid the food? Do they get worse when you reintroduce it? If you find a problem food, ask your doctor whether you may have a food intolerance.

●**What are the major sources of stress in your life?** Our bodies' nerves, hormones and immune cells work together to help us cope with emotional stress. In people who experience chronic stress, this network becomes overwhelmed and stops working efficiently.

Why it matters: The body is designed to respond to stress and often benefits by becoming stronger. However, when people have high levels of stress on a daily basis, the cost of responding to this stress exceeds the benefit. This results in an increased risk for cardiovascular disease, infection, depression and other illnesses.

What you can do: It's impossible to eliminate stress altogether, but we can learn to manage it more efficiently.

Example: Daily exercise—30 minutes of walking at a moderate to brisk pace—diminishes the effects of stress-related hormones.

●**Do you feel close to your family and/or friends?** Doctors are often reluctant (or too busy) to ask about patients' personal lives. However, personal relationships are among the most important factors in preventing and treating disease.

Why it matters: Patients who are diagnosed with serious illnesses, including cancer and heart disease, live longer when they have a strong social network. Research also shows that people who are active in their communities or close to family and friends are less likely to get sick in the first place. A social support network also eases depression and protects you from the effects of daily stress.

What you can do: Take stock of your relationships with other people and nourish them by spending time with people you care about. If you are isolated, get involved in activities that help others.

●**How much personal control do you believe you have over your health?** There are two primary ways that you can approach your health—you can rely on your doctor to tell you what to do…or you can actively participate in your health care.

Why it matters: Research shows that people are healthier and actually have better medical outcomes when they take responsibility for their own care…make important lifestyle changes… and generally put themselves in charge of their own health.

What you can do: The first step is to motivate yourself and make a commitment to yourself and to those you love that you will be proactive in advocating for your own health. The second step is to learn what you can about the health conditions that affect you.

•Do you have physical problems or certain personality traits that remind you of someone in your family? Your family medical history can help identify diseases that you may be predisposed to develop. Family history is an especially important risk factor for depression, heart disease, diabetes, high blood pressure and allergic and autoimmune disorders. Most cancers are not due to genetic risk factors, but to environmental exposures or diet.

Why it matters: A family history of a disease doesn't mean that you will develop that illness—but knowing your history (or just noticing similarities) makes it easier to predict and prevent future problems.

Example: If you experience unexplained fatigue, weight gain or mood disturbances, and there is a history of thyroid problems in a close family member, such as a parent or sibling, your symptoms may be thyroid-related.

What you can do: Maintain a family tree that includes the health status and cause of death of grandparents, parents, aunts, uncles and siblings and show it to your doctor.

■ ■ ■ ■

90% of Doctors and Nurses Don't Speak Up

When they see patients have received treatment that could jeopardize their health, 90% of doctors and nurses don't speak up.

Reasons for their silence: Fear of confrontation, lack of time, feeling that the problem is not his/her job.

Joseph Grenny, president, VitalSmarts, a research and training firm, Provo, UT, and coauthor of *Crucial Conversations: Tools for Talking When Stakes Are High.* McGraw-Hill.

Doctors Quick to Prescribe Unproven Drugs

Sharon Giordano, MD, MPH, assistant professor of medicine, department of breast medical oncology, M.D. Anderson Cancer Center, University of Texas, Houston.

Lisa Schwartz, MD, codirector, VA Outcomes Group, Department of Veterans' Affairs, White River Junction, VT, and associate professor of medicine, Dartmouth Medical School, Hanover, NH.

Journal of the National Cancer Institute.
The Journal of the American Medical Association.

Many American doctors are switching to new—and largely unproven—therapies on which there is only early, incomplete data, according to the results of a study.

The danger is that many drugs or therapies that look promising in the early trials prove useless—or even harmful—as more complete data emerges over time.

THE STUDY

In the study, Dr. Sharon Giordano, an assistant professor of medicine in the department of breast medical oncology at the University of Texas M.D. Anderson Cancer Center in Houston, and her colleagues tracked changes in breast cancer treatment after researchers announced preliminary findings on *paclitaxel* (Taxol) at the 1998 annual meeting of the American Society of Clinical Oncology (ASCO). The presentation introduced early data suggesting that Taxol improved survival in women who had breast cancers that had spread to the nearby lymph nodes, if the drug was given after a lumpectomy or mastectomy.

"We found that very, very quickly after the meeting, physicians began prescribing [Taxol]," Giordano says.

In fact, before the ASCO presentation, only 5% of patients were using Taxol and other taxanes as adjuvant breast cancer therapy. That rate rose to nearly 24% soon after the conference.

More alarming was that doctors gradually extended Taxol's use to breast cancer cases that did not involve the lymph nodes—even though there was no data to support the drugs' efficacy against these malignancies.

Fortunately, longer-term data, published in 2003, found Taxol to be of real benefit to women who had lymph node-positive breast cancers.

NOT ALWAYS A HAPPY ENDING

But not all stories end so well, the study authors warn. They list examples such as hormone replacement therapy (HRT), the now-banned Cox-2 inhibitors Vioxx and Bextra, as well as Iressa, a lung cancer drug that physicians turned to based on early findings, only to find out later that it might do more harm than good.

"Our message is for physicians in the community to be aware of the potential risks of adopting therapies too early, and also for physicians presenting early results at meetings to be aware of how dramatically practice can change based on their presentations," says Giordano.

> *There's a lot of hyping of results—some of it comes from industry, where they're often magnifying the benefit and minimizing the harms.*
>
> *Lisa Schwartz, MD*

"When things are reported at scientific meetings, those are often preliminary results," notes Dr. Lisa Schwartz, an associate professor of medicine at Dartmouth Medical School.

"That means that the study might not even be complete—they are reporting on interim findings," says Schwartz. "So, we just don't know whether those results will hold up over time."

A Canadian study found that 41% of the preliminary trial results that were presented as "highlights" at medical meetings had disappointing conclusions when the final findings were actually published in medical journals at a later date.

No one is advocating that researchers withhold early results from their peers or the public, however. "If there are breakthroughs in the field and new treatments that are truly showing a benefit, then we want to know about that as soon as possible, to be able to pass that on and change our practice," Giordano says.

CONSUMER, BEWARE

Schwartz says that doctors and patients need to "bring a little skepticism" to data that is reported outside of major, peer-reviewed journals. She points out that studies that are presented at meetings are simply not subject to the same kind of review as studies that are published in a journal.

"There's a lot of hyping of results—some of it comes from industry, where they often present results using relative terms, magnifying the benefit and minimizing the harms," Schwartz says.

A drug company's stock can also spike upward on the basis of preliminary trial results, she adds. "So, there are all these other interests that are [pushing] drugs to be portrayed in a very favorable light."

It's easy to see how doctors and patients can get swept up in all the hype. But Schwartz suggests that people investigate the results of a new study or drug by asking a few questions. "Is there really a big difference in something that patients [in the trial] experienced—how long they lived, what their quality of life was? Is this [information] coming from the gold standard—a big, randomized trial with a control group? What about side effects?" she says.

In addition, Schwartz says that "new" drugs are not necessarily "improved." "There's the assumption that the newest drug is the latest and greatest," she says, "but that's not always the case. And if there are already existing treatment options that have better science behind them, it's often better for people to take those proven options instead."

info For more information on clinical trials, visit the National Institutes of Health Web site at *www.clinicaltrials.gov.*

Making Sense of Confusing Medical News

Charles B. Inlander, health-care consultant and president, People's Medical Society, a nonprofit consumer health advocacy group, Allentown, PA. He is author of more than 20 books, including *Take This Book to the Hospital with You: A Consumer Guide to Surviving Your Hospital Stay.* St. Martin's.

What does a medical consumer do when new scientific research contradicts long-standing health advice? In previous years, we've confronted this problem as new major studies called into question the use of aspirin, sunscreen and vitamin E. Doctors were left scrambling, and consumers felt utterly confused. Because I advocate on behalf of medical consumers in all health matters, I followed up on these issues by reviewing the studies and consulting leading experts. *My findings...*

●**Aspirin.** For more than a decade, doctors have prescribed a daily baby aspirin to help prevent heart attack and stroke, especially in older people. A major study published in *The New England Journal of Medicine* found that low-dose aspirin reduces heart attack risk in all men, but only in women age 65 or older. The *British Medical Journal* reported that baby aspirin does not save lives or add years to life in people older than age 70 who did not already have cardiovascular disease. In fact, daily baby aspirin increased the risk of gastrointestinal bleeding. Where does this leave us?

What to do: Because the risks–benefits of aspirin therapy are highly individualized, speak to your doctor. Ask if he/she believes that these recent findings in any way change your need for aspirin therapy.

●**Sunscreen.** For decades, medical experts have strongly recommended the liberal use of sunscreen to help prevent skin cancer. However, researchers are now realizing that sunscreen blocks the ultraviolet (UV) sun exposure that's necessary for the formation of vitamin D. Four recent studies have found that vitamin D helps protect against lymphoma, cancers of the prostate, lung and even the skin! There is stronger evidence that it helps prevent colon cancer. Unfortunately, we cannot get as much vitamin D as we need from diet and supplements alone.

What to do: Do *not* throw away your sunscreen. Recent studies suggest that limited sun exposure (10 to 15 minutes, a few times a week) on the face, arms, hands or back without sunscreen can do you a great deal of good. Ideally, this sun exposure should occur before 10 am and after 4 pm, when damaging UV rays are the least intense.

●**Vitamin E.** Researchers at Johns Hopkins University analyzed 19 previous clinical trials of vitamin E and discovered that people taking daily doses of 400 international units (IU) or more per day had a higher risk of dying from any cause than people not taking the vitamin. As you probably know, vitamin E had been highly touted as a preventive for heart disease. However, none of the recent clinical trials have shown this to be true. Research on other potential benefits of vitamin E is ongoing.

What to do: If you take vitamin E, talk to your doctor. This study in no way suggests that lower doses of the vitamin—or vitamin E from food—are harmful. There simply may be better ways to prevent heart disease, such as changing your diet, exercising more and losing weight.

■ ■ ■ ■

TV News Offers Fuzzy Picture on Health

There's room for improvement by both TV stations and the experts who appear in medical and health-related news stories, according to a study by researchers from the University of Michigan and the University of Wisconsin-Madison.

During a one-month period, health and medical stories comprised 11% of the news portion of late-evening newscasts.

There were 1,799 medical and health stories carried on 2,795 news broadcasts that were aired on 122 stations in the top 50 media markets in the United States.

The average medical or health story was 33 seconds long. Most of the stories did not provide specifics about the source of the information.

The study also found that when reporting on specific diseases, the experts often failed to give the viewers recommendations or information about the prevalence of the disease, which could help them put the story into perspective.

In addition, the researchers note that there were errors in the stories that could lead to serious consequences.

Example: Several stations aired a story on lemon juice's effect on sperm. Nearly all of the stories failed to mention that this was a laboratory study that did not involve humans. One story misinterpreted the research altogether and reported that lemon juice may be a substitute for costly HIV medications.

info The National Institutes of Health has more information about medical and health news at *www.nih.gov/news/WordonHealth/apr 2004/risk.htm.*

University of Michigan Health System news release.

Simpler CPR Guidelines May Save More Lives

Mary Fran Hazinski, RN, clinical nurse specialist, pediatric emergency and critical care, Vanderbilt University Medical Center, Nashville, and senior science editor, American Heart Association.

Robert O'Connor, MD, MPH, director of education and research, Christiana Care Health System, Newark, DE, and vice chairman, emergency cardiac care committee, American Heart Association.

Michael Sayre, MD, associate professor of emergency medicine, Ohio State University, Columbus, and volunteer chairman, basic life support subcommittee, American Heart Association.

New, simplified guidelines for *cardiopulmonary resuscitation* (CPR) now place more emphasis on pushing on the chest than on breathing into a person's mouth. The revised guidelines are aimed at everyone—from bystanders and police to doctors and nurses.

"We're starting to get more scientific evidence, and this year we reached the [turning] point to make changes," says Mary Fran Hazinski, senior science editor for the American Heart Association and a clinical nurse specialist in pediatric emergency and critical care at Vanderbilt University Medical Center in Nashville.

Dr. Robert O'Connor, vice chairman of the American Heart Association's emergency cardiac care committee and director of education and research at Christiana Care Health System in Newark, Delaware, adds, "We have tried to tighten the chain of survival."

THE NEW GUIDELINES

In total, 380 international scientists analyzed approximately 20,000 studies and came up with recommendations that emphasize a simplified, "back-to-basics" approach.

"The most common reason people die is because no one nearby knows CPR or [they don't] actually do it after cardiac arrest happens," says

Dr. Michael Sayre, volunteer chairman of the American Heart Association's basic life support subcommittee, and associate professor of emergency medicine at Ohio State University.

"One of the reasons for that is that the skill has been very complicated," he adds. "We believe that the first step toward bystanders taking action is to improve the accessibility and quality of CPR training and to simplify instructions."

The biggest change in the guidelines is in the ratio of chest compressions to breaths. The new guidelines recommend 30 compressions for every two breaths, compared with 15 compressions for every two rescue breaths in the 2000 guidelines.

The rate of compressions (100 per minute) has not changed.

"The more times someone pushes on the chest, the better off the patient is [because] more blood flows to the heart and brain and other vital organs," Sayre explains.

The most common reason people die is because no one nearby knows CPR. One of the reasons for that is that the skill has been very complicated.

Michael Sayre, MD

When blood flow is increased in this way, it is not as crucial for oxygen to be delivered through breaths. Some health experts have advocated eliminating breaths in CPR altogether, but the breaths have been shown to be effective for cardiac arrest in infants, children and some adults.

The new guidelines eliminate some steps, including checking a victim's pulse if it has already been ascertained that he/she isn't moving and breathing.

Another change is the timing of heart rhythm analysis and CPR when using *automatic external defibrillators* (AEDs). The previous guidelines called for an AED to analyze the heart rhythm before and after delivering a shock, with this sequence being repeated up to three times before beginning CPR, thus losing precious time.

The new guidelines recommend one shock, followed by two minutes of CPR before going back to an AED. "It really requires choreography," O'Connor says.

At a minimum, the American Heart Association guidelines urge more people to learn CPR. "We're stressing the importance of the public taking CPR classes," O'Connor says.

INCREASING SURVIVAL

At the heart of the new guidelines is a desire to increase survival rates for cardiac arrest—when the heart suddenly stops beating. "We have been concerned that the overall survival rates from cardiac arrest in the US have not budged in the last several years," Hazinski says.

The chance that a victim of cardiac arrest will be successfully resuscitated and go on to live a normal life ranges from 2% to 70% in the United States and Canada, depending on the location.

info For more about the new CPR guidelines as well as emergency cardiovascular care, visit the American Heart Association Web site at *www.americanheart.org*. Click on "CPR & ECC."

How to Tell What Your Lab Tests Really Mean

Kandice Kottke-Marchant, MD, PhD, section head, hemostasis and thrombosis, department of clinical pathology, The Cleveland Clinic, and professor of pathology, The Cleveland Clinic Lerner College of Medicine, Case Western Reserve University.

Even if they're otherwise health-savvy, few patients know as much as they should about diagnostic blood and urine tests.

Result: Patients are less able to help spot errors that could lead to a physician's misdiagnosis and/or inappropriate treatment. *Key facts...*

LABORATORY TESTS

The *complete blood count* (CBC) measures the number of cells in your blood. Hundreds of diseases can cause abnormalities in these counts, including infections, some cancers and blood disorders.

Urinalysis evaluates the appearance and chemistry of your urine. Abnormalities can signal kidney disease, urinary tract infections, some types of cancer or diabetes.

You should review your lab reports with your physician. Keep a copy of each report in your files to compare it with past or future results.

Printouts of lab reports include a *reference range*, the statistically normal values for a person your age.

What most people don't know: Some people are what pathologists call *outliers*—that is, even though healthy, they have slightly higher or lower values in one or more categories. Further testing typically is required.

INTERPRETING THE CBC

A CBC may be ordered prior to surgery and/or for evaluation of an infection, fatigue, fever, anemia, cancer or heart disease. The CBC analyzes white blood cells (WBCs), red blood cells (RBCs) and platelets, all of which are produced in the bone marrow. *Most important measurements...*

●**WBC count.** WBCs battle viruses, bacteria and any other infectious agents. They are measured in thousands per cubic millimeter (K/mm3) of blood.

Normal range: 4.0 to 11.0.*

●**WBC differential.** This measures the relative percentage of five different types of WBCs—*neutrophils* (which fight bacterial infection)...*basophils* and *eosinophils* (they play a role in allergic responses)...and *lymphocytes* and *monocytes* (which develop when there is an immune response to many infections). Ask your doctor for your normal ranges.

●**Absolute neutrophil count (ANC).** This uses a formula involving *polys* (mature neutrophils) and *bands* (young neutrophils). A decreased ANC can signal bone marrow failure, while a high ANC is seen when there are infections and some leukemias.

Normal range: 38% to 78% of all WBCs.

What your results may mean: WBCs that fall outside the normal range could signal an infection...a disorder of the bone marrow...or an allergy.

●**RBC count.** RBCs carry oxygen to and remove carbon dioxide from the tissues. They are measured in millions per cubic millimeter (mil/mm3) of blood.

Normal range: 4.5 to 6 for men...4.2 to 5.4 for women.

●**Hemoglobin (HGB) value.** Hemoglobin is the protein that carries oxygen. It is measured in grams per deciliter (g/dL) of blood.

*Normal ranges vary slightly from lab to lab.

Normal range: 13.5 to 17.5 for men...12 to 16 for women.

•**Hematocrit (HCT) value.** HCT is the percentage of your blood that consists of RBCs. A decrease in HCT indicates anemia, which can result in not enough oxygen being delivered to the tissues.

Normal range: 40% to 52% for men...37% to 47% for women.

What your results may mean: RBCs that fall outside the normal range are a sign of anemia, bleeding, some cancers, bone marrow disease or a drug side effect, typically from chemotherapy.

•**Platelet count.** Platelets form clots and stop bleeding. They're measured in thousands per cubic millimeter (K/mm3) of blood.

Normal range: 150 to 400.

What your results may mean: Platelet counts that fall outside the normal range can be a sign of leukemia, *thrombocytopenia* (too few platelets), rare congenital disorders or a drug side effect.

INTERPRETING URINALYSIS

If you complain of low back pain, painful or frequent urination, or discover that you have dark or bloody urine, your physician should order a urinalysis. *Most important components...*

•**Protein.** Normally, the kidneys do not allow protein to leak into the urine. The presence of high levels of protein—greater than 10 milligrams (mg) per 100 milliliters (mL)—suggests an abnormality, such as kidney disease. If a high protein level is found, other kidney function tests, such as creatinine, should be ordered.

•**Glucose.** Excess levels of glucose indicate diabetes. If you have high glucose, your doctor should order a blood glucose test and other diabetes screening tests, such as *hemoglobin A1C.*

•**Nitrite.** High levels of this compound indicate a urinary tract infection.

•**Leukocyte esterase.** When present in the urine, this enzyme (produced by white blood cells) may indicate an infection.

•**Casts.** The presence of casts (cellular deposits that are formed in the kidneys) and their specific type can indicate many problems, including kidney disease and diabetes.

•**Crystals.** When present in small numbers, most crystals, such as those made of *calcium oxalate,* are not significant. Others, such as crystals of the amino acid *leucine,* can indicate severe liver disease.

•**RBCs.** High levels of RBCs in the urine can indicate trauma to the kidney or urinary tract, cancer or urinary tract infections.

PREVENTING ERRORS

The automated instruments that are used to analyze blood are precise, and most CBCs are accurate. Similarly, few mistakes are made in a typical urinalysis, but errors can occur.

Best ways to avoid lab errors...

•**Make sure your doctor or hospital uses an accredited lab.** Yearly inspections are required for labs that are accredited by various organizations, such as the College of American Pathologists. To find out if a lab is accredited, ask the lab or hospital administrator.

•**Don't assume that your tube is labeled correctly.** Mix-ups can occur. Ask the lab technician, *How did you label the tube?*

Even better: Ask politely to see the tube, so you can be sure it has your name on it.

•**Check for clots.** If blood takes more than two minutes to fill the tube, it will clot in the process. This renders it useless for a CBC. Ask the lab technician, *Does my tube have any clots in it?*

Even better: Ask to see the tube, and tilt it gently. If there's a large clot, you'll see it.

Medicine Coming to The Shopping Mall

Sharon Weber, spokeswoman for Wal-Mart, Bentonville, AR.

Larry Fields, MD, president, American Academy of Family Physicians.

Michael Howe, chief executive officer, MinuteClinic, Minneapolis.

Increasingly, major American merchandisers are partnering with health-clinic chains to provide routine medical services in a mall-like setting.

This retail health-care trend is being led by conglomerates such as Wal-Mart and Target; by national pharmacy chains such as Brooks-Eckerd, Rite Aid, Osco Drug and CVS; and even by regional grocers such as Albertson's.

For both logistical and legal reasons, the retailers do not own, operate or directly profit from the clinics that are on their premises. Instead, outside medical providers—including InterFit Health Services (operating the RediClinic chain), Solantic, Quick Quality Care, MinuteClinic and Take Care Health Care Systems—rent space from their brand-name landlords.

There's certainly no place for these clinics in complicated diagnoses, long-term management or even a second visit for the same problem.

Larry Fields, MD

These appointment-free clinics—now operating in Arkansas, Florida, Georgia, Indiana, Maryland, Minnesota, New York, North Carolina, Oklahoma, Rhode Island, Tennessee and Texas—typically charge a $25 to $60 up-front fee (only some clinics take insurance) to address a limited range of 25 to 30 acute medical conditions and common ailments—allergies; bronchitis; colds; flu; eye, ear, skin and sinus infections; headaches; and gastrointestinal issues.

Preventative care is also available, including checking blood pressure, cholesterol and body fat; providing vaccinations, physicals and weight-management advice; testing for asthma and diabetes; and screening for prostate cancer and heart disease.

THE BENEFITS

Both retailers and health-care tenants say the clinic-within-a-store concept can be a win-win for everyone.

"We're a very customer-focused company, and customers are busy, and this will just add one more thing to their shopping list that they can do," says Sharon Weber, a spokeswoman for Wal-Mart, the world's largest retailer, with more than 3,600 stores in the United States alone.

"And these facilities will be open the same hours as our pharmacies," she adds. "This means including Sundays. So when Junior needs a physical for the football or basketball team, the family can drop by the Wal-Mart on a Sunday afternoon and get that taken care of."

CONVENIENCE, BUT NO DOCTORS

This easy-to-use approach has the potential to reshape the American medical landscape by establishing a store—rather than a doctor's office—as a patient's first place of medical contact.

And that may be a problem. Many physicians' groups have expressed concern that not only are patients not being cared for in a doctor's office, but in most cases, they are not being cared for by a doctor at all.

With the exception of the Solantic organization, which maintains an in-store staff of only board-certified physicians, clinics are typically operated by registered nurse practitioners and physician assistants—with physician advice limited to phone consultations.

"There's certainly no place for these clinics in complicated diagnoses, long-term management or even a second visit for the same problem," says Dr. Larry Fields, president of the American Academy of Family Physicians. "Certainly, if any of these situations arise, patients should be sent to a physician," he advises.

"It's not a solution—or even a part of the solution—for a lack of insurance," Fields adds. "In most cases, for what these places will be charging, you can see a family physician for the same problem. But, of course, these clinics are going to be open nights and weekends when the doctor's office is not open. So it's a convenience factor."

Michael Howe, chief executive officer of Minneapolis-based MinuteClinic, which operates 51 clinics throughout the United States, agrees with Fields that in-store clinics are best viewed as a convenient supplement to, rather than a replacement for, the traditional doctor's office.

"We make it very clear to our patients that this is not a medical home," he says. "The medical home is a critical part of managing their health on an ongoing basis. We gather a list of primary-care providers in the area who are accepting new patients, and we actually are involved in establishing medical homes for our patients outside of MinuteClinic.

"As we move to more consumer-managed health care, you're going to see more and more the role that these retail-based health clinics will play," Howe adds.

info To learn more, visit the California Health-Care Foundation Web site at *www.california healthline.org*, and do a search for "in-store clinics."

The Doctor Will See You... If You Have the Right Insurance

Brent R. Asplin, MD, MPH, head, department of emergency medicine, Regions Hospital, St. Paul, MN.
Mark Murray, MD, MPA, principal, Mark Murray and Associates, Sacramento, CA.
The Journal of the American Medical Association.

What happens to people who have potentially serious health conditions after they're treated and released from the emergency room with explicit instructions to seek an appointment for follow-up care? It may depend on the type of health insurance they have, a new study suggests.

THE STUDY

Eight graduate students posing as new patients in urgent need of care called 499 randomly selected ambulatory clinics in nine US cities. The calls were made to community clinics and private doctors' offices.

Callers read from one of three clinical scenarios that would require follow-up care—pneumonia, high blood pressure or possible ectopic pregnancy. Women using the latter vignette called only obstetrics and gynecology and family medicine clinics. Each caller contacted each clinic twice using the same scenario but saying they had different types of insurance on each of the calls.

RESULTS

Although the clinics rigorously screened the callers for their insurance status, they were not as careful about the medical screening process. Of the clinics contacted, 98% screened the callers for a source of payment, but only 28% attempted to determine the severity of the caller's condition.

"In some respects, financial screening has trumped medical triage," notes lead researcher Dr. Brent R. Asplin, head of the emergency medicine department at Regions Hospital in St. Paul, Minnesota.

The results showed that 47% of all the callers were offered appointments within a week, compared with 64% of privately insured callers.

Privately insured callers had much greater success in booking appointments than those who said they were uninsured but could pay $20 at the time of their visit. However, callers claiming to be uninsured but offering to pay for the visit in cash were just as likely to get a timely appointment as the privately insured callers. In addition, a caller claiming to have private insurance was almost twice as likely to get a timely appointment as someone who said they had Medicaid (63% vs. 32%).

IMPLICATIONS

"What we were interested in understanding was how big a role health insurance plays in patients' ability to get access to care after they leave us," Asplin says. He concludes, "Health insurance matters—that's the basic message from this study. If you are not a card-carrying member of our health-care system, you have a very difficult time getting access to care."

Still, even having private insurance did not guarantee timely follow-up care, the researchers found.

> *If you are not a card-carrying member of our health-care system, you have a very difficult time getting access to care.*
>
> Brent R. Asplin, MD, MPH

"Over one-third of the callers who claimed to have private insurance coverage could not get a follow-up appointment within one week in our study," notes Asplin. "And that finding really begs the question of whether there is adequate capacity in our ambulatory care system to see people who most need to be seen."

RECOMMENDATIONS

But what can Medicaid recipients and the more than 45 million uninsured Americans do to boost the odds of getting to see a health-care professional promptly?

"Lie," says Dr. Mark Murray, a consultant and authority on patient access to care.

However, he agrees with Asplin that it's not just those who lack private insurance or those who have no insurance at all who find it difficult to get timely appointments. Because most health systems are backlogged with work, it is difficult for many Americans—even those who do have insurance—to get appointments within a reasonable amount of time.

"So, I suppose, don't get sick or lie is the best approach," he adds.

info Visit The Commonwealth Fund at *www. cmwf.org* for more information on health-care coverage and access.

What to Do If You Lose Insurance While You're Sick

Michelle M. Doty, PhD, senior analyst, The Commonwealth Fund.
Alwyn Cassil, spokeswoman, Center for Studying Health System Change.
Seeing Red: Americans Driven into Debt by Medical Bills. The Commonwealth Fund.
"Rising Health Costs, Medical Debt and Chronic Conditions." Center for Studying Health System Change.
Health Affairs.

Millions of American families are struggling to pay their medical bills, while others are drowning in the debt accrued by doctor and hospital visits, according to recent studies. What's troubling is that a significant percentage of these people have health insurance.

As the cost of medical care continues to rise, consumers are bearing a greater share of their medical expenses. The additional cost comes in many forms, including higher deductibles and copayments, separate deductibles for hospital admissions, and the move from fixed-fee co-payments to percentage-based "coinsurance." In some cases, health plans are widening the limits on coverage for certain treatments.

The resulting cost-shift can be a real strain on family budgets, particularly for low-income Americans, who are pinching pennies to begin with, and for people who have chronic or multiple health conditions.

Michelle M. Doty, a senior analyst at The Commonwealth Fund and author of a study examining insurance trends, and her colleagues report that almost two out of five adults in the US—an estimated 77 million people—have difficulty paying medical bills or are struggling with medical debt. Surprisingly, 70% of the people who are overwhelmed by medical debt and 57% of those who have current bill-paying problems said they were insured at the time their difficulties began, the study found.

"We're looking at the tip of what's happened with the erosion of benefits, as employers and plans start to share the costs with employees. We're going to see more of this," Doty predicts.

RECENT STATISTICS

In 2003, one in five working-age Americans who had chronic health problems—approximately 12.3 million people—lived in families that had problems paying medical bills, according to an analysis by the Washington, DC-based Center for Studying Health System Change (HSC).

For some families, filing for personal bankruptcy may be the only way to escape the debt they've piled up. However, the recent overhaul of federal bankruptcy laws makes it even tougher to extinguish those debts.

According to a Harvard study, illness and medical bills contributed to approximately half of the personal bankruptcy filings in 2001. More than 75% of the filers were insured when they incurred the debt that set them back, yet many lost coverage during their illness.

WHAT YOU CAN DO

If you have health insurance, there are a few things you can do to help avoid financial trouble. "Here's the best advice I can give every American who has health insurance—understand how your policy works. Understand the limits and understand where the 'carrots' are," says Alwyn Cassil, a spokeswoman for HSC.

For example, if you are enrolled in a preferred provider organization (PPO), try to use doctors and hospitals that participate in the provider network. You'll get a substantial discount on "in-network" services and your out-of-pocket costs will be lower than if you were to see out-of-network providers, she says.

If you're having an elective procedure, try not to get stuck with bills from hospital-based physicians who don't contract with your health plan. Find out ahead of time whether the anesthesiologist, radiologist or pathologist who will participate in your care is a member of the provider network. These specialists may not have agreements with your insurer, Cassil warns, even if your hospital and surgeon do.

To save money on drugs, investigate alternatives. "Oftentimes, you can save significant money by going mail-order or generic, or switching from a nonpreferred brand to a preferred brand," she notes.

If your health plan imposes an annual limit on, say, physical therapy or mental health visits, try to schedule your care so you will not have to pay for extra visits out of pocket.

As for patients who are already in debt, "Don't stick your head in the sand," Cassil urges. "Talk to the people you owe money to and see what you can negotiate. See what you can work out."

info The National Health Law Program offers advice on how to control your healthcare costs at *www.healthcarecoach.com.*

Medicating the US: How Drug Companies Are Turning Us into Patients

Alan Cassels, drug policy researcher, University of Victoria, British Columbia, and coauthor of *Selling Sickness: How the World's Biggest Pharmaceutical Companies Are Turning Us All into Patients.* Nation.

How many pills did you and your family take today? It seems that there is a prescription drug for every condition now, no matter how benign.

In fact, the US has become the most medicated society in the world. We make up 5% of the world's population, but we buy 50% of all prescription medicine. Conflicts of interest abound—from your doctor, who may be on the payroll of a pharmaceutical firm, to your favorite celebrity, who may get a kickback for hawking powerful meds.

To help you make the best health-care choices, we interviewed Alan Cassels, a pharmaceutical policy researcher. *He believes that we need to protect ourselves from a culture that insists on "medicalizing" every problem in our lives...*

●**Why has our society become overmedicated?** We all just want a quick fix, even if we aren't sick but just feel vulnerable or at risk. The trouble is that vast commercial forces are exploiting this desire.

Much of the health information that we get is distorted so that drugs are the first choice we consider for, say, depression, high cholesterol or high blood pressure—even if there are safer effective alternatives, such as exercise or a healthy diet.

Drug ads use statistical gimmicks to exaggerate benefits. I saw an ad that claimed a certain pill would lower your risk of a heart attack by 33%. Technically, that's correct, but the actual clinical study indicated a drop in risk from 3% to 2%. In absolute terms, that's only a one-percentage-point reduction.

●**What's an example of a drug that is prescribed too often?** Look at the multibillion-dollar sales of antidepressants in the past few years. If you walk into a doctor's office complaining of mild to moderate depression, you often are given a prescription for a *selective serotonin reuptake inhibitor* (SSRI), such as Paxil, Prozac or Zoloft—drugs that may have significant side effects—despite evidence that behavioral and talk therapy can be equally effective.

What happened: Marketing campaigns from pharmaceutical firms have transformed the way we think about physical and mental health, convincing us that our problems are best cured by using medication. Alternative views of the illness and treatment get short shrift.

●**Are these drug companies really the problem?** Drug companies make wonderful products that extend lives and ameliorate suffering. However, they are aggressively targeting the healthy as well as the sick in pursuit of profits. One of their strategies is to broaden the boundaries of what constitutes an illness.

Example: In the 1990s, only approximately 13 million Americans warranted treatment under the National Institutes of Health's (NIH) cholesterol guidelines. Then, in 2003, a panel of experts rewrote the guidelines and lowered the numbers so much that now 36 million more people have "high" cholesterol. Many of the doctors on that panel had served as paid speakers, consultants or researchers for the large pharmaceutical companies that manufacture cholesterol-lowering drugs known as *statins.*

It's not surprising that high cholesterol has become an obsessive concern for everyone. We all know our "numbers," but high cholesterol isn't an illness. It's just one of many risk factors for a future illness—heart disease. While there's extensive evidence that statins are valuable for people who have had heart attacks, there often are much cheaper, safer and equally effective treatments for the rest of us, including an improved diet, more exercise and not smoking.

Even more insidious is that drug companies don't just market blockbuster pills through advertising—they market conditions for their medications to cure.

Example: Formerly, Paxil was one of many popular antidepressants on the market, but in the past five years, its manufacturer, GlaxoSmithKline, took a rare psychiatric condition known as *social anxiety disorder* and helped transform it into an often-diagnosed condition for which Paxil is the cure.

●**Who is the primary target for this kind of advertising?** Every segment of the population is targeted.

Women are told that they should take medication for "illnesses" such as menopause and premenstrual syndrome, which actually are natural cyclical changes. Children who simply can't sit still or who drift off in, class are diagnosed with *attention deficit hyperactivity disorder* (ADHD) and given Ritalin.

Older people who do not have high blood pressure are told they have a condition called *prehypertension* (a systolic blood pressure of 120 to 139, or a diastolic pressure of 80 to 89) that may warrant drug intervention. There is no evidence that giving medication to people who have this blood pressure reading will result in any alteration in the length or quality of life.

Prehypertension is a verbal tactic designed to cast the net wider, creating more patients and selling more pills. Maybe we should rename life itself and call it "predeath." Then we would all need to be taking drugs of some kind.

●**Aren't these drugs helpful and warranted in many cases?** Of course. I'm not saying that you should ignore symptoms or that every diagnosis is being blown out of proportion. There may be many times in your life when you need drug intervention. But we have become too comfortable popping pills. We assume that as long as it's advertised on TV or recommended by our doctors, it must be safe.

●**Isn't my doctor supposed to be the gatekeeper for all this information? Can't he/she see through these marketing tactics?** Doctors may be very responsible and hard to manipulate, but they still are under enormous pressure to prescribe drugs. Patients come into their offices asking for the drugs they see advertised on TV. Pharmaceutical representatives bombard doctors with sales pitches—the typical doctor averages at least one visit from a rep every day.

●**What should I be doing to protect myself as a patient?** Be skeptical. Ask your doctor if a drug has been tested on people like yourself (your age, sex and physical condition). What are the benefits and dangers? Would lifestyle changes work instead? *Also, seek out reputable sources of independent information, including...*

●*Consumer Reports'* free Web site, *wwwcrbestbuydrugs.org,* which provides information to help make cost-effective prescription drug choices.

●*The Medical Letter,* a publication for physicians and other health-care professionals that publishes critical appraisals of new drugs and comparative reviews of older drugs. 800-211-2769, *www.medicalletter.org.*

●*Public Citizen,* a nonprofit advocacy organization that has information on hundreds of drugs in its book, *Worst Pills Best Pills,* and on its free Web site, *www.worstpills.org.*

●**Is overmedicating the wave of the future?** Not necessarily. The thousands of lawsuits pending against pharmaceutical giant Merck over the side effects of its painkiller Vioxx may have a profound effect on our public and private regulatory systems. The US Food and Drug Administration (FDA) already has tightened its protocols.

Influential medical journals are now calling for an international clinical trial medical registry. This is crucial. Right now, a pharmaceutical company can conduct a dozen trials for a new drug…only publish the positive-result trials…and then use those as evidence for drug approval or marketing. Drug companies should be required to register every study in a central database and publish all results so that we can judge for ourselves what to allow into our medicine cabinets.

How to Save Hundreds of Dollars Buying Drugs Online

Rick Melcher, RPh, registered pharmacist, Yakima, WA, and coauthor of *Smart Buys Drug-Wise*. Harbor. *www.smartbuysdrugwise.com*.

Internet pharmacies can provide big savings for people who need prescription drugs. Prices average 18% less than even discount retail store prices. For some drugs, the savings are as high as 45%.

How it works: A patient orders a drug online. The patient or his/her doctor sends a written prescription to the Internet pharmacy. A pharmacist reviews and fills the prescription, which then is shipped through the mail.

Many over-the-counter (OTC) products are available at Internet pharmacies, too. Most Internet pharmacies also accept phone orders if you do not have computer access…or you can go to your library and use the computer there.

The convenience and savings of Internet pharmacies have led many patients to abandon brick-and-mortar stores—but you must make sure the pharmacy is reputable and shop wisely to get the best deals. *Here's how…*

•**Look for the VIPPS seal.** Internet pharmacies that advertise themselves as Verified Internet Pharmacy Practice Sites (VIPPS) have been inspected by the National Association of Boards of Pharmacy (NABP). NABP evaluates participating pharmacies on the quality and consistency of their procedures.

Caution: Some unscrupulous Internet companies display the VIPPS seal even though they have not been inspected. Check a company's status at *www.nabp.net*. Some reputable pharmacies, such as AARP's and Costco's, are not VIPPS members—be sure you are familiar with the company's reputation.

•**Check insurance participation.** Most Internet pharmacies work with a limited number of insurance companies. Some bill the insurers directly…others do not.

You can find this information on the pharmacy Web sites or you can call your insurance company to find out which, if any, Internet pharmacies are part of its network.

•**Figure in extra costs.** Some Internet pharmacies offer free shipping for standard ground delivery. This usually takes two weeks, so order well in advance. Fees for overnight delivery can be high.

A few Internet pharmacies, such as AARP's, charge patients annual membership fees. If you need many prescriptions over a year, the savings can more than offset the extra fee.

•**Buy in bulk.** Some insurance companies allow people to get a three-month supply of medication for a single copayment when they order from Internet pharmacies, cutting costs by 67%.

Patients can also save by buying up to a year's supply at a time.

Example: One man ordered a year's supply of the thyroid hormone *levothyroxine*. He skipped his insurance company entirely—and still saved $80.

In addition, some pharmacies offer free shipping on big orders.

•**Pick a company that has a "live" pharmacist.** Avoid any Internet pharmacies that don't provide customer support. Look for one that has a pharmacist available to answer questions, either via E-mail or telephone.

•**Ask a pharmacist.** Some drugs, such as the anticoagulant *warfarin* and the heart drug *digoxin*, are sensitive to extremes in temperature and so can degrade while they are in the mail. Ask the Internet pharmacist whether your medications can withstand the rigors of mail travel before ordering on the Internet.

■ ■ ■ ■

Online Pharmacy Pros and Cons

Online pharmacies offer convenience, privacy, easy comparison shopping and bargains. But their risk is that you may not know who you are dealing with—and prescription drugs are too dangerous to buy from a dubious seller.

Safety: Before buying drugs online, visit the Web site of the National Association of Boards of Pharmacy (NABP) at *www.nabp.net*, to determine whether the prospective seller is a licensed pharmacy in good standing. These are named in the NABP's listing of Verified Internet Pharmacy Practice Sites (VIPPS).

info For more tips on the smart and safe use of Internet pharmacies, visit the FDA's online buying page at *www.fda.gov/buyonline*.

UC Berkeley Wellness Letter.

US Pharmacist Shortage Looms

David A. Mott, PhD, associate professor, School of Pharmacy, University of Wisconsin, Madison.
Sharlea Leatherwood, past president, National Community Pharmacists Association, and pharmacy owner, Kansas City, MO.
American Pharmacists Association annual meeting, San Francisco.

There could be fewer US pharmacists in the next decade, as aging male practitioners retire and workers of both genders choose part-time instead of full-time work, a survey reveals. The shortage looms even as the demand for prescription services rises, and pharmacists themselves call for more time to focus on patient care (such as immunization and drug counseling), beyond just dispensing medications.

THE SURVEY

Researchers reviewed written questionnaires that were completed in 2004 by 1,470 randomly chosen pharmacists throughout the United States. The surveys collected information on the pharmacists' demographic and employment status, the number of hours worked per week, the type and quality of work environment and his/her future work plans. The answers showed a shrinking workforce and the potential for a real shortage in the coming decade.

LESS HOURS, MORE PRESCRIPTIONS

The researchers also found that, overall, both full- and part-time pharmacists—whether stationed in a chain, supermarket, independent business or hospital—are working less than they did four years ago, while earning an average 38% more for their time.

Pharmacists may not have enough time to spend with patients answering questions about how to take their medications.

David A. Mott, PhD

More than 25% of women pharmacists are working part-time, as are approximately 15% of male pharmacists. Yet, despite a cutback in their work week, pharmacists are actually handling more prescriptions now than they had been in the past—presumably taking advantage of an increase in the number of nonpharmacist technicians who now assist customers.

TECHNOLOGY'S ROLE—GOOD AND BAD

Technology may also play a role in pharmacists' ability to maintain service levels despite the increasing number of prescriptions. More than 60% of those surveyed said new equipment—such as refill phone systems, bar coding and medication counters—have improved both productivity and quality of care, while simultaneously boosting job satisfaction.

However, there may be a downside to this technology. While it has allowed the faster dispensing of drugs, it has also discouraged other types of patient-care services, such as face-to-face consultations.

Patient consultations account for 19% of pharmacists' time, followed by business management (16%) and drug-use management (13%). The pharmacists surveyed indicated that nearly half of their time is still spent filling prescriptions, much as it was in 2000.

They said that this emphasis on filling prescriptions takes away from consultation and drug-use management.

More than one out of every two pharmacists said their workload was high or excessively high, and 58% said that their workload had increased (sometimes greatly) during the prior year.

"The key message is that there is a shortage of pharmacists," concludes survey project director David A. Mott, an associate professor in the School of Pharmacy at the University of Wisconsin. "Certainly, pharmacists are busier than ever, and they may not have enough time to spend with patients, answering questions about how to take their medications."

Almost 46% of practicing pharmacists are now female, the survey revealed—up from 31% in 1990 and slightly higher than in 2000. In addition, male pharmacists are an aging group, with more than 40% of them older than 55, compared with just 10% of female pharmacists.

THE GOOD NEWS

The survey did uncover several positive indicators. Most of the pharmacists, particularly those employed by independent stores, said their attitude toward their job has improved since 2000.

More than 77% said they have a high level of job satisfaction, up from 66% in 2000.

Mott's team believes that the nation's pharmacy schools need to emphasize this good news, while acknowledging that the industry is changing.

"We're looking 10 or 15 years down the road at a real change in our pool of pharmacists," says Mott. "There are only approximately 100 pharmacy schools in the country, which graduate approximately 80 to 100 students each year, so there's a limit to how we can deal with a shortage."

Sharlea Leatherwood, a past president of the National Community Pharmacists Association and a pharmacy owner in Kansas City, Missouri, agrees that the problem is real and looming.

"We are experiencing a very large growth in the boomer population, and they are the ones who are taking a very large number of the meds," she notes. "So, the need for filling prescriptions grows just as we are losing pharmacists. This makes for a very serious situation."

info For more information on pharmacy issues, visit the American Pharmacists Association Web site at *www.aphanet.org.*.

Don't Be Fooled by Food Label Lies

Suzanne Havala Hobbs, DrPh, RD, clinical assistant professor, department of health policy and administration, University of North Carolina at Chapel Hill. She is author of *The Natural Kitchen: The Complete Guide to Buying and Using Natural Foods and Products.* Berkley.

I f you are confused about the claims that manufacturers are now making on food labels, you are not alone.

"ORGANIC"

The term organic is hotly debated. The US Department of Agriculture's (USDA) current definition states that organic foods are those plants produced without the use of pesticides, sewage sludge (for fertilization) or synthetic fertilizer…or those animals raised without hormones or antibiotics.

To read the complete definition, go to the USDA's Web site at *www.ams.usda.gov/nop/NOP/standards.html.*

Organic foods, including produce, meat, milk and other dairy products, typically cost more than nonorganic varieties.

The FDA has linked pesticides to some types of cancer, and numerous other studies have linked them to Parkinson's disease. There's also strong evidence from the American Medical Association that bacteria are becoming resistant to some antibiotics because they are used in meat production.

What you may not know: In October 2005, the Agricultural Appropriations Conference Committee voted to allow synthetic ingredients into foods labeled "organic." Therefore, yogurt, pudding and other items may be considered organic even if they contain synthetic additives.

What you can do: Whenever possible, buy organic meats and dairy products.

For produce, choose organic varieties if you're buying one of the items found by the Environmental Working Group (a nonprofit group of researchers who investigate environmental health threats) to be among the most contaminated (see chart on page 293).

If you must buy nonorganic, choose produce that is least likely to be contaminated. Wash the nonorganic produce vigorously under running water to remove as much potentially harmful residue as possible. (Organic produce also should be washed.)

If you must buy nonorganic meat, choose the leanest cuts available and, whenever possible, remove the skin from poultry (toxins from hormones and antibiotics tend to accumulate in fatty tissue).

"NATURAL"

"Natural" is a word used for marketing purposes—it is not a term that is defined by the government.

What you may not know: Natural does not mean that a food product is necessarily "healthful."

Example: Breyers labels its ice cream "all natural," but it is high in fat and saturated fat.

What you can do: Read food labels carefully to determine the levels of fat and saturated fat as well as other ingredients in products that are labeled natural.

"LOW"

Many dairy products and some processed foods, such as soup, frozen entrees and snacks, use the term "low" or some variation thereof. *What these terms mean…*

Low fat: 3 grams (g) or less of total fat per serving.

Low saturated fat: 1 g or less of saturated fat per serving.

Low calorie: 40 calories or less per serving.

Low cholesterol: 20 milligrams (mg) or less of cholesterol and 2 g or less of saturated fat per serving.

Low sodium: 140 mg or less of sodium per serving.

Very low sodium: 35 mg or less of sodium per serving.

Nonfat: Less than 0.5 g of fat per serving.

"LEAN" AND "EXTRA-LEAN"

"Lean" and "extra-lean" refers to the fat content of meat, poultry and seafood. *What these two terms mean…*

Lean: Less than 10 g of fat, including no more than 4 g of saturated fat and less than 95 mg of cholesterol per 3.5-ounce serving.

Extra-lean: Less than 5 g of fat, including no more than 2 g of saturated fat and less than 95 mg of cholesterol per 3.5-ounce serving.

OTHER TERMS

Reduced: The food contains at least 25% less of an ingredient (such as fat, cholesterol, sodium or added sugar) or calories than the regular product.

Example: Reduced Fat Fig Newtons have at least 25% less fat than the original recipe.

High: The food contains at least 20% of the Daily Value (recommended daily intake) for a particular nutrient.

Example: The Daily Value for fiber is 25 g. If a food product contains 5 g of fiber per serving, it might say "high fiber" on its label.

■ ■ ■ ■

When Organic Is Worth the Price

MOST CONTAMINATED PRODUCE
(best to buy organic)

Apples	Peaches
Bell peppers	Pears
Celery	Potatoes
Cherries	Red raspberries
Imported grapes	Spinach
Nectarines	Strawberries

LEAST CONTAMINATED PRODUCE
(buy nonorganic, if desired, but wash vigorously)

Asparagus	Kiwi
Avocados	Mangoes
Bananas	Onions
Broccoli	Papaya
Cauliflower	Peas (sweet)
Corn (sweet)	Pineapples

Environmental Working Group. *www.ewg.org.*

What You Must Know About Food 'Sell-By' Dates

Suzanne Havala Hobbs, DrPh, RD, clinical assistant professor, department of health policy and administration, University of North Carolina at Chapel Hill. She is author of *The Natural Kitchen: The Complete Guide to Buying and Using Natural Foods and Products.* Berkley.

Many states require food manufacturers to put a date on perishable foods so that customers can gauge product freshness. However, because there are no federal regulations requiring products to be dated, there isn't a uniform system. *Here is a guide to the most commonly used terms and what they really mean...*

●**"Sell-by" dates** let stores know how long products can remain on the shelves. They also are used as guides for rotating stock. The sell-by date takes into consideration the length of time a product typically sits on the shelf at home after purchase. Perishable foods remain good for a period of time after the sell-by dates, assuming that they have been stored properly. Use your eyes and nose to judge product freshness.

Example: Milk, cheese and yogurt that are starting to smell sour or have turned color should be thrown out.

General guidelines for shelf life beyond sell-by dates...

●Eggs are usually good for three to five weeks past the sell-by date.

●Milk is typically good for up to seven days past the sell-by date.

●Fresh chicken and turkey should be cooked or frozen within two days of the date.

●Fresh beef, pork and lamb should be cooked or frozen within three to five days of the date.

●Ground meats should be cooked or frozen within two days of the date.

●Unopened processed meats, such as bacon, hot dogs and luncheon meats, should be used within two weeks of the sell-by date.

●Unopened canned meats, such as tuna and sardines, will keep for approximately two years beyond the sell-by date.

●**"Best if used by" and "use by" dates** refer to the point after which peak quality—flavor or texture—begins to decline. These are not safety or purchase dates.

Caution: Shelf life depends on the handling and storage conditions. Fresh perishable foods should be kept at 38°F to 40°F for maximum safety and quality.

14

Stroke Prevention

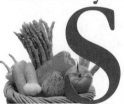

Best Ways to Prevent Stroke

Stroke is now the third-leading cause of death and a common reason for disability in older adults. That's the bad news. There's good news, too — the stroke mortality rate is declining. In 1950, approximately 89 per 100,000 people died of stroke. By 1994, it had dropped to 27 per 100,000. Today, it is even lower due to improvements in preventive and treatment strategies.

WHAT HAPPENS

A stroke occurs when blood flow to part of the brain slows or stops. Brain cells, called *neurons*, begin to die within minutes as levels of oxygen and nutrients decline.

Approximately 80% of strokes are *ischemic*—blood clots or other debris block circulation through cerebral arteries.

Other strokes are *hemorrhagic*—a blood vessel in the brain leaks or ruptures and impairs normal circulation. The leakage of blood also damages surrounding brain tissue.

A full-fledged stroke is often preceded by a *transient ischemic attack* (TIA). This temporary interruption of blood flow results in the same symptoms as a stroke. Symptoms of a TIA disappear within a few minutes to 24 hours—but don't ignore them. People who have had a TIA are at least nine times more likely to have a stroke than those who have not had a TIA.

PREVENTION

The American Heart Association advises everyone 20 years of age and older to have early risk-factor screenings for stroke. These include measuring blood pressure, pulse rate, body mass index (BMI) and cholesterol and glucose levels.

Most stroke risk factors can be dramatically reduced through changes in lifestyle. Medications also can cut the risk.

•**Manage hypertension.** High blood pressure is a major cause of ischemic and hemorrhagic strokes.

David Chiu, MD, medical director, stroke unit, The Methodist Hospital; director of the Eddy Scurlock Stroke Center; neurologist at The Methodist Hospital Neurological Institute; and associate professor of neurology, Baylor College of Medicine, all in Houston.

Daily exercise reduces hypertension. So does maintaining a healthy weight. A weight loss of as little as 10 pounds can lower blood pressure. Also, limit your sodium intake.

In addition, your doctor may recommend the use of diuretics, ACE inhibitors and/or other blood pressure-lowering drugs.

Take a daily multivitamin that contains B-complex vitamins. This group of vitamins lowers levels of *homocysteine*, an amino acid that increases the risk of stroke.

Beware: Few doctors routinely test for homocysteine. Insist on the test. An average reading is approximately 10—but lower is better.

People who have elevated homocysteine are two to three times more likely to have a stroke than those who have lower levels.

●**Take aspirin daily.** People who have had a stroke or who are at high risk of having one should consider taking a daily aspirin to inhibit blood clots in the arteries. An 81-milligram (mg) baby aspirin and a 325-mg adult aspirin appear to be equally effective, but the smaller dose is less likely to cause intestinal bleeding. Other blood-thinning drugs, such as *warfarin* (Coumadin) or *clopidogrel* (Plavix), also significantly reduce stroke risk for some people.

●**Ask your doctor about statins.** This class of cholesterol-lowering drugs appears to reduce stroke risk by approximately 25%, even in people who have normal cholesterol. Side effects can include muscle pain, nausea and diarrhea or constipation.

●**If you smoke, quit.** Smokers are several times more likely than nonsmokers to have a stroke. Within 10 years of quitting smoking, the risk of having a stroke is almost the same as for someone who has never smoked.

SCREENING

People who have had a TIA or stroke require a number of screening tests to identify the type of stroke and where in the brain it occurred.

New finding: Magnetic resonance imaging (MRI) is more effective than traditional *computed tomography* (CT) scans for stroke diagnosis. MRI reveals areas of the brain that have been damaged by ischemic stroke and also gives information about cerebral blood flow.

TREATMENTS FOR ISCHEMIC STROKE

Neurologists say, *time is brain.* If given intravenously within three hours of a stroke, *tissue plasminogen activator* (tPA) can dissolve blood clots, restore normal circulation and minimize tissue damage. Any delay in treatment greatly reduces survival and increases the likelihood of post-stroke disability.

New research: Studies have found that only approximately 3% of stroke victims receive tPA, usually because they don't seek help until it's too late for the drug to do any good.

New finding: Research has also shown that tPA can be injected directly into a blood clot in the brain via a catheter threaded through an artery. Catheter-directed delivery might extend the window for using tPA to six hours.

Another technique removes clots in the brain but does not use tPA. A catheter is inserted in the groin and guided upward until it reaches the clot. A corkscrew-shaped device, called the MERCI (*mechanical embolus removal in cerebral ischemia*) Retriever, is then used to snare the clot and remove it from the artery.

●**Carotid endarterectomy** is a surgical procedure in which the carotid artery is opened and plaque is removed to promote better blood flow.

New technique: Carotid stenting, in which a mesh tube is inserted inside a carotid artery to maintain blood flow. The stent acts like scaffolding to prevent the artery from collapsing or being closed by plaque. Early studies suggest that stenting is as effective as surgery—and possibly safer for some high-risk patients.

TREATMENT FOR HEMORRHAGIC STROKE

Surgery to repair blood vessels is the primary approach doctors use. Scientists are developing drugs to minimize brain tissue damage following a hemorrhagic stroke, but these drugs are still experimental.

Botox Takes the 'Wrinkle' Out of Stroke Recovery

Allison Brashear, MD, professor and chairman of neurology, Wake Forest University Baptist Medical Center, Winston-Salem, NC.

Todd Schlifstein, MD, physical medicine and rehabilitation, New York University Medical Center, New York City.

American Association of Physical Medicine and Rehabilitation annual meeting, Philadelphia.

Perhaps best known for its wrinkle-banishing ability, Botox can also help stroke patients recover some functioning, according to a new study.

Repeated injections of Botox, or *botulinum toxin* type A, helped stroke survivors regain enough function to perform everyday activities, such as dressing themselves, without pain, says Dr. Allison Brashear, a professor and chairman of neurology at Wake Forest University Baptist Medical Center in Winston-Salem, North Carolina.

THE STUDY

Brashear's team injected Botox into the wrists, fingers and elbow flexors of 279 patients who had post-stroke muscle spasticity. Treatments were spaced at least 12 weeks apart during the year-long study.

*The new study is additional
proof of the benefit of
Botox for reducing spasticity
in stroke patients.*

Todd Schlifstein, MD

The team measured muscle tone as well as disability in hygiene, dressing, limb posture and pain, and asked the patients which area they most wanted to improve. None of the participants experienced serious side effects from the Botox injections, and muscle tone greatly improved by week six, Brashear says.

The improvement lasted throughout the study period, and at the end of the study, at least half of the survivors achieved an improvement in the area they deemed most important.

The study was funded by Allergan Inc., the company that developed Botox.

REACTION

"We all agree that Botox relaxes muscles," Brashear says. "What this paper tried to get a handle on is what does that mean to the [stroke] patient."

From the results of the study, "It's evident that Botox makes a difference in function," Brashear concludes.

Another expert says this study of stroke survivors confirms what some clinicians have long known. "I've been using it for years for patients with spasticity," says Dr. Todd Schlifstein, a physical medicine and rehabilitation physician at New York University Medical Center.

The new study, he says, is "additional proof of the benefit of Botox for reducing spasticity in stroke patients."

BOTOX BACKGROUND

Botox was first approved by the US Food and Drug Administration (FDA) in 1998 to treat eye problems such as "lazy eye." Next, it received FDA approval for the treatment of a movement disorder that causes neck and shoulder contractions. Then it was approved for cosmetic use.

Botox has been used "off-label" for stroke patients for approximately five years, according to Brashear. Off-label use refers to the common practice of prescribing a drug or treatment for a purpose that has not been specifically approved by the FDA.

Botulinum toxin type A, a protein complex produced by the bacterium *Clostridium botulinum*, contains the same toxin that causes botulism, a potentially deadly form of food poisoning. However, sterile, purified botulin toxin in small doses also blocks the release of *acetylcholine*, a chemical released by nerve cells that signals muscles to contract.

Other studies have found Botox effective for a variety conditions, including excessively sweaty palms and feet.

MANY CAN BE HELPED

According to the American Stroke Association, 700,000 people in the United States have a stroke each year. Approximately 4 million Americans are stroke survivors, and one-third of them experience spasticity, Brashear estimates.

Schlifstein estimates that up to 10% of stroke survivors could benefit from Botox injections.

Typically, a stroke survivor who experiences spasticity is referred to a neurologist or a physical medicine rehabilitation specialist, Brashear says. They can assess whether the condition warrants Botox treatment.

■ ■ ■ ■

Know the Symptoms

Up to one-half of all Americans cannot name a single stroke symptom. Many victims don't seek emergency care because they don't take their symptoms seriously.

Warning: Some people who have a stroke experience brain damage that makes it impossible for them to recognize symptoms. It's critical for family members, friends or coworkers to recognize the first signs of stroke.

●**Sudden numbness, weakness and/or paralysis** in the face, an arm or a leg. The symptoms usually affect one side of the body.

●**Difficulty in talking or understanding words…confusion.**

●**Sudden changes in vision,** such as blurring or double vision.

●**Dizziness or a loss of balance.**

●**Severe headache** that occurs without warning, possibly accompanied by vomiting.

Cut Your Stroke Risk

Patrick Lyden, MD, professor of neurosciences and director, Stroke Center, University of California, San Diego. He is chief of the Stroke Clinic, San Diego VA Medical Center.

Stroke is the most *preventable* cause of death and disability in the US. Yet more than 750,000 Americans experience strokes each year…approximately 160,000 of these people die …and 200,000 live with lasting disability. What are we doing wrong?

You can't change some risk factors, such as family history. If you have a parent or sibling who has had a stroke, you are at greater risk yourself. Your age also plays a role. While strokes can occur even in young children, overall risk steadily increases as we grow older. That's why more than two-thirds of strokes occur in people older than age 65.

Beyond these factors, whether we have a stroke is largely up to us.

STROKE PREVENTION

What most affects stroke risk…

●**Smoking.** Everyone knows that smoking increases heart disease risk, but did you know that smoking is actually more likely to cause a *stroke* than a heart attack? Not only does smoking promote the development of fatty deposits that narrow arteries (*atherosclerosis*), but the nicotine in tobacco causes blood vessels in the brain to constrict.

Result: Smokers have up to a four times greater risk of stroke than nonsmokers.

What you can do: Quit smoking. If you've tried but can't kick the habit, consider using nicotine-replacement patches or gum…or the prescription drug *bupropion* (Zyban).

●**Blood pressure.** High blood pressure gradually damages blood vessels and substantially increases the risk for both *ischemic* and *hemorrhagic* strokes. The risk is greater because high blood pressure rarely causes symptoms, so the problem goes unrecognized in 30% of people who have hypertension.

What you can do: If your blood pressure is higher than 120/80, take steps to reduce it. Weight loss and exercise may be enough, but you also may need medication, such as diuretics or beta blockers.

●**Cholesterol.** To prevent a stroke, maintain the same cholesterol levels that are recommended to reduce heart disease risk—total cholesterol less than 200…LDL ("bad") cholesterol less than 100…HDL ("good") cholesterol greater than 40.

What you can do: Weight loss and exercise help control cholesterol levels. If these strategies are not sufficient, cholesterol-lowering medication may be needed.

●**Diabetes.** Maintaining tight control of blood sugar (glucose) will minimize small blood vessel damage that can lead to stroke.

What you can do: With your doctor, create a treatment plan that keeps your *hemoglobin A1C* (blood sugar over time) level at less than 7.

●**Diet.** Stroke risk, like heart disease risk, can be related to diet.

What you can do: Maintain a diet that's low in saturated fats (no more than 30% of total fats per day) and high in fruits and vegetables (five to nine one-half cup servings per day).

Research shows that people who are deficient in potassium are 1.5 to 2.5 times more likely to have a stroke. Aim for the government's recommended potassium intake of 4,700 milligrams (mg) daily. Although bananas are a popular source of potassium (one medium banana contains 457 mg of potassium), cantaloupe can be an even richer source (one cup of cantaloupe balls contains approximately 547 mg).

If you determine that sodium raises your blood pressure, limit your daily sodium intake to 2.4 grams (g) (slightly more than one teaspoon of salt).

●**Exercise.** Physical activity reduces the risk of heart disease, diabetes and hypertension—and may offer stroke protection as well.

What you can do: Work with your doctor to create an exercise program based on your history of heart disease, smoking, etc.

●**Daily aspirin.** Aspirin reduces the tendency of platelets to clump, which helps prevent blood clots that can lead to ischemic stroke.

What you can do: If you're older than 55 and have diabetes, high cholesterol or other stroke risk factors, ask your doctor about starting daily low-dose (81-mg) aspirin therapy. In patients who have never had a stroke or heart attack, and who do *not* have hypertension, diabetes or elevated cholesterol, the risk of hemorrhage may outweigh the potential benefits of aspirin.

●**Alcohol.** Moderate alcohol consumption has been shown to benefit the heart, but it does *not* curb stroke risk.

What you can do: Men should limit their alcohol intake to two drinks per day...one drink per day for women. A drink is defined as 1.5 ounces of hard liquor, 4 ounces of wine or 12 ounces of beer. The risk of hemorrhagic stroke jumps substantially if you exceed this amount.

OTHER RISK FACTORS

Some medical conditions significantly raise your stroke risk...

●**Atrial fibrillation.** Approximately 2.2 million Americans are affected by atrial fibrillation (AF), a heart rhythm disturbance that increases stroke risk five- to sixfold.

AF can cause dizziness, shortness of breath, constriction or other uncomfortable sensations in the chest. Or it may cause no symptoms and be found during a routine examination or when you have an electrocardiogram.

What you can do: Taking a blood-thinning drug, such as *warfarin* (Coumadin), can virtually eliminate AF's added stroke risk by preventing the formation of blood clots. Aspirin may be nearly as effective.

●**Transient ischemic attack (TIA).** If you have had one or more of these brief stroke-like episodes, your risk for a full-blown stroke increases dramatically. A TIA can cause dizziness, numbness or paralysis on one side of the body, difficulty speaking, double vision or other stroke symptoms that disappear after minutes or hours.

What you can do: After a TIA, ask your doctor about taking antiplatelet medication, such as aspirin, *clopidogrel* (Plavix) or *dipyridamole* along with aspirin (Aggrenox).

●**Carotid stenosis.** When fatty deposits accumulate in the carotid artery, which carries blood up through the neck, they can impede brain circulation enough to cause a stroke. Up to half of all ischemic strokes are associated with carotid stenosis.

What you can do: If you have had a stroke or TIA, get an ultrasound of your carotid artery. If this artery is at least 70% blocked, ask your doctor about surgery.

■ ■ ■ ■

Types of Stroke

A stroke occurs when the blood supply to a part of the brain is interrupted. Without oxygen and nutrients, brain cells die within minutes, potentially damaging areas that control movement, speech and even involuntary activities, such as breathing. *There are two types of stroke...*

●**Ischemic.** Approximately 80% of strokes are *ischemic*—a blood clot stops the blood supply to an area of the brain.

•**Hemorrhagic.** An estimated 20% of strokes are *hemorrhagic*—a broken or leaking blood vessel causes bleeding into or around the brain.

Most Stroke Patients Miss Out on Clot-Busting Drug

Mathew J. Reeves, PhD, assistant professor of epidemiology, Michigan State University, Lansing. *Neurology*.

According to a US survey, only a very small percentage of stroke patients are getting *tissue plasminogen activator* (tPA), a powerful clot-busting drug that must be administered within three hours of the start of a stroke to have a beneficial effect.

THE SURVEY

Researchers reviewed the records of nearly 2,100 people treated at 15 hospitals in Michigan who had an *ischemic* stroke, the type of stroke caused by a blood clot. Only approximately 2% of the patients received tPA according to the survey.

The survey found that 41% of the stroke patients did not receive tPA because they got to the hospital after the crucial three-hour time frame, according to study author Mathew J. Reeves, an assistant professor of epidemiology at Michigan State University.

WHY THE DELAY?

"There are lots of reasons why a patient doesn't arrive in time," Reeves says. "The first problem is people don't recognize the warning signs of a stroke, and don't act on those warning signs."

This was borne out by the survey, which found that the medical records of 38% of the patients had no information on exactly when the stroke started.

Warning signs of a stroke include dizziness, sudden weakness on one side of the body and headache.

Another reason tPA may not have been given is that hospitals need time to diagnose stroke patients before administering any drugs.

"Ideally, the target is that when patients arrive at the hospital, tPA should be given within an hour," Reeves says. "That requires diagnostic tests to make sure it is a stroke, and an ischemic stroke, and determining that there are no contraindications to giving tPA. Our data show that most hospitals take between one and two hours to do those things."

While the findings point out the need to educate the public to call 911 at the first sign of a stroke, it is also necessary that hospitals evaluate patients much more quickly than they are doing, Reeves says.

There are lots of reasons why a patient doesn't arrive at the hospital in time. The first problem is people don't recognize the warning signs.

Mathew J. Reeves, PhD

The value of calling 911 was illustrated by the recent finding that patients arriving by ambulance were seven times more likely to be given tPA than those arriving on their own. The paramedics in the ambulance can not only notify the hospital that a stroke patient is on the way, but they can also perform preliminary tests that allow the patient to be fast-tracked through the emergency department, Reeves says.

info For more information on the warning signs of a stroke, visit the American Heart Association Web site at *www.americanheart.org*.

■ ■ ■ ■

Get Treatment Fast

Stroke victims often don't receive appropriate treatment fast enough. Those patients treated with tissue plasminogen activator (tPA)—which dissolves stroke-causing clots—within three hours of the onset of symptoms are three times more likely to have a good outcome as those who are not given tPA. Yet only between 2% and 3% of stroke patients receive this treatment.

Reasons: Victims and bystanders may not call for help immediately because they do not recognize stroke symptoms. Hospital phone operators may not recognize stroke symptoms and so discourage callers from coming in for help.

Larry B. Goldstein, MD, director, stroke program, Duke University, Durham, NC.

Breakthrough Strategies Help Prevent Death or Disability

Cathy Sila, MD, associate medical director of the Cerebrovascular Center, The Cleveland Clinic.

If you have a stroke, one of the most common—and devastating—mistakes is failing to seek treatment fast enough. When blood supply to the brain is cut off by a clot (*ischemic* stroke) or there is bleeding in or around the brain (*hemorrhagic* stroke), damage starts within minutes. Getting help *right away* could save your life —or profoundly improve your recovery.

IS IT A STROKE?

The onset of stroke symptoms is sudden and consists of episodes of neurological dysfunction. *Transient ischemic attacks*, or TIAs, are stroke warning symptoms that usually last 15 minutes to several hours and are not associated with permanent damage. Approximately 10% of patients who experience a TIA go on to have a stroke within the next three months. If you think that you may be having a stroke, call 911. Studies have shown that treatment may be delayed if you first call your doctor or hospital. While waiting for emergency help, lie down in a comfortable position that allows you to breathe freely.

Caution: It is not recommended that you take aspirin for a suspected stroke. While its clot-fighting ability may help if you are having an ischemic stroke (or heart attack), it could make things worse if you are actually having a hemorrhagic stroke.

THE RIGHT DIAGNOSIS

At the hospital, brain imaging is one of the first tests performed to help diagnose a stroke and determine its type. Usually, this is done using a standard *computed tomography* (CT) scan. This painless, noninvasive test takes multiple detailed images of the brain.

A hemorrhagic stroke, in which blood pools in or around the brain, is easy to identify because blood looks different on a CT scan than brain tissue. In an ischemic stroke, the brain can appear normal on a CT scan if swelling or damage has not yet occurred. In this case, the scan rules out other causes, and ischemic stroke is diagnosed by a clinical history and exam. A follow-up CT scan is performed a few days later to confirm the diagnosis.

ISCHEMIC STROKE

During the period immediately following an ischemic stroke, medication may be needed to stabilize blood pressure and heart rate. If the stroke patient has a fever, it is treated with *acetaminophen* (Tylenol) or a cooling blanket— even a slight fever can worsen brain damage. *Other treatments...*

●**Medication.** The clot-dissolving drug *alteplase* (Activase) is the most effective emergency treatment for ischemic stroke. Also known as a *tissue plasminogen activator,* or tPA, the drug works with the body's own chemicals to dissolve the clot that is blocking circulation to the brain. To be effective, tPA must be given within three hours of the first stroke symptoms. However, tPA also has risks. As a potent "clot buster," it can cause bleeding. Approximately 6% of the patients who receive it develop bleeding into the stroke-damaged area of the brain, which can be fatal.

Latest development: Administering clot-busting drugs via an intra-arterial route through a catheter threaded up to the blocked artery itself may extend the treatment window to six hours. This approach requires special imaging, such as angiography, to pinpoint the blockage and can be performed only at centers that have such equipment and personnel trained in the technique. Although studies have shown this technique to be effective for some patients, the bleeding risk is higher (10% to 12%) than standard tPA.

●**Surgery.** After a TIA or minor stroke due to a blockage of the carotid (neck) artery, other options include clearing the carotid artery to prevent another stroke. Called *carotid endarterectomy,* the blocked artery is opened and the clot is removed to restore circulation. Another option is *angioplasty* and *stenting,* in which a balloon is inserted via a catheter, and then expanded at the site of the clot to widen the blood vessel. A wire mesh framework, called a stent, is then placed in the artery to keep it open.

Latest development: Another new approach uses a corkscrew-shaped device called the MERCI (*mechanical embolus removal in cerebral ischemia*) Retriever. It is approved by the US Food and Drug Administration (FDA) for removing stroke-causing clots from brain arteries. The device looks promising, but it has not been definitively shown to improve the outcomes of patients. It also carries a risk of bleeding into the brain.

HEMORRHAGIC STROKE

Hemorrhagic stroke treatment first focuses on stabilizing the patient—using a ventilator, if necessary, to restore breathing and treating life-threatening heart problems that have been caused by the stroke, such as heart rhythm disturbances (fibrillation). *Other treatments...*

•**Medication.** Blood pressure needs to be brought down quickly to prevent additional bleeding in other parts of the brain. Blood pressure medications are often administered intravenously so they can take effect rapidly.

Bleeding in the space between the inner layer and the middle layer of the tissue covering the brain (subarachnoid hemorrhage) is usually caused by a *ruptured aneurysm*—a burst bubble in a brain artery. Your doctor may prescribe *nimodipine* (Nimotop), a calcium channel blocker that prevents arteries from going into spasm and causing more damage. After the first hemorrhage, rebleeding can occur unless corrective steps are taken.

•**Surgery.** The standard treatment for a brain aneurysm is *clipping*—a surgical procedure in which a small clip is placed at the base of the aneurysm to close it off from blood flow. It is the preferred form of treatment for aneurysms in certain areas of the brain, particularly in medically stable patients.

Latest development: For aneurysm patients who are not medically stable, a new technique known as *coiling* may be the best form of treatment. In coiling, a catheter is guided up through a blood vessel to place a collection of tiny platinum coils in the aneurysm. This causes a clot to form within the aneurysm. The procedure is less invasive and safer than clipping, but some aneurysms cannot be completely treated using this technique. The risks of both procedures include rebleeding from the aneurysm.

ONGOING CARE

Perhaps the most frustrating aspect of stroke recovery is waiting to determine the extent of brain damage. During this time, an antidepressant may be needed if there are signs of depression.

For most stroke suvivors, physical and/or occupational therapy over a period of months—or indefinitely—is essential to optimize functions, such as speech and the physical capacities that were impaired by brain damage.

Latest development: Nutrition has only recently been fully recognized as an important factor for stroke patients. In a 2005 update, the American Stroke Association recommended assessing and correcting nutritional problems, such as malnutrition, in stroke survivors.

New Stroke Treatment Is 'Hot and Cold'

Fu-Zen Shaw, associate professor of biological science and technology, National Chiao Tung University, Hsinchu, Taiwan.
Stroke.

A technique called *thermal stimulation*—the alternate application of hot and cold—improved the functioning of stroke patients' paralyzed arms and hands.

Up to 85% of stroke patients have impairment of an upper limb, and while existing rehabilitation techniques can be effective, they tend to be costly and complicated.

THE STUDY

The Taiwanese study included 46 stroke patients, half of whom received standard rehabilitation therapy; the other half received standard treatment plus thermal stimulation.

The thermal stimulation patients had five 20- to 30-minute sessions every day for six weeks. Cold packs chilled to just above freezing and hot packs heated to 167°F were alternately applied to the hand and wrist.

"We looked at whether a simple, easily used and inexpensive technique could improve motor and sensory recovery in stroke patients within a short time," says lead author of the study, Fu-Zen Shaw, an associate professor of biological science and technology at National Chiao Tung University.

The thermal stimulation patients had significantly better recovery on four of six measures of function, including changes in sensation, grasping strength and the ability to bend the wrist, according to the researchers.

Although thermal stimulation is used in orthopedic rehabilitation and to treat *dysphagia*, or difficulty swallowing, this is the first time it has been tried in stroke rehabilitation, Shaw says.

HOW IT WORKS

"Thermal stimulation can simultaneously activate large brain areas," Shaw explains. "This great activation of brain areas may be beneficial for functional reorganization of the brain, which may be helpful" for improving motor control.

The treatment also has a psychological effect, he says. Thermal stimulation may cause reflexive movements or actually enhance voluntary movements of the paralyzed hand, creating hope for stroke patients, Shaw says. "This psychological driving force...cannot be ignored."

GREAT IMPROVEMENTS

Because of the small number of patients, "the same experiment should be performed in a large population to demonstrate the effect of thermal stimulation," Shaw says. "In fact, we are going to collect data from a larger population," he adds.

But even before that happens, Shaw and his colleagues are using the technique to treat stroke patients. "We see great improvements in our patients now," he reports.

Natural Stroke Care

Rebecca Shannonhouse, editor, *Bottom Line/Health*, 281 Tresser Blvd., Stamford, CT 06901.

Naturopathic physician Andrew Rubman, ND, medical director of the Southbury Clinic for Traditional Medicine in Southbury, Connecticut, believes that more people could benefit from the use of supplements to help prevent and treat stroke.

In addition to regular visits to a neurologist...a physical and occupational therapy regimen... and anticoagulant medication, the following nutritional supplements may be helpful...

• **L-carnitine.** This amino acid allows the brain to burn fat instead of carbohydrates, which conserves oxygen.

• **Calcium/magnesium butyrate.** This is a single product containing a highly absorbable form of these important minerals. It prevents arteries from going into spasm and causing more brain damage.

• **Omega-3 fatty acid.** This "good" fat helps curb the inflammation that is associated with "mini-strokes," known as *transient ischemic attacks* (TIAs)—a significant danger for people who experience a stroke for the first time and for people who have recurrent strokes.

• **B-12 and B-complex.** These vitamins help support neurological function.

Before using supplements to help prevent or treat stroke, be sure to consult a naturopathic physician who will work with your neurologist or primary-care physician to create a full treatment regimen.

■ ■ ■ ■

Aspirin vs. Stroke

Because aspirin can cause bleeding, it is typically avoided by people who have had a hemorrhagic stroke, which occurs when a blood vessel bursts in the brain.

New finding: In a study of 207 hemorrhagic stroke survivors, those who took an antiplatelet drug, such as aspirin, were not at increased risk for another hemorrhage.

Implication: Aspirin therapy may be appropriate for hemorrhagic stroke survivors who are at high risk for heart attack or ischemic stroke, in which a blood clot blocks the blood flow to the brain.

Anand Viswanathan, MD, PhD, clinical research fellow, neurology clinical trials unit, Massachusetts General Hospital, Boston.

Aspirin–Drug Combo Better at Preventing Second Strokes

Cathy Sila, MD, associate medical director of the Cerebrovascular Center, The Cleveland Clinic.

The Lancet.

Recent European research suggests that combining aspirin and a second drug, *dipyridamole*, may be better than aspirin alone in helping stroke survivors ward off another cardiovascular event.

Both medications prevent clotting individually, and the combination has been available in the United States in the prescription drug Aggrenox. Current guidelines for what is called "secondary prevention of stroke" recommend aspirin alone, the combination of aspirin and dipyridamole, or a third clot-preventer, *clopidogrel* (Plavix), depending on individual patient characteristics.

STUDY RESULTS

Dr. Ale Algra, a Dutch neurologist and lead author of the European/Australasian Stroke Prevention in Reversible Ischemia Trial (ESPIRIT), says, "The results of ESPIRIT, combined with the results of previous trials, provide sufficient evidence to prefer the combination therapy of aspirin and dipyridamole over aspirin [alone]" for stroke survivors.

During the more than three years of the study, 13% of the 1,363 patients who took the combination of drugs had circulatory events such as second strokes, compared with 16% of the 1,376 patients who took aspirin alone.

The reduction in risk is "a modest difference but a significant difference," says Dr. Cathy Sila, associate director of the Cerebrovascular Center at The Cleveland Clinic. "We're always looking for something that eats away at the problem more," she adds.

FACTORS TO CONSIDER

While the study supports current US guidelines, "I don't think combined therapy is going to replace aspirin" for all people who have had strokes or mini-strokes, formally called *transient ischemic attacks* (TIAs), Sila says.

Physicians must consider a number of factors before deciding which medication(s) is best for their patients, Sila says.

First, the physician must consider the source of the clot that caused the stroke, Sila says. If the clot is caused by *atrial fibrillation*—the abnormal heartbeat that promotes clot formation—the preferred treatment is *warfarin* (Coumadin), a clot-preventing drug that is potent but difficult to manage.

If the clot did not originate in the heart, a patient's potential reaction to dipyrimadole must be considered, Sila says. Approximately one-third of the people who were put on combination therapy in the European trial stopped taking the medication because of side effects, most notably headaches.

In addition, the benefit of the combined therapy was apparent only after approximately 2.5 years of treatment, she notes.

Finally, cost must be considered. Sila says a one-month supply of Aggrenox is $122 and the same amount of Plavix is $117. A one-month supply of aspirin would cost less than $2.

The final word on secondary prevention is not in, Sila says. Several studies are under way, including one that compares Aggrenox with Plavix.

What is clear is that "the vast majority" of people who have had strokes should be on some kind of clot-preventing medication, Sila says.

info For more information on preventing stroke, visit the American Stroke Association Web site at *www.strokeassociation.org*.

∎ ∎ ∎ ∎

Stroke Prevention Surgery Improves Brain Function

In a recent study, 29 patients who had *carotid stenosis* (narrowing of the artery in the neck) underwent carotid artery stenting, in which the narrowed artery is expanded with a balloon and a metal tube known as a *stent*. All of the patients were given neuropsychological tests 24 hours before the procedure and 48 hours after.

Result: Cognitive function increased by nearly 6% after stenting.

Theory: Stenting increases blood flow to the brain, which improves cognitive function. This finding contradicts previous studies that suggested that stenting may cause a slight decrease in cognitive function. More research is under way.

Iris Q. Grunwald, MD, consultant physician, department of interventional and diagnostic neuroradiology, Saarland University Clinic, Hamburg, Germany.

■ ■ ■ ■

Foods that Reduce Stroke Damage

Blueberries, spinach and spirulina (a type of green algae) may reduce stroke damage. These foods have high levels of antioxidants that help neutralize damaging free radicals.

Recent study: Rats that were fed diets enriched with these foods for one month prior to an induced stroke had only half as much brain damage as rats that were not fed these foods.

This study suggests that including these foods —one cup of blueberries, a big spinach salad or a few teaspoons of spirulina powder—in your daily diet may make a difference in the severity of a stroke.

Paula C. Bickford, PhD, professor of neurosurgery, University of South Florida, and James A. Haley VA Hospital, both in Tampa.

15

Women's Health

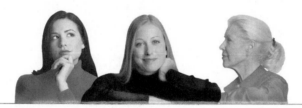

Cervical Cancer Vaccine 100% Effective For Most Types

The US Food and Drug Administration (FDA) has approved the first vaccine that protects against the *human papillomavirus* (HPV), known to cause most cervical cancers. The vaccine, Merck & Co.'s Gardasil, was approved for girls and women ages nine to 26. The National Advisory Committee on Immunization Practices will now decide whether to include the vaccine in routine vaccination schedules.

IMPRESSIVE RESULTS

In a two-year study that involved more than 12,000 women, the vaccine was found to be *100% effective* against four types of human papillomavirus—HPV 16 and HPV 18, which are responsible for approximately 70% of cervical cancer cases, and HPV 6 and HPV 11, which cause 90% of genital wart cases.

The study also showed that the Gardasil vaccine was 100% effective against vulvar and vaginal precancerous lesions caused by HPV 16 and HPV 18.

"This study shows that the prophylactic vaccine developed to prevent cervical cancer could actually also prevent vulvar and vaginal cancer as well," says Dr. Jorma Paavonen, the author of the study and chief physician in the department of obstetrics and gynecology at the University of Helsinki in Finland.

REACTION

The FDA action was hailed by experts. "It's huge!" says Dr. Michael A. Bookman, director of medical gynecologic oncology at Fox Chase Cancer Center in Philadelphia. "The thing that is incredible is the global possibilities. In the

Jorma Paavonen, MD, professor and chief physician, department of obstetrics and gynecology, University of Helsinki, Finland.

Michael A. Bookman, MD, director, medical gynecologic oncology, Fox Chase Cancer Center, Philadelphia.

US Food and Drug Administration statement.

Merck & Co. news release.

American Society for Clinical Oncology annual meeting, Atlanta.

US, we have done a good job of implementing screening and testing. In the rest of the world, this is a much more serious problem."

"Today is an important day for public health and for women's health, and for our continued fight against serious life-threatening diseases like cervical cancer," says Alex Azar, deputy secretary at the US Department of Health and Human Services.

LIFESAVING POTENTIAL

Merck has said that this vaccine has the potential to reduce the annual number of new cervical cancer cases around the world from 500,000 to approximately 150,000, and to reduce the number of deaths by more than two-thirds to approximately 90,000.

This is an opportunity to get in and educate people at an early age, have them accept the vaccine as part of their culture.

Michael A. Bookman, MD

Officials at Merck have said that the vaccine would work best when given to girls before they become sexually active.

Most experts agree that the earlier the vaccine is given, the better. "Young kids respond better to vaccines. They're immunologically poised to respond better," Bookman explains.

"You also want to get the vaccine into girls and boys before they are sexually active—not just intercourse but oral sex and any way the virus might spread," he adds.

"This is an opportunity to get in and educate people at an early age, have them accept the vaccine as part of their culture," Bookman says. Like many other vaccinations that are given in a series, Gardasil will require three shots during the course of six months.

THE FUTURE

Despite the vaccine, women will still need to be screened for cervical cancer that is caused by other types of HPV, experts note. This is most often accomplished by a Pap test, which is still a very accurate indicator of a woman's cervical condition.

■ ■ ■ ■

What Is Cervical Cancer?

Cervical cancer is the second most common malignant disease in women globally, causing an estimated 290,000 deaths worldwide each year. In the United States, approximately 10,400 new cases will be diagnosed each year, and 3,700 women will die from the disease.

The main cause of cervical cancer is continuous infection with HPV, especially HPV 16 and 18, which are spread by sexual contact.

The virus also causes precancerous and benign cervical lesions and genital warts, and may be implicated in some anal and oral cancers.

An estimated 20 million men and women in the United States are infected with HPV, but for most, the virus shows no symptoms.

info For more information on a second cervical cancer vaccine, Cervarix from GlaxoSmithKline, read the following article.

Second Cervical Cancer Vaccine Is On the Horizon

Diane M. Harper, MD, MPH, professor of community and family medicine and obstetrics and gynecology, Dartmouth Medical School, Lebanon, NH.
Rachel Winer, PhD, research scientist, University of Washington, Seattle.
The Lancet.

Another cervical cancer vaccine—Cervarix, developed by GlaxoSmithKline—has demonstrated positive results in a recent trial. The vaccine was found to still be effective after nearly five years, and may protect women against more types of cancer-causing viruses than originally thought, researchers report.

A specific type of infectious pathogen, called the *human papillomavirus* (HPV), causes most cervical cancers. Cervarix is designed to protect against HPV 16 and HPV 18, which account for approximately 70% of cervical malignancies, Harper says.

THE STUDY

This study is a follow-up on some of the women who participated in a previous study that measured the effectiveness of the Cervarix vaccine.

Study author Dr. Diane M. Harper, a professor of community and family medicine and obstetrics and gynecology at Dartmouth Medical School, and her team tracked 776 of these women for up to 53 months. The women had received either three doses of the vaccine or three doses of placebo.

The researchers found that not only did the vaccine provide protection against HPV 16 and HPV 18, but also against two other HPV types—HPV 45 and HPV 31, which can also trigger cervical cancer.

After 4.5 years, all of the women still tested positive for having been immunized with HPV 16 and HPV 18.

And, Harper notes, "Their antibody levels [which develop after a vaccine is administered], on average, did not decrease," indicating that the vaccine was still working and offering ongoing protection against these cancer-causing viruses.

PROMISING

The vaccine's apparent long-term effectiveness is promising, says Rachel Winer, a research scientist and HPV researcher at the University of Washington, Seattle.

Once a cervical cancer vaccine hits the market, young women in their late teens or early 20s would be the most likely candidates to receive it, she says.

The multistrain cross-protection that Cervarix offers is a bonus, Winer adds, and "worth investigating further" to find out the mechanism behind it.

info For more information on cervical cancer, visit the National Cancer Institute at *www. cancer.gov/cancerinfo/types/cervical.*

Common Cervical Cancer Treatments Raise Risk of Problems in Pregnancy

Maria Kyrgiou, MD, department of obstetrics and gynecology, Royal Preston Hospital, London.
Steven R. Goldstein, MD, professor of obstetrics and gynecology, New York University School of Medicine, New York City.
The Lancet.

Some of the most common methods used to treat precancerous cells of the cervix may greatly increase the risks for problems in pregnancy, researchers report.

In recent years, cervical screening programs and treatment of precancerous cells have dramatically reduced the incidence of cervical cancer.

If you hear your doctor mention LEEP, perhaps you should question him or her about the alternatives.

Steven R. Goldstein, MD

Using *cold knife* (or *laser*) *conization* (where a cone-shaped piece of cervical tissue is removed), laser ablation (in which a laser is used to remove the tissue) or the *loop electrosurgical excision procedure*, or LEEP (where cervical tissue is removed using a fine wire loop and a low-energy current), doctors have been able to successfully remove or destroy abnormal cells while preserving cervical function, the researchers explain.

All of these techniques are equally successful in preventing the progression of precancerous cells to cervical cancer. However, their effect on future fertility and pregnancy has been unclear until now.

THE STUDY

A British study found that several of these techniques may be responsible for a variety of problems during pregnancy.

In the study, lead researcher Dr. Maria Kyrgiou, from the department of obstetrics and gynecology at Royal Preston Hospital in London, and her colleagues analyzed data from 27 previous studies. They found that cold knife conization more than doubled a woman's risk of both preterm delivery and of delivering a low-birth-weight baby, and tripled the risk of Cesarean section, compared with women who did not have the procedure.

In addition, LEEP—the procedure that is used most often to remove precancerous cells—increased a woman's risk of both preterm delivery and of delivering a low-birth-weight infant by between 70% and 80%, and nearly tripled the risk for premature rupturing of the cervical membranes, compared with women who did not undergo this procedure. Laser conization showed similar but not as severe results, the researchers say.

Of all the methods used, only laser ablation did not increase the risk of pregnancy complications.

"All the conservative excisional methods of treatment that remove part of the cervix together with…the abnormal precancerous cells have more or less similar unfavorable effects on future pregnancy, while laser ablation was not associated with an increased risk of pregnancy-related morbidity," says Kyrgiou.

REACTION

"This epidemic of LEEP procedures is virtually as dangerous as the cold knife procedure," says Dr. Steven R. Goldstein, a professor of obstetrics and gynecology at New York University School of Medicine. "The abandonment of laser vaporization and cryosurgery for early surgical disease is scary and dangerous," he adds.

Currently, doctors are using LEEP because that's what they were trained to do, Goldstein says. "In young women, you start cutting on their cervix instead of freezing or vaporizing on the cervix and you are going to see adverse obstetrical outcomes," he says. "Lasering or freezing of the cervix doesn't have any of the risk."

Goldstein's advice to women is to avoid LEEP during childbearing years. "If you hear your doctor mention LEEP, perhaps you should question him or her about the alternatives," he says. "In addition, mild lesions don't always have to be treated; they can be watched," he adds.

Kyrgiou agrees that invasive surgeries are not always required for less suspicious lesions. "The treatment of precancerous lesions is necessary for the prevention of cervical cancer," she says. "However, it should be performed when it is necessary and appropriate by experienced clinicians, as a large proportion of low grade-mild lesions will eventually regress back to normal."

"Women should seek detailed information on efficacy, but also on long-term pregnancy-related morbidity before they consent," she adds.

Goldstein's advice for doctors is to think twice about using LEEP on young women. "Think about whether you would want your daughter to have this procedure before you do it," he says. "The pendulum needs to swing back."

Abdominal Chemo May Be Lifesaving Treatment For Ovarian Cancer

Deborah Armstrong, MD, associate professor of oncology, gynecology and obstetrics, Johns Hopkins Kimmel Cancer Center, Baltimore.

Stephen Cannistra, MD, professor of medicine, Harvard Medical School, and director, gynecologic medical oncology, Beth Israel Deaconess Medical Center, both in Boston.
The New England Journal of Medicine.

Chemotherapy that is delivered through an abdominal catheter may prolong the lives of women who have ovarian cancer.

Intraperitoneal chemotherapy is infused directly into the abdomen through a catheter that is surgically placed under the skin, usually beneath the lower left rib cage. Because the medicine is going directly to the area affected by the cancer, rather than throughout the entire body, higher doses of chemotherapy can often be used. The medications do eventually enter the bloodstream and spread throughout the body, hopefully killing any cancer cells that may have spread beyond the abdominal region, explains Dr. Deborah Armstrong, an associate professor of oncology, gynecology and obstetrics at Johns Hopkins Kimmel Cancer Center in Baltimore.

THE STUDY

A recent study looked at 415 women who had stage III ovarian cancer tumors and had all or most of their tumor removed. The American Cancer Society defines stage III as cancer that is in one or both ovaries and has spread to the lining of the abdomen (*peritoneum*) and/or the lymph nodes.

The study volunteers were randomly assigned to one of two groups: One group received standard intravenous chemotherapy, consisting of the drugs *paclitaxel* and *cisplatin*. The other group received intravenous and intraperitoneal paclitaxel and intraperitoneal cisplatin in higher doses than what was given to the intravenous-only group. Paclitaxel was delivered through both methods in this group because it doesn't spread throughout the body as well as abdominally delivered cisplatin, according to Armstrong, the author of the study.

Patients in both groups were scheduled for six cycles of treatments, to be given approximately every three weeks.

Women in the intraperitoneal group were more likely to experience side effects, such as gastrointestinal difficulties, hematological problems, infection, fatigue, pain and neurological problems. Less than half of the women completed all six cycles of the intraperitoneal therapy, although most completed the intravenous portion. The most common reason for discontinuing the intraperitoneal therapy was catheter-related problems, according to the researchers.

Study participants in the intraperitoneal group also reported a lower quality of life during and soon after chemotherapy. However, when quality of life was assessed one year after treatment, the results were similar for both groups.

Average survival times were significantly higher for women who received the intraperitoneal therapy. While women who received intravenous chemotherapy had a median survival time of 49.7 months, women who got the combination of intravenous and intraperitoneal chemotherapy had a median survival of 65.6 months—25% longer, the researchers say.

"This is the longest survival reported to date for advanced ovarian cancer," says Armstrong.

The average time before the disease recurred was also longer for women who received the combination therapy—23.8 months compared with 18.3 months for women on the intravenous therapy alone, the study found.

NOW THE STANDARD TREATMENT AT HOPKINS

Armstrong says the results are so encouraging that intraperitoneal chemotherapy is now Johns Hopkins' standard treatment for stage III ovarian cancer with surgically removed tumors.

Dr. Stephen Cannistra, director of gynecologic medical oncology at Beth Israel Deaconess Medical Center in Boston, says, "The regimen used in the Armstrong study has produced the largest survival advantage to date for patients with newly diagnosed stage III epithelial ovarian cancer. We are slowly but surely making progress against this terrible disease."

Cannistra says he is now offering this option to his patients, but added that it might not be widely available yet because it requires additional training to administer.

Both Armstrong and Cannistra say this therapy probably would not be used for more advanced ovarian cancers, because they have spread throughout the body.

RECOMMENDATIONS

Armstrong recommends that any woman who has a suspicious mass that could be cancerous either have the initial surgery done by a surgeon who is a gynecological oncologist, or make sure a gynecological oncologist is on-call during the surgery. If cancer is found, the oncologist can take over because outcomes are generally much better if tumors are surgically removed by these specialists, she says.

If stage III cancer is found, both Armstrong and Cannistra recommend discussing intraperitoneal chemotherapy with your physician. If intraperitoneal chemotherapy isn't available, ask for a referral to a center that is experienced in this treatment.

■ ■ ■ ■

Ovarian Cancer Statistics

Ovarian cancer affects one in every 57 American women, according to the National Cancer Institute. Most cases occur in women older than 50, although younger women can also be affected. Because ovarian cancer rarely produces noticeable symptoms in its early stages, the disease often isn't found until it is advanced and more difficult to treat successfully.

info The American Cancer Society has more information on the different types of treatment available for ovarian cancer at *www. cancer.org.*

Standard Test Misses Heart Disease Signs in Women

Nieca Goldberg, MD, former chief, women's cardiac care, Lenox Hill Hospital, New York City, spokeswomen, American Heart Association, and author of *The Women's Healthy Heart Program*. Ballantine.

George Sopko, MD, cardiologist, National Institutes of Health, and project officer, Women's Ischemia Syndrome Evaluation, National Heart, Lung, and Blood Institute. *Journal of the American College of Cardiology.*

Because plaque tends to collect in smaller blood vessels in women rather than in major arteries as it does in men, standard diagnostic testing of women can miss the warning signs of heart disease, a large US government study suggests.

STANDARD TESTS MAY NOT WORK FOR WOMEN

As many as 3 million women in the US have *coronary microvascular syndrome*, a condition in which small blood vessels are blocked by plaque, putting them at an increased risk of heart attack and even death, experts say.

> *When women go for an angiogram and they don't find blockages, it doesn't mean they don't have a problem.*
>
> *Nieca Goldberg, MD*

Unfortunately, routine angiographies usually find only significant blockages in major arteries, according to results from the Women's Ischemia Syndrome Evaluation (WISE) study, initiated in 1996 and sponsored by the National Institutes of Health.

"We're learning more and more about women [and heart disease] every day. This is a mechanism of heart disease that frequently goes undiagnosed," says Dr. Nieca Goldberg, former chief of women's cardiac care at Lenox Hill Hospital in New York City and author of *The Women's Healthy Heart Program*.

"Women and physicians should pay attention to symptoms related to the heart," adds Dr. George Sopko, WISE project officer for the National Heart, Lung, and Blood Institute (NHLBI).

THE NUMBERS

Despite an awareness of the increasing number of women who have heart disease, *coronary angiography*—an X-ray examination of the blood vessels and chambers of the heart—is not specific enough to detect these problems in women, the researchers say.

WISE investigators found that a majority of women who were given an "all-clear" on their angiograms continued to have symptoms in addition to hospitalizations and a declining quality of life.

"We found that women who have no significant blockages but have evidence of ischemia are at a high risk for future heart attacks, repeat hospitalization or even death," says Sopko. "That was noted in small studies before but nobody had such a big [study group]."

DON'T IGNORE SYMPTOMS

"When women go for an angiogram and they don't find blockages, it doesn't mean they don't have a problem. It means the problem isn't caused by a build-up of plaque," Goldberg says. "It doesn't mean that the symptoms aren't coming from the heart. They can come from very small blood vessels that we don't see in standard testing."

If women have symptoms, but no significant blockages, Sopko says you can't ignore the problem. "We're saying if you don't have the big blockages but you've got some problems, let's go look," Sopko says. "You don't neglect or deny medical therapy to these women."

An added problem, however, is that there aren't many ways to detect these kinds of problems, Goldberg says.

"Unfortunately, for this particular mechanism we don't yet have all the tools we need," Goldberg notes. "Clearly, when it comes to women and heart disease, we can't take for granted that it's going to be exactly the same script as for men."

Ischemic heart disease (IHD) is the leading cause of death in the United States, and women bear a disproportionate burden of the illness. Approximately 250,000 women die each year from IHD and its related conditions, according to the report. More than two-thirds (38%) of all deaths in women are related to coronary heart disease. And, since 1984, more women than men have died each year from IHD. It is the leading killer of women of all ages, the report adds.

311

info For more information on heart disease in women, visit the National Heart, Lung, and Blood Institute Web site at *www.nhlbi.nih. gov/health/hearttruth/index.htm.*

▪ ▪ ▪ ▪

Women Have Different Heart Attack Warning Signs than Men

Women may experience heart attack warning symptoms more than a month before the attack. The most common symptom is overwhelming fatigue, reported by 71% of women. Other reported symptoms are sleep disturbance (48%), shortness of breath (42%), indigestion (39%) and anxiety (35%). Only 30% experience chest discomfort.

Self-defense: If you are experiencing these or any suspicious symptoms, contact your doctor.

Jean McSweeney, PhD, RN, professor, University of Arkansas for Medical Sciences, Little Rock.

Facing the Midlife Crisis

Sue Shellenbarger, author of *The Breaking Point: How Female Midlife Crisis Is Transforming Today's Women.* Holt.

We all know about the male midlife crisis, a turbulent time of questioning lifelong values and goals. But slightly *more* women than men report going through a stressful midlife transition by age 50, according to a Cornell University study.

Whereas a man's midlife turmoil is more likely to be driven by work or career issues, a woman's more often begins because of family events or problems, such as divorce, a parent's death or difficulties with children.

I interviewed women around the country who have gone through a midlife crisis. I found that although the process was difficult and painful, most came to view it as a positive experience. They emerged with a greater sense of personal control and freedom…a fulfilling new sense of direction…a deeper connection to family and friends…and a richer, more creative life.

If you are a woman facing a midlife transition, watch out for these traps…

Trap: Avoiding risk. Midlife is a time when long-buried desires resurface and just won't go away. A successful manager longs to quit her job at a big corporation and start her own business. A woman who always prided herself on being diplomatic wants to speak more directly. Pay attention to these urges, no matter how awkward or frightening. Ask yourself what risks you need to take to honor the parts of yourself that you have been ignoring.

Example: A woman who has a lifelong fear of heights heard about a friend who had gone bungee jumping. At age 48, she decided to try it herself. She was absolutely terrified, but when the jump was over, she felt profound relief at having faced her fear. She then decided to confront her fear of failure by pursuing her lifelong dream of running for political office.

The women I spoke with who had the most regrets were those who were too afraid to try anything new. Even those who did make changes wished that they had taken still more risks.

Not all midlife changes are dramatic. Some women discovered their adventurous side by traveling. Some tested themselves physically by participating in sports. Some took up artistic pursuits, such as photography. Others found ways to enrich existing parts of their lives, from planting a lush garden to training the family dog to being a hospice visitor.

Trap: Not setting limits. During turbulent times, strong feelings can obscure good judgment. As you take risks, be realistic about your physical and financial boundaries. Instead of taking out a second mortgage to fund a Ferrari, buy a snazzy Volkswagen that doesn't jeopardize your financial security. If you want to try snowboarding, get an instructor until you are ready to go out on your own.

One of my midlife passions was driving all-terrain vehicles (ATVs). During one reckless ride, I flipped the vehicle and nearly died. Now I have a permanently dislocated collarbone.

If I had it to do over again, I would still get the ATV, but I would take a safety course first.

Trap: Scapegoating. The feeling that everything you have done up until now is wrong is a common symptom of midlife. You may be tempted to blame your unhappiness and confusion on your spouse or your employer.

Some couples do outgrow their marriages, just as some workers outgrow their jobs. Yet in my interviews, I found that many marriages emerged stronger from the crisis. A number of women regretted making impulsive choices that damaged their relationships, such as having affairs. Before plunging into an affair or quitting your job, look for less drastic ways to "get away."

Examples: See if your best friend wants to join you on a trip to Europe. Research the steps involved in starting a part-time business. Seek the advice of a counselor or clergy member.

Trap: Going it alone. Support is crucial to successfully navigating a midlife crisis. Women who didn't tell friends about the "crazy" feelings they were experiencing lacked valuable perspective and support.

Families can be powerful sources of encouragement. However, not all family members have the sensitivity and confidence to play this role. Recognize that your spouse and children may be puzzled and unnerved by the changes that they're seeing in you. Explain what you are going through as best you can and ask for their patience and forbearance.

Some of the best support comes from people who are experiencing similar crises. If you're part of a book club, investment club or other group, devote a few meetings to midlife issues.

Or form your own group. Nine years ago, a dozen Manhattan friends in their 40s and 50s started a "Dream Salon." At twice-monthly meetings, each participant has 20 minutes to talk about something she dreams of doing, no matter how outlandish. Then the other women respond by offering encouragement and help. Members have started businesses, earned degrees and exhibited artwork, thanks to the group's support.

One of the greatest rewards of successfully navigating a midlife crisis is the opportunity to support those who come after you. Look for ways to pass on what you have learned. When you mentor younger colleagues, volunteer in the community or act as a role model for your children, you demonstrate that a passionate second half of life is something to look forward to.

■ ■ ■ ■

Sex After 50 Can Be Better than Ever

You can get better at sex and enjoy it more—at any age. With retirement's gift of time, you can learn how your body works differently from its younger self, what pleases you and how to please each other in new ways.

PRACTICAL MATTERS

Yes, bodies change with age. Many women start to feel old and asexual at menopause. Men may develop erectile problems. But most difficulties can be overcome.

Physical change: Chronic conditions, such as diabetes, thyroid disease, cancer, Parkinson's disease and depression, can affect sexual function. With heart disease, sex can cause chest pain, and with asthma, breathlessness.

Remember, intercourse is the equivalent of walking two city blocks. Check with your doctor first.

Physical change: Joint pain and stiffness from arthritis makes sex difficult.

Solution: Relax in a Jacuzzi or bath before sex...vacation together in a warm climate...find new positions that won't stress your sore spots.

Physical change: Many drugs—antidepressant, hypertension and some cancer medications, as well as alcohol—can affect sexual function.

Solution: Ask your doctor if switching medications might help.

Dagmar O'Connor, PhD, a sex therapist for more than 30 years, and creator of a self-help sex therapy video and book packet, *How to Make Love to the Same Person for the Rest of Your Life—and Still Love It*. Dagmedia.

■ ■ ■ ■

Ladies—Even Your Testosterone Can Be Too Low

Approximately 30 million American women are thought to have low levels of the androgens (so-called male hormones) they need, including testosterone and DHEA.

Common causes of these low levels include diminished ovarian function, estrogen supplementation (either by birth control pills or by hormone replacement therapy) and impaired adrenal function.

Symptoms include: Osteoporosis, reduced sex drive (which could be due to diminished libido or lack of interest due to pain or dryness), loss of muscle tone, low energy, lack of mental clarity and decreased enjoyment of life.

Diagnosis: To check for androgen deficiency in women, it's best to measure levels of testosterone and DHEA-sulfate (DHEA-S), another androgen. Total testosterone less than 30 nanograms per deciliter (ng/dL) and/or DHEA-S levels less than 100 micrograms per deciliter (mcg/dL) may be reason to consider supplementation.

Treatment: Among women who have sexual dysfunction due to low androgens, treatment using low-dose testosterone or low-dose DHEA significantly increases sex drive—approximately 70% of the time. Although the US Food and Drug Administration (FDA) has not yet approved testosterone supplements for use in women, many doctors are prescribing them anyway.

Warning: Unnecessary supplementation can lead to excessive androgen levels, resulting in heavier pubic hair growth, clitoral enlargement, acne, increased facial hair growth, lowered voice, and reduced levels of HDL ("good") cholesterol. Close monitoring of testosterone levels is advised.

Culley Carson, MD, Rhodes Distinguished Professor and chief of urology, University of North Carolina Medical Center, Chapel Hill.

Natural Ways to Ease Menopause Symptoms

Ann Louise Gittleman, PhD, nutritionist and author of *Hot Times: How to Eat Well, Live Healthy, and Feel Sexy During the Change.* Avery.

For decades, women relied on *hormone replacement therapy* (HRT) to relieve symptoms of menopause—hot flashes, sleep disturbances, anxiety and mood swings. But several large studies have linked long-term HRT with an increased risk of breast cancer, dementia, heart attack and stroke.

Fortunately, there are safer, natural alternatives to HRT.

MORE THAN JUST ESTROGEN

People typically attribute menopausal symptoms to the declining production of the female hormones *estrogen* and *progesterone*. But poor eating and lifestyle habits also play a role by overtaxing the adrenal glands. For women who are going through menopause, the adrenal glands are nature's backup system. When the ovaries decrease their production of estrogen and progesterone, the adrenals have the ability to produce hormones to compensate for this. Poor diet and lifestyle choices put stress on the adrenals, creating an imbalance in body chemistry and contributing to the uncomfortable symptoms that we associate with menopause.

If you are a woman who has menopausal symptoms, adopting healthier habits can help to even out these imbalances.

If you are a man and the woman you love is going through menopause, you can help by understanding that she is experiencing a profound physiological change. Your kindness and patience can ease her transition through a time that is confusing—for her as well as for you.

Common symptoms and natural solutions…

HOT FLASHES

As many as 80% of women experience hot flashes during menopause. One theory is that the *hypothalamus*, which controls body temperature, is somehow triggered by hormonal fluctuations.

●**Avoid spicy foods.** Foods containing cayenne or other peppers have a *thermogenic* effect, meaning that they raise body temperature.

●**Cook using garlic, onion, thyme, oregano and sage.** These seasonings contain very small amounts of *phytoestrogens* (plant-based estrogens, such as *lignans* and *isoflavones*, that occur naturally in certain foods) and can help restore hormone balance.

●**Cut down on caffeine.** Caffeine stimulates the adrenal glands, leading to a spike in blood sugar levels followed by a plunge in blood sugar to levels even lower than before. This stresses the body and aggravates menopausal woes.

If you don't want to give up coffee completely, have one cup a day with food. Don't use coffee as a stimulant between meals. Instead, eat frequent small meals for energy.

Better than coffee: Green, white and black teas have less caffeine and are high in disease-fighting antioxidants. Try substituting tea for coffee. Then transition to herbal tea or hot water with lemon.

●**Add flaxseed.** Ground flaxseed contains lignans, which seem to modulate fluctuating estrogen and progesterone levels. Aim for two tablespoons a day. Ground flaxseed has a pleasant nutty flavor—sprinkle it on cereal, yogurt and salads.

Bonus: Flaxseed reduces cholesterol, helps prevent certain cancers and relieves constipation (be sure to drink plenty of water).

●**Eat soy foods in moderation.** Some countries that have diets containing large amounts of soy report low rates of menopausal symptoms and breast cancer. But I'm cautious about soy. Preliminary research suggests that while the isoflavones in soy appear to protect against some breast cancers, they also may stimulate the growth of other types of breast cancer.

I'm especially concerned about isolated soy protein, which is often added to protein powder, energy bars and supplements. This puts far more soy isoflavones into the diet than other cultures typically consume—and these high amounts may not be healthful.

If you enjoy soy foods, limit your consumption to two servings per week, and eat them in their whole-food form—as tofu, tempeh, miso and edamame.

●**Be wary of herbal remedies.** I'm cautious about black cohosh, red clover and other plant remedies that have estrogen-like properties. Research has not demonstrated clearly that they help, and some can have harmful side effects if not properly monitored. However, some women do report good results when they use these remedies. Check with your doctor first. If you don't notice a clear change in symptoms after two to three weeks of trying a new remedy, ask your doctor about trying something else.

What men can do: Buy a dual-control electric blanket so that both of you will be comfortable. Make her a cup of herbal tea. Join her in eating flaxseed—it's good for your colon and prostate, too.

INSOMNIA

During menopause, elevated levels of the stress hormone *cortisol* make it difficult to fall asleep and can trigger intermittent awakening throughout the night. *Natural sleep aids…*

●**Wild yam cream.** This topical cream, extracted from yams grown in Mexico, is a source of natural progesterone. It's available at most health-food stores and at some pharmacies. Applying small amounts of wild yam cream daily may help balance cortisol levels and enhance sleep. (It also helps reduce anxiety and hot flashes.)

Apply ¼ teaspoon once in the morning and once at night. Rub the cream on areas where you see capillaries, such as the wrist, back of the knee and neck—these are where the skin is thinnest and the cream is easily absorbed. Alternate where you apply the cream on a daily basis.

●**Magnesium.** Levels of magnesium, a natural sleep aid, are depleted when you consume too much coffee, cola, alcohol, sugar or salt. Foods that are high in magnesium include halibut…whole-wheat bread…leafy green vegetables such as spinach…nuts…and dried beans (soaked and cooked). If your diet is low in magnesium, take 200 to 400 milligrams (mg) in supplement form at bedtime.

●**Zinc.** This mineral can help quiet an overactive mind. Foods that are rich in zinc include poultry, red meat and nuts, but it is hard to get enough zinc from food. Take 25 to 45 mg in supplement form before bed.

●**Exercise.** One study found that women older than age 50 who walked, biked or did stretching exercises every morning fell asleep more easily. Try to perform 30 minutes of exercise most mornings. Avoid working out in the evening—you may have trouble winding down. And don't go to extremes—overexercising (more than two hours of strenuous, nonstop activity every day) can lead to a hormonal imbalance.

What men can do: Exercise with her in the morning. Make sure there is a bottle of magnesium tablets by the bedside.

MOOD SWINGS

Drinking less coffee and eating frequent, small meals will go a long way toward balancing your moods by reducing spikes in blood sugar and stress on the adrenals. *In addition…*

●**Eat a balanced diet.** The emotional and mental stress of menopause can lead to a vicious cycle in which stress depletes important mineral stores, further taxing the adrenals.

Among the minerals depleted by stress are copper, calcium, magnesium, potassium, sodium and zinc. To restore these minerals, eat an adrenal-supportive diet that is rich in bright-colored fruits and vegetables, legumes, lean meats and whole grains. Avoid sugar and other refined carbohydrates.

Recommended: Sea vegetables, such as *nori, arame, wakame* and *hijiki.* These are especially high in key minerals. Health-food stores sell these vegetables in dried form. They can be crumbled into soup, salad and vegetables.

●**Get the right kind of fat.** Although you should avoid saturated fats (in pork, beef and high-fat dairy products) and hydrogenated fats (in margarine, shortening and many packaged baked goods), certain fats are necessary for hormone regulation and the proper functioning of the nervous system. Known as *essential fatty acids* (EFAs), these healthy fats help to stabilize blood sugar.

Try to consume two tablespoons of healthy oil every day (use it in cooking, salad dressings, etc.). Olive, sesame, almond, macadamia and flaxseed oils are especially high in EFAs. (Flaxseed oil does not cook well.)

●**Take B-complex vitamins.** B vitamins are known as the antistress vitamins because they nourish the adrenals. Good sources of B vitamins include whole grains and dried beans (soaked and cooked). Most diets are too low in these vitamins, so a 50- to 100-mg B-complex supplement is usually needed.

What men can do: Make it easy for her to avoid sugar and caffeine by cutting back on them yourself—your health will benefit, too. If she seems distant or on edge, don't take it personally. Remind yourself that it is not you—it is her biochemistry that is acting up.

WEIGHT GAIN

One reason so many women gain weight during menopause is that the ovulation process burns calories—as much as 300 calories per day during the first 10 days of the menstrual cycle. When ovulation stops, fewer calories are burned and metabolism slows. *Foods that will counter the slowdown...*

●**Protein.** Aim for 3 to 4 ounces of lean protein from fish, poultry, beef or lamb twice a day. Eggs and beans are also good sources.

●**Healthy carbohydrates.** Whole grains, vegetables and fruits metabolize slowly and give you energy throughout the day. Try to consume at least two servings of fruits, three servings of vegetables and three servings of whole grains daily.

What men can do: Don't nag her about her weight. Support her by not buying high-calorie foods, such as potato chips and rich desserts.

Better Alternatives to Hysterectomy

Esther Eisenberg, MD, MPH, professor of obstetrics and gynecology, and director of reproductive endocrinology and infertility, Vanderbilt University School of Medicine, Nashville. She is coauthor of *Hysterectomy: Exploring Your Options.* Johns Hopkins.

During the past 25 years, advances in gynecologic surgery have caused a steady decline in the number of hysterectomies (removal of the entire uterus) performed in the US.

Now: A variety of new surgical techniques are giving women even more options for treating abnormal uterine bleeding and fibroid tumors.

ABNORMAL UTERINE BLEEDING

This condition typically occurs in women older than age 45. It results from a high level of estrogen that is not balanced by progesterone. Ovulation does not occur, but the *endometrium* (lining of the uterus) thickens and is then shed incompletely and irregularly, causing bleeding.

In the past, abnormal uterine bleeding was treated by a complete hysterectomy.

Alternatives to hysterectomy...

●**Endometrial ablation.** This approach, requires no incision and is performed on an outpatient basis. It stops uterine bleeding in up to 80% of women.

How it works: A *hysteroscope* (a thin, lighted telescope) is inserted through the vagina and cervix into the uterus. An electric current or laser is then used to heat and destroy the endometrium. Scar tissue may develop, which is likely to impair a woman's ability to become pregnant. Other potential risks include perforation of the uterine wall and injury to adjacent structures, such as burns to the bowel.

• **Thermal balloon ablation.** This newer technique appears to be as effective as endometrial ablation, and typically, has fewer risks. However, not all hospitals have the equipment that is needed to perform thermal balloon ablation.

How it works: A balloon that is filled with fluid is placed in the uterus and heated until it destroys the endometrium without damaging surrounding tissue.

UTERINE FIBROIDS

Up to 40% of hysterectomies are performed to remove uterine fibroids. Although the cause of these tumors is unknown, recent research has linked them to a genetic mutation. Fibroids are almost always benign and often produce no symptoms.

However, fibroids can cause extremely heavy or frequent menstrual flow (sometimes leading to anemia)...chronic pain...bloating...pressure on the bladder and other internal organs...infertility...and/or abdominal swelling. In these cases, surgery is often the best solution. *Procedures to consider...*

• **Myomectomy.** Currently the preferred treatment for women who want to keep their reproductive options open, this procedure removes fibroids but retains the woman's uterus to allow for pregnancy.

How it works: A surgeon makes an abdominal incision, cuts the fibroid out and repairs the wall of the uterus using sutures.

• **Laparoscopic myomectomy.** This procedure is less invasive than the standard myomectomy, but it may not be advisable if the fibroid is too large.

How it works: A *laparoscope* (a thin, lighted viewing tube) and other instruments are introduced through a small (less than 1 inch) abdominal incision. The fibroids are cut into fragments small enough to be removed through the ab-

dominal incision or another small incision made through the vaginal wall. Most women can sustain a pregnancy after they have undergone laparoscopic myomectomy.

However, there is increased risk of uterine rupture at delivery because the laparoscopic closure of the uterine muscle may not be as effective as in a standard myomectomy.

In one out of three women who receive standard or laparoscopic myomectomy, fibroid tumors eventually recur.

• **Hysteroscopy.** An even less invasive technique than laparoscopic myomectomy, hysteroscopy is now being used for some submucus fibroids, which protrude inside the uterine cavity. (Many fibroids are embedded in the uterine muscle.)

How it works: After the cervix is dilated, a hysteroscope is passed through the cervix into the uterus, which is inflated with gas or fluid to provide a better view. Because dilation is painful, a local or regional anesthetic is usually administered.

In a hysteroscopy, fibroids are removed using an electrosurgical tool that burns the tissue so that the fibroids can be removed in pieces. The procedure, which requires no incision, is performed on an outpatient basis, and recovery takes two to three days.

• **High-frequency ultrasound.** This is a promising experimental procedure.

How it works: While the patient lies in a *magnetic resonance imaging* (MRI) scanner, a doctor uses the image to aim heat-producing, high-frequency ultrasound beams at the tumor to destroy it.

The patient is awake throughout the high-frequency ultrasound, and no incisions are required. Currently available at The Johns Hopkins Hospital in Baltimore, Brigham and Women's Hospital in Boston and the Mayo Clinic in Rochester, Minnesota, this procedure has been found to be safe and effective in preliminary studies.

NEW HYSTERECTOMY OPTIONS

Despite the availability of newer treatments, up to 600,000 women each year still choose to have a hysterectomy.

Reason: A hysterectomy provides a permanent cure for abnormal uterine bleeding and fibroid tumors and also eliminates the risk of uterine cancer.

Newer, less invasive types of hysterectomy have sharply reduced hospitalization—to just two to three days for many patients—and hastened recovery to as little as a week.

•**Supracervical hysterectomy.** The uterus, but not the cervix, is removed through an abdominal incision. This surgery has fewer complications than total hysterectomy, but it still leaves a woman at risk for cervical cancer.

•**Laparoscopic hysterectomy.** The uterus is removed using a laparoscope inserted through a small abdominal incision.

•**Vaginal hysterectomy.** The uterus is removed through an incision inside the vagina. This procedure includes removal of both the cervix and the uterus. It can only be performed on fibroids that are small enough to pass through the vagina. Vaginal hysterectomy can also be performed with laparoscopic assistance.

■ ■ ■ ■

Reducing Fibroid Risk

Fibroids—benign tumors of the uterus—are dependent on the hormone *estrogen* for growth. *To minimize risk...*

•**Keep your body-fat percentage down** through good diet and exercise. The more body fat you have, the higher your estrogen levels are likely to be.

•**Eat a high-fiber diet** that includes lots of cruciferous vegetables, such as broccoli and cauliflower. They contain a nutrient called *indole 3 carbinol* that helps the liver lower estrogen levels.

•**Eat certain foods,** such as miso and tempeh (from fermented soy)...ground flaxseed...and the herb chasteberry—take 40 drops of tincture or 180 to 240 milligrams in capsule form daily.

•**Have your hormone levels tested** by a naturopathic or holistic doctor—who will use a saliva test to determine whether you need additional hormone-balancing foods or supplements.

Mark A. Stengler, ND, naturopathic physician, La Jolla Whole Health Clinic, La Jolla, CA.

Low-Fat Diet Lowdown for Postmenopausal Women

Jacques E. Rossouw, MD, project officer, Women's Health Initiative, National Heart, Lung, and Blood Institute.

Michael Thun, MD, vice president, epidemiology and surveillance research, American Cancer Society.

Elizabeth G. Nabel, MD, director, National Heart, Lung, and Blood Institute.

Nieca Goldberg, MD, former chief, women's cardiac care, Lenox Hill Hospital, New York City, spokeswoman, American Heart Association, and author of *The Women's Healthy Heart Program.* Ballantine.

The Journal of the American Medical Association.

American Heart Association statement.

A large US government study has found that a diet low in fat and high in vegetables, grains and fruits does *not* reduce the risk of cardiovascular disease, breast cancer or colorectal cancer in postmenopausal women. The results, from the Women's Health Initiative (WHI), are not likely to be the last word on the subject, however.

It's about a balance—how we exercise and how we eat—and balancing the stress as well. Nobody wants to hear it. We all want the quick fix.

Nieca Goldberg, MD

Previous research has suggested that low-fat diets might protect against cancer and heart disease, but no other studies have been as large or as well-designed as this one.

THE STUDY

The WHI is a large, 15-year study that is designed to identify the most common causes of death, disability and poor quality of life in postmenopausal women.

The study looked at 50,000 postmenopausal women, who were randomly assigned to one of two groups. The first group followed a reduced-fat diet (20% of total calories) and ate large quantities of vegetables and fruits (five or more servings per day), as well as grains (six or more servings per day). The second group served as a control group in which the women did not change their diets. The participants were followed-up for approximately eight years.

The women in the low-fat group had a 9% lower risk of breast cancer than the women in the control group, but this difference is not statistically significant, the researchers say.

However, women in the low-fat group who had eaten a higher fat diet before the study began *did* have a significant reduction in their risk of breast cancer, indicating that such a diet might indeed confer a benefit.

The low-fat diet did not reduce the risk of colorectal cancer, but there was a reduction in the incidence of polyps, a precursor to this type of cancer, allowing for the possibility that some benefit may appear in the future.

"It's possible that with longer-term adherence to such a diet, a benefit might emerge," says Dr. Jacques E. Rossouw, WHI project officer at the National Heart, Lung, and Blood Institute (NHLBI).

The low-fat diet did not appreciably reduce the risk of coronary heart disease, stroke or cardiovascular disease, achieving only modest effects on triglyceride levels.

However, LDL ("bad") cholesterol levels and diastolic blood pressure were significantly reduced.

The researchers also note that a high intake of carbohydrates did not increase body weight, but rather, tended to maintain it.

INTERPRETATIONS

Dr. Michael Thun, vice president of epidemiology and surveillance research at the American Cancer Society says, "This is by far the most definitive study showing that a concerted effort to reduce fat intake to 20% of total [calories] over an eight-year period did not reduce the incidence of breast or colorectal cancer in these women. But it's unlikely to end the debate completely."

It is possible that a diet that is lower in particular types of fat might be beneficial. "Reducing total fat didn't make any difference to heart disease, but women who chose to reduce their saturated fat or trans fat had a significant reduction" in heart disease, Rossouw says.

"With heart disease, it's very clear that total fat isn't enough. We've got to focus on specific types of fat," he adds.

Dr. Elizabeth G. Nabel, director of the NHLBI, says, "We really think these findings are good news. This study was the most comprehensive study of this kind, and the findings are very consistent with current US dietary recommendations about following a diet low in saturated and trans fats and cholesterol and keeping fat calories to approximately 20% to 35% of total calories."

It's also not clear if starting a low-fat diet earlier in life can confer a greater reduction in heart disease risk. All of the women in the study were postmenopausal when they changed their eating habits.

CAUTIONS

Despite the somewhat surprising findings, experts still believe women should follow a healthy lifestyle.

"We have to be very careful. The last thing I want is someone to go out eating a high-fat, high-calorie diet," says Dr. Nieca Goldberg, former chief of women's cardiac care at Lenox Hill Hospital in New York City and a spokeswoman for the American Heart Association (AHA).

"It would be easy to misinterpret the results of this study," adds Dr. Robert H. Eckel, president of the AHA.

"Reducing the risk of cardiovascular disease is about following an integrated lifestyle program, rather than concentrating solely on dietary composition," he says.

"It's a combination of things that lowers cardiovascular risk. It's no one diet, no one exercise, no one pill," Goldberg adds. "We have to avoid extremes. Really, it's about a balance—how we exercise and how we eat—and balancing the stress level as well. Nobody wants to hear it. We all want the quick fix."

THE STUDY CONTINUES

"The issue isn't over," Rossouw says. "We plan to follow these women for another five years because it's quite possible that a benefit for both breast cancer and colorectal cancer will emerge over time."

More examination will be done on the existing data to determine if specific dietary components have a beneficial effect on health, experts say.

info To find out more information about the Women's Health Initiative, visit *www.nhlbi.nih.gov/whi.*

Daily Aspirin
A Smart Move
After Menopause

Jeffrey S. Berger, MD, cardiology fellow, Duke University Medical Center, Durham, NC.

Nieca Goldberg, MD, former chief, women's cardiac care, Lenox Hill Hospital, New York City, spokeswoman, American Heart Association, and and author of *Women Are Not Small Men.* Ballantine.

American Heart Association annual meeting, Dallas.

Simply taking aspirin appears to be a lifesaving measure for millions of women who have heart disease.

New research has found that aspirin significantly reduces the death rate for postmenopausal women who have cardiovascular disease.

The dosage does not seem to matter, as long as it is taken regularly.

THE STUDY

For this study, the authors analyzed data from the Women's Health Initiative (WHI), funded by the National Institutes of Health.

The researchers focused on 8,928 women between the ages of 50 and 79, who had cardiovascular disease, including those who had experienced a heart attack, stroke, mini-stroke, cardiac chest pain or a procedure to open clogged coronary arteries.

During approximately six-and-a-half years of follow-up, postmenopausal women who were taking aspirin on a regular basis had a 17% lower risk of death from any cause, compared with women who were not taking aspirin.

The women taking aspirin also had 25% fewer deaths from cardiovascular disease.

The results were identical for the women taking 81-milligrams (mg) and those taking 325 mg.

A SURPRISING FIGURE

The study also found that only 46% of the participants actually took aspirin regularly, despite ample previous research demonstrating that aspirin reduces both fatal and nonfatal vascular events in people who have existing cardiovascular disease.

"This was rather surprising," says Dr. Jeffrey S. Berger, first author of the study and a cardiology fellow at Duke University Medical Center in Durham, North Carolina.

"Unfortunately, we don't know why, although there are a few things to think about. Although we know that aspirin is effective, there's not much data on aspirin in women, so the message may not have come across as strong as it should have," he says.

"Also, because aspirin is over-the-counter, people do not look at it as a lifesaving medication.

"Hopefully, this study will really demonstrate that aspirin is effective, and hopefully, more women will use it," he says.

"The results are consistent, and make it clear that women who have cardiovascular disease benefit from aspirin," says Dr. Nieca Goldberg, former chief of women's cardiac care at Lenox Hill Hospital in New York City. "It doesn't change any of our guidelines."

> *Because aspirin is over-the-counter, people do not look at it as a lifesaving medication.*
>
> *Jeffrey S. Berger, MD*

Because the trial was observational and not randomized, it's not possible to say with certainty whether it was the aspirin that actually caused the benefit.

However, Berger says, "We have biological plausibility and we have size, so we're pretty comfortable saying that aspirin therapy is associated with this, and perhaps it does cause this" reduced risk.

For women who decide to begin aspirin therapy, Berger suggests choosing the lower dose. "The lower dose is just as effective, and we already know there are fewer side effects," he says.

info The American Heart Association's Go Red For Women movement has more information on women and heart disease at *www.americanheart.org.*

Menopause May Increase Salt-Linked Hypertension

Ivonne Hernandez Schulman, MD, Veterans Affairs Medical Center, and assistant professor of clinical medicine, Miller School of Medicine, University of Miami.

Howard Weintraub, MD, codirector, Lipid Treatment Program, New York University, and associate professor of medicine, NYU School of Medicine, New York City

Ana Paula Dantas, PhD, assistant professor of medicine, division of nephrology and hypertension, and Center for the Study of Sex Differences in Health, Aging and Disease, Georgetown University, Washington, DC.

American Heart Association's Council for High Blood Pressure Research conference, Washington, DC.

Doctors have long known that a sensitivity to salt can lead to high blood pressure in some people. Now, a new study has found that hormonal changes following menopause can trigger this sensitivity in women previously unaffected by salt.

In fact, within four months, levels of salt sensitivity doubled for younger women who had hysterectomies with ovary removal, the researchers report.

THE STUDY

Researchers studied 40 women, who had an average age of 47, who had normal blood pressure and no history of diabetes. All of the women underwent hysterectomy and ovary removal, which induced menopause.

The researchers found that the number of women who were sensitive to salt was significantly higher after menopause. Four months after surgery, 21 women (52%) were salt-sensitive compared with just nine women (22.5%) who were salt-sensitive before surgery.

While the women in the study who developed salt sensitivity did not show an increase in blood pressure, other studies indicate that most women will not develop high blood pressure for five to 10 years after menopause, according to lead researcher Dr. Ivonne Hernandez Schulman, an assistant professor of clinical medicine at the University of Miami's Miller School of Medicine.

"Among women who undergo surgical menopause, there is an increase in their sensitivity to salt, potentially raising their blood pressure," says Schulman.

According to Schulman, some women will naturally develop salt sensitivity after menopause, and therefore, run the risk of developing high blood pressure and the ensuing risks of cardiovascular disease and stroke.

"Approximately 50% of people with high blood pressure are considered to be salt-sensitive," Schulman says. "Even people with a normal blood pressure who are salt-sensitive have a higher risk of developing high blood pressure and possibly cardiovascular disease," she adds.

STUDY LIMITATIONS

However, Dr. Howard Weintraub, codirector of the New York University Lipid Treatment Program and associate professor of medicine at NYU School of Medicine, says, "These findings need to be taken with a grain of salt."

The study did not take into account the weight or ethnic makeup of the participants. Obesity and some ethnic heritages can predispose a woman to salt sensitivity, he notes. Both of these factors could have influenced the results.

> *These findings need to be taken with a grain of salt.*
>
> *Howard Weintraub, MD*

"Everything we know now about postmenopausal hypertensive women is that the problem is not salt sensitivity," Weintraub says. "The problem that we are looking at is the impact of women who develop obesity. Salt sensitivity is an added problem that goes on top of [that]."

In addition, Weintraub is concerned that the study sends the wrong message. "I don't want people thinking that a 55-year-old woman's blood pressure can be adequately handled by just diuretics, which reduce salt," Weintraub says.

IMPORTANT QUESTIONS

Despite these limitations, the study does raise important questions.

"The observation that a high percentage of women who were salt-resistant before the removal of ovaries became salt-sensitive suggests that salt sensitivity may be partially responsible for the increase in the progression of hypertension after menopause," says Ana Paula Dantas, an assistant professor of medicine in the division of nephrology and hypertension and the Center for the Study of Sex Differences in Health, Aging and Disease at Georgetown University.

"This study raises some important questions —should postmenopausal women be more concerned about dietary salt intake than men? Would diuretics be more effective in menopausal women than in men?" she asks.

OTC Painkillers Push Blood Pressure Higher

Clarence Grim, MD, professor of clinical medicine, Medical College of Wisconsin, Milwaukee.
Gary C. Curhan, MD, associate professor of medicine, Harvard Medical School, Boston.
Hypertension.

Women who take daily high doses of the over-the-counter (OTC) painkillers *ibuprofen* and *acetaminophen* are much more likely to develop high blood pressure than women who do not use these drugs, according to new research.

THE STUDY

The study looked at the medical records of more than 5,000 women—ages 34 to 77—for up to eight years, and found that those who took 500 milligrams (mg) or more of acetaminophen daily were twice as likely to develop high blood pressure as women who did not take the drug.

Women ages 51 to 77 who took an average of 400 mg of ibuprofen daily were 80% more likely to develop high blood pressure than women of the same age who did not take this drug. Younger women (ages 34 to 53) who took the same dose were 60% more likely to develop high blood pressure, according to the study.

Interestingly, the researchers did not find that aspirin increased women's chances of developing high blood pressure.

POSSIBLE EXPLANATIONS

The mechanism by which the medications could raise blood pressure is uncertain, explains Dr. Clarence Grim, a professor of clinical medicine at the Medical College of Wisconsin, and an expert on high blood pressure. There is a "general hypothesis" that they might increase blood levels of sodium by affecting kidney metabolism, he says.

Ibuprofen and acetaminophen are used so frequently and so widely that they could be one reason why the incidence of high blood pressure is so high.

Gary C. Curhan, MD

Another possibility, says Dr. Gary C. Curhan, an associate professor of medicine at Harvard Medical School and a member of the research team, is that the painkillers may influence blood vessel relaxation. Acetaminophen is known to affect levels of nitric oxide, a substance that is important in blood vessel control, he says.

Ibuprofen and acetaminophen "are used so frequently and so widely that they could be one reason why the incidence of high blood pressure is so high," Curhan says.

RECOMMENDATIONS

Grim suggests that people who take the painkillers frequently make sure they tell their physicians how often they are taking them. And, he advises, "Be sure to keep an eye on your blood pressure. Even small changes in blood pressure can be very significant.

"This is another thing we need to add to the list of items that raise blood pressure, at least for women," Grim says.

The new research involved only women because men generally use painkillers less often. However, studies of a possible relationship between these drugs and high blood pressure in men are just beginning, and Curhan says he expects the results will be the same as for women.

"Call me back in four or five years and I'll have some information for you," Curhan says.

info For more information on high blood pressure, visit the American Society of Hypertension, Inc. at *www.ash-us.org.*

Boning Up:
Calcium, Vitamin D
Not as Effective as Hoped

Andrea LaCroix, PhD, coprincipal investigator, Women's Health Initiative Clinical Coordinating Center, Fred Hutchinson Cancer Research Center, Seattle.

Joel S. Finkelstein, MD, endocrinologist, Massachusetts General Hospital, and associate professor of medicine, Harvard Medical School, both in Boston.

The New England Journal of Medicine.

Council for Responsible Nutrition.

Taking daily calcium and vitamin D supplements does not result in the significant health benefits for older women that many had hoped for. According to results from the Women's Health Initiative (WHI), healthy postmenopausal women older than age 50 who took the supplements achieved a small but significant improvement in hip bone density but not a significant reduction in their risk of hip fracture until they reached their 60s.

Previous research had suggested that calcium and/or vitamin D supplements might slow bone loss and reduce the risk of falls in older women, but the evidence of any reduction in fracture risk has been scanty.

THE FIRST STUDY

The current study involved more than 36,000 postmenopausal women, ages 50 to 79, all of whom received daily either 1,000 milligrams (mg) of elemental calcium as calcium carbonate plus 400 international units (IU) of vitamin D-3 or a placebo. Calcium is a major component of bone, and vitamin D helps the body properly absorb calcium through the intestines.

The women took the calcium supplement in addition to their average daily calcium intake of 110 mg from food or multivitamins, for a total calcium intake of 1,110 mg, which "is close to the national recommendation" for women older than 50, according to Andrea LaCroix, coprincipal investigator of the WHI Clinical Coordinating Center at Fred Hutchinson Cancer Research Center in Seattle.

After tracking the women's bone health for seven years, the researchers found that hip bone density rose an average of 1.06% in the group taking the supplements compared with the placebo group. And, although women who took the supplements had an average 12% reduction in their incidence of hip fracture, this finding was not considered statistically significant, according to the researchers.

In addition, the women taking calcium plus vitamin D had an increased risk of kidney stones.

The studies showed disappointing outcomes inconsistent with the large body of scientific evidence about the beneficial effects of these two nutrients.

John Hathcock

The news did look slightly better for women older than 60, who had a 21% reduction in hip fractures. Calcium plus vitamin D "looked more effective in women over 60 who adhered to the study medication," LaCroix says.

LOOKING AT THE RESULTS

The results were not surprising, say some experts. "The study looked at a large number of postmenopausal women who weren't specifically selected to be at risk for fractures, so the deck was largely stacked against the study," says Dr. Joel Finkelstein, an endocrinologist at Massachusetts General Hospital in Boston. "In that setting, there was no overall effect on fracture risk, which wasn't terribly surprising because calcium and vitamin D are relatively weak therapies for osteoporosis.

"The message is it's a fairly mild to moderate effect," Finkelstein says. "I recommend that women should take calcium and vitamin D, but shouldn't rely on it as adequate protection for osteoporosis."

THE SECOND STUDY

A second study found that daily calcium plus vitamin D had no effect whatsoever on colorectal cancer risk in the same group of women. The incidence of invasive colorectal cancer did not differ appreciably between women taking the supplements and those taking the placebo. The incidence of colon polyps—a precursor to cancer—was also similar in both groups.

"For colorectal cancer, this means that we can't count on calcium for prevention," explains LaCroix. She stresses that, despite the disappointing results, calcium is "just one avenue that looked promising" for the prevention of colon cancer. "It [still] leaves women with other avenues, such as early detection," she notes.

Representatives of the supplements industry downplayed the results. The studies "showed disappointing outcomes inconsistent with the large body of scientific evidence and the prevailing wisdom about the beneficial effects of these two nutrients," according to John Hathcock, vice president for scientific and international affairs at the Council for Responsible Nutrition.

info To learn more about vitamin D, visit the National Institutes of Health's Office of Dietary Supplements at *http://ods.od.nih.gov/fact sheets/vitamind.asp.*

Women Still Missing Critical Folic Acid

Tsunenobu Tamura, MD, professor of nutrition science, University of Alabama at Birmingham.

Kathleen Yadrick, PhD, professor of nutrition and food systems, University of Southern Mississippi, Hattiesburg.

Siobhan Dolan, MD, associate medical director, March of Dimes.

Despite years of public health campaigns telling women of child-bearing age to take enough folic acid every day to prevent birth defects, the message doesn't seem to be getting through.

NUMBERS ARE DROPPING

The number of women in the US taking folic acid supplements dropped from 40% in 2004 to 33% in 2005, according to a report from the March of Dimes.

A daily supplement of 400 micrograms (mcg) of folic acid, a vitamin crucial for proper cell growth, can dramatically reduce birth defects of the brain and spine, such as spina bifida. Such problems occur in approximately 3,000 pregnancies every year, according to the Centers for Disease Control and Prevention (CDC).

Getting that much folic acid isn't difficult—you can take a single vitamin pill or you can get it from folate-rich foods, such as leafy green vegetables and citrus fruits, or from folate-fortified foods, including enriched breads and cereals. Fortifying foods with folic acid has been mandated in the US since 1998, in an effort to boost folate intake.

TAKE A MULTIVITAMIN

Other than repeating the message about the importance of folic acid, most public health officials can't figure out what else might persuade women to follow the advice.

Dr. Tsunenobu Tamura, a professor of nutrition science at the University of Alabama at Birmingham, says the focus of the message should be to encourage women to take their vitamins daily, since most contain adequate folate.

A recent study, led by Kathleen Yadrick, a professor of nutrition and food systems at the University of Southern Mississippi in Hattiesburg, seems to support Tamura's theory.

Yadrick and her colleagues studied 100 African-American, female college students. "The [result] of this research is that women are more likely to pay attention to things that encourage them to take supplements in general rather than just folic acid," Yadrick says.

Dr. Siobhan Dolan, associate medical director of the March of Dimes, says women need to make taking a multivitamin a daily habit. Taking a multivitamin at the same time every day or leaving the bottle near something associated with a morning ritual, such as a coffee cup or a box of cereal, might help boost compliance, she says.

It's important that all women of child-bearing age follow the advice about multivitamins and folic acid because many pregnancies are unplanned, Dolan says.

info To learn more about folic acid, visit the Centers for Disease Control and Prevention Web site at *www.cdc.gov/ncbddd/folicacid.*

■ ■ ■ ■

Diabetes Drug May Boost Fertility

The drug *metformin* (Glucophage), which is used to make the tissues of diabetics more insulin-sensitive, can help treat the type of infertility that is caused by a failure to ovulate.

In some women who are not diabetic, excess insulin levels interfere with ovulation. For these women, metformin may restore normal ovulation. It is considered safe for use by women trying to get pregnant. See your doctor for more information.

Marguerite Shepard, MD, reproductive endocrinology specialist and professor emerita of obstetrics and gynecology, Indiana University School of Medicine, Indianapolis.

Everything's Faster—Even Pregnancy—Now Just 39 Weeks!

Nancy Green, MD, medical director, March of Dimes.
Michael J. Davidoff, manager of informatics, research and development, March of Dimes.
Amanda Cotter, MD, assistant professor of obstetrics and gynecology, Miller School of Medicine, University of Miami.
Seminars in Perinatology.

The average length of a pregnancy in the United States is getting shorter, with the most common duration now 39 weeks, rather than the full term 40 weeks, according to a recent report.

Babies born close to full term—five to six weeks early, called *late preterm*—now account for most of the premature births in the US. And those babies, like very premature babies, face greater health risks.

"Most of the rise in premature [births] is related to these so-called late preterm babies," says Dr. Nancy Green, medical director of the March of Dimes in White Plains, New York.

THE NUMBERS

Approximately one in eight babies is born prematurely, and 70% of those are late preterm, accounting for more than 355,000 births each year, says Michael Davidoff, manager of informatics, research and development at the March of Dimes and lead author of the study.

Between 1992 and 2002, births at or after 40 weeks declined by nearly 21% while births occurring between 34 and 36 weeks increased by 12%, according to the new report.

Preterm births represent a steadily rising proportion of all births in the US, increasing from 9.4% of live births in 1981 to 12.3% in 2003, a 31% increase. Healthy People 2010, a federal health initiative, has established a target rate of no more than 7.6%.

During this period, the rate of very preterm births remained relatively constant—1.8% compared with 2%. These babies have been the focus of much attention in the past because they have high complication rates. Prematurity and low birth weight are the leading causes of infant mortality among African-American infants and the second-leading cause of mortality among all infants.

However, attention is now shifting to the late preterm babies because they, too, can experience similar complications, such as respiratory distress syndrome, hypoglycemia and longer stays in the neonatal intensive care unit (ICU).

"They certainly have more complications at birth, and end up anywhere from a few days to a few weeks in the neonatal ICU," Green says.

> *If everything is going well, and everything is uncomplicated, go to term. Don't deliver early, because there are consequences.*
>
> Nancy Green, MD

"Nobody has been focusing on the babies at more than 34 weeks—are we doing the right thing by not bringing them to full term?" asks Dr. Amanda Cotter, assistant professor of obstetrics and gynecology at the University of Miami's Miller School of Medicine.

Although the impact on one infant may not be huge, the public health ramifications are considerable. "The total hospital cost for these [late preterm] infants is about the same as it is for the extremely preterm babies because there are fewer of the extremely preterm infants," Green says.

WHY THE CHANGE?

The study authors speculate that the rise of Caesarean sections and induced labor may partly explain the trend toward more preterm infants. She suspects that some early deliveries may not be medically necessary.

On the other hand, early delivery isn't always a bad thing. "Some of this is a success story—better maternal and fetal monitoring, detecting problems early and intervening before calamities happen," Green says. "We know that mortality rates have gone down over time, which largely reflects better management," she adds.

Green advises expectant parents to make their pregnancy as healthy as possible, starting before conception by adopting proper nutrition and lifestyle habits. Try to detect and treat underlying maternal health conditions, whether it's hypertension, asthma or diabetes.

Finally, Green says, "If everything is going well for a singleton pregnancy, and everything is uncomplicated, go to term. Don't deliver early, because there are consequences."

info For more information on a healthy pregnancy, visit the March of Dimes Web site, *www.marchofdimes.com/pnhec/pnhec.asp.*

Stress Near Conception May Affect Pregnancy

Pablo A. Nepomnaschy, PhD, postdoctoral fellow, National Institute of Environmental Health Sciences, National Institutes of Health.

Mary Stephenson, MD, MSc, professor of obstetrics and gynecology, and director, Recurrent Pregnancy Loss Program, University of Chicago.
Proceedings of National Academy of Sciences.

Pregnant women who are stressed in the first three weeks after conception are nearly three times as likely to miscarry as those who are not stressed, according to a new study.

THE STUDY

A research team evaluated 61 women for 12 months, collecting each woman's urine three times a week to check for pregnancy and levels of *cortisol,* a stress-linked hormone.

Of the 61 women, 22 became pregnant; nine carried to term and 13 miscarried. The women who had higher cortisol levels during the first three weeks of pregnancy were 2.7 times more likely to miscarry than the women whose cortisol levels were normal, the researchers report.

In all, miscarriages occurred in 90% of the women who had increased cortisol levels and in only 33% of those who had normal cortisol levels.

Lead researcher Pablo A. Nepomnaschy, a postdoctoral fellow at the National Institute of Environmental Health Sciences, part of the National Institutes of Health, says the testing was done very early in the pregnancy because "most pregnancy losses take place in the first three to four weeks after conception."

The women studied were all residents of a rural area of Guatemala. "This population is more alike than any population in the United States," Nepomnaschy says. By choosing women of the same ethnicity who had similar diets and activity levels, Nepomnaschy was trying to rule out any other factors that might influence miscarriage rates.

POSSIBLE EXPLANATIONS

Nepomnaschy says it's unclear why a boost in cortisol might raise miscarriage risks, but he speculates, "The body might interpret that [increased cortisol level] as conditions deteriorating, and that might trigger an abortion mechanism."

Another expert, Dr. Mary Stephenson, a professor of obstetrics and gynecology, who runs the Recurrent Pregnancy Loss Program at the University of Chicago, says, "It's an intriguing [study]. Certainly more research is needed. But it is a potential mechanism by which miscarriage may occur."

Other studies have looked at the cortisol–miscarriage link, Stephenson says. "The results have been conflicting. There are some studies in animals that suggest that stress increases the risk of miscarriage. And doctors have long suspected that stress does the same in people."

Approximately 15% of recognized pregnancies end in miscarriage, according to the March of Dimes. But Stephenson says that statistic usually includes the pregnancies that survive for six weeks. "When you count the ones that occur before six weeks, up to half of the pregnancies end in miscarriage," she notes.

ADVICE: DE-STRESS

The best advice for women trying to get pregnant is to de-stress your life before you conceive, Stephenson suggests. "I talk about this a lot with my patients," she says. "I recommend that before they get pregnant, they take a serious look at their lifestyle."

"Try to provide yourself with what you consider a good environment. The less stress, the better," advises Nepomnaschy.

info To learn more about miscarriages, visit the March of Dimes Web site at *www. marchofdimes.com.*

Mom's Antidepressant Use Raises Newborn's Risk for Lung Condition

Christina D. Chambers, PhD, assistant professor of pediatrics, University of California, San Diego.
Sandra L. Kweder, MD, deputy director, Office of New Drugs, Center for Drug Evaluation and Research, US Food and Drug Administration.
Jennifer Wu, MD, obstetrician/gynecologist, Lenox Hill Hospital, New York City.
The New England Journal of Medicine.

Compared with women who do not take antidepressants late in their pregnancies, women who do have a higher risk of delivering infants who have serious breathing problems, a recent study shows. The condition, which could be fatal, is called *persistent pulmonary hypertension of the newborn* (PPHN) and occurs when a newborn's circulation system does not adapt to breathing outside the womb.

THE STUDY

The study compared 377 women whose infants had PPHN with 836 women whose infants did not have the disorder.

In all, 14 of the infants who had PPHN had been exposed to *selective serotonin reuptake inhibitors* (SSRIs), a group of antidepressants that includes Celexa, Paxil, Prozac and Zoloft, after the 20th week of gestation. Only six of the infants who did not have PPHN had been exposed to SSRIs.

That means that PPHN "occurred approximately six times more frequently in women taking SSRIs," says Christina D. Chambers, lead author of the study and assistant professor of pediatrics at the University of California, San Diego. "It's highly unlikely that that would have happened by chance, although this study doesn't tell you for sure that the drug caused that outcome."

Using SSRIs before the 20th week or using non-SSRI medications at any time during pregnancy was not associated with an increased risk of PPHN.

IMPLICATIONS

"This appears to be a very well-conducted study and we find the results to be very concerning," says Dr. Sandra L. Kweder, deputy director of the Office of New Drugs at the US Food and Drug Administration's (FDA) Center for Drug Evaluation and Research.

The small risks suggested by the study may be outweighed by women's own personal need for treatment of a mental health condition.

Sandra L. Kweder, MD

However, the new research provides no clear indication of what pregnant women should do when it comes to using SSRIs.

"These are very small numbers and it's hard to know exactly what this means," adds Dr. Jennifer Wu, an obstetrician/gynecologist at Lenox Hill Hospital in New York City. "I think that there are a certain number of patients who have severe depression for whom SSRIs do work, who need to continue them during pregnancy. Other patients with less severe depression may want to go off" their medication, she says.

"Pregnant women with depression or other conditions that need treatment have to make decisions, with their clinicians, about what medications they can be best treated with and which medications are the safest," says Chambers.

Kweder adds, "This isn't a cause for panic among women who are taking these medicines, and they should not stop their medication on their own. Stopping these medications on your own can sometimes create more problems than it solves. Also, for many women, the small risks suggested by the study may be outweighed by their own personal need for treatment of a mental health condition."

The researchers stress that PPHN remains a rare condition, with only an estimated one to two infants per 1,000 live births developing it. In fact, 99% of women taking SSRIs during pregnancy will deliver a healthy infant.

PREVIOUS RESEARCH

Both depression and taking SSRIs during pregnancy pose risks to the mother and child.

A recent study found that pregnancy does not appear to confer a protective effect on women who have major depression, as experts previously thought. Quite the opposite—pregnant women who discontinued their antidepressant medication were found to be at five times the risk of having a relapse of depression than women who continued taking their medication.

However, in September 2005, the FDA issued a warning about possible birth defects in infants born to women who took Paxil during their first trimester. A number of studies have also shown that approximately 20% to 30% of babies born to women taking SSRIs in late pregnancy will develop "neonatal complications," which can include jitteriness and respiratory difficulties, Chambers says. In addition, a small study found that newborns whose mothers had used SSRIs during their pregnancy were at an increased risk of experiencing withdrawal symptoms.

More studies are needed "to see if there truly is a risk, what factors affect that risk, when you need to stop medication and what dosages are best," Wu says.

info For more information on PPHN, visit the Nemours Foundation Web site at *http://kids health.org/parent/medical/lungs/pphn.html.*

'Morning-After' Pill Approved for Over-the-Counter Sales

Steven Galson, MD, director, Center for Drug Evaluation and Research, US Food and Drug Administration
American Society for Reproductive Medicine

After three years of delay, the US Food and Drug Administration (FDA) has approved the over-the-counter (OTC) sale of the emergency contraceptive *Plan B*, sometimes called the *morning-after pill*. However, the drug can only be dispensed over-the-counter by a licensed pharmacist.

The pill is an extra-high dose of regular birth control that is effective only if it is taken within 72 hours of unprotected intercourse. The drug prevents pregnancy by delaying ovulation, but it does not interrupt an already-implanted pregnancy.

"Emergency contraception is a method of preventing pregnancy after contraceptive fails or after unprotected sex," explains Dr. Steven Galson, director of the FDA's Center for Drug Evaluation and Research. "Plan B acts primarily by stopping the release of an egg from the ovary. It's important to note that Plan B is not intended for routine use. It's an emergency contraception."

RESTRICTION

Although approved, the approval was accompanied by the restriction that women younger than age 18 cannot purchase the pills without a doctor's prescription. This condition was set to respond to the concerns of conservative groups that said the contraceptive's easy availability would encourage premarital sex.

"Our assessment is that this younger age group would strongly benefit from consultation with a health-care provider before using the product," says Galson. "The application [for approval] did not contain enough information about this age group to make us comfortable to do the switch fully for those younger people."

BACKGROUND ON THE CONTROVERSY

The announcement "concludes an extensive process that included getting expert advice from two of the FDA's advisory committees, and [allowing] an opportunity for public comment," according to Galson.

The FDA originally approved Plan B as a prescription drug in 1999. In 2001, more than 60 health groups petitioned the US government to make emergency contraceptives available without a prescription. In December 2003, the FDA advisory committees concluded that Plan B was both safe and effective. They overwhelmingly recommended that the agency make Plan B available without a prescription.

But in an unusual move, the FDA ignored the advice of the committees, and delayed making its decision.

Soon after, the FDA added another condition for approval, informing Barr Pharmaceuticals, the drug's manufacturer, that the morning-after pill could not be sold OTC until more studies were done. The FDA denied that this move was politically motivated, and said it arose from concern that teenage girls would not be able to use the product safely.

REACTION

Reaction from groups that advocate the OTC sale of this contraception was swift in coming.

"The American Society for Reproductive Medicine [ASRM] is pleased that the FDA has approved making emergency contraception available to women age 18 and over," says ASRM President Dr. Joseph S. Sanfilippo. "We are encouraged that the FDA has heeded the advice of its Reproductive Health Drugs Advisory Committee and the Over-the-Counter Advisory Committee, and has recognized that the morning-after pill is a safe and effective way to protect against pregnancy in an emergency."

However, other supporters of Plan B, such as Planned Parenthood, say the FDA's decision to require age restrictions will hamper efforts to reduce the nation's 3 million annual unplanned pregnancies, and consequently, the number of abortions.

"While we are glad to know the FDA finally ended its foot-dragging on this issue, Planned Parenthood is troubled by the scientifically baseless restriction imposed on teenagers," says Cecile Richards, president of Planned Parenthood. "The US has one of the highest rates of teen pregnancy in the Western world. Anything that makes it harder for teenagers to avoid unintended pregnancy is bad medicine and bad public policy."

Plan B opponents fear that requiring a doctor's prescription for women younger than 18 will do little to limit teen promiscuity.

"If the FDA thinks that enacting an age restriction will work, or that the drug company will enforce it...then they are living in a dream world," says Wendy Wright, president of Concerned Women for America, which led the opposition to the contraceptive.

info For more information on Plan B, visit the US Food and Drug Administration at *www.fda.gov/cder/drug/infopage/planB/default.htm.*

C-Section Infants Have Twice the Risk Of Death

Blackwell Publishing, news release.

Among American women who have low-risk pregnancies, those who opt for Caesarean section have higher infant and neonatal death rates than women who deliver vaginally, according to a new study.

THE STUDY

Researchers at the Centers for Disease Control and Prevention (CDC) analyzed data from more than 5.7 million live births and nearly 12,000 infant deaths during a four-year period. Overall, neonatal (younger than 28 days) deaths were rare for infants born to low-risk women. The rate was approximately one death per 1,000 live births.

However, the study found that the death rate among neonatal infants who were delivered by Caesarean section was more than twice that of infants who were delivered vaginally. This held true even after the researchers adjusted for sociodemographic and medical risk factors.

The researchers note that between 1996 and 2004, there was a 41% increase in the number of Caesarean sections in the US. According to the National Center for Health Statistics, nearly 1.2 million C-sections—29.1% of all births—were performed in the United States in 2004.

IMPLICATIONS

"These findings should be of concern for clinicians and policy makers who are observing the rapid growth in the number of primary Caesareans to mothers without a medical indication," says lead researcher Marian MacDorman, a CDC statistician and senior social scientist, and co-chair of the SIDS and Infant Mortality Committee for the American Public Health Association.

"While timely Caesareans in response to medical conditions have proven to be lifesaving interventions for countless mothers and babies, we are currently witnessing a different phenomenon—a growing number of primary Caesareans without a reported medical condition," MacDorman says.

Health Resources

- **Administration on Aging**
  Washington, DC 20201
  202-619-0724
  www.aoa.gov

- **Alzheimer's Association**
  225 North Michigan Ave., Fl. 17
  Chicago, IL 60601-7633
  800-272-3900, 312-335-8700
  www.alz.org

- **American Academy of Allergy, Asthma & Immunology**
  555 East Wells St., Suite 1100
  Milwaukee, WI 53202
  800-822-2762, 414-272-6071
  www.aaaai.org

- **American Academy of Dermatology**
  PO Box 4014
  Schaumburg, IL 60168-4014
  847-330-0230
  www.aad.org

- **American Academy of Neurology**
  1080 Montreal Ave.
  Saint Paul, MN 55116
  800-879-1960, 651-695-2717
  www.aan.com

- **American Board of Medical Specialties**
  1007 Church St., Suite 404
  Evanston, IL 60201-5913
  847-491-9091
  Board Certification Verification:
  866-ASK-ABMS (275-2267)
  www.abms.org

- **American Cancer Society**
  1599 Clifton Rd. NE
  Atlanta, GA 30329

  800-ACS-2345 (227-2345)
  www.cancer.org

- **American Chiropractic Association**
  1701 Clarendon Blvd.
  Arlington, VA 22209
  800-986-4636
  www.amerchiro.org

- **American Chronic Pain Association (ACPA)**
  PO Box 850
  Rocklin, CA 95677
  800-533-3231
  www.theacpa.org

- **American College of Obstetricians and Gynecologists**
  409 12th St. SW
  PO Box 96920
  Washington, DC 20090-6920
  202-638-5577
  www.acog.org

- **American College of Rheumatology**
  1800 Century Place, Suite 250
  Atlanta, GA 30345
  404-633-3777
  www.rheumatology.org

- **American Council for Headache Education**
  19 Mantua Rd.
  Mt. Royal, NJ 08061
  856-423-0258
  www.achenet.org

- **American Council on Alcoholism**
  1000 E. Indian School Rd.
  Phoenix, AZ 85014
  800-527-5344
  Alcoholism Treatment HelpLine: 800-527-5344
  www.aca-usa.org

- **American Council on Exercise (ACE)**
  4851 Paramount Dr.
  San Diego, CA 92123
  800-825-3636, 858-279-8227
  www.acefitness.org

- **American Dental Association**
  211 E. Chicago Ave.
  Chicago, IL 60611
  312-440-2500
  www.ada.org

- **American Diabetes Association**
  National Call Center
  1701 North Beauregard St.
  Alexandria, VA 22311
  800-DIABETES (342-2383)
  www.diabetes.org

- **American Dietetic Association**
  120 South Riverside Plaza, Suite 2000
  Chicago, IL 60606-6995
  800-877-1600
  www.eatright.org

- **American Urological Association Foundation**
  1000 Corporate Blvd.
  Linthicum, MD 21090
  866-746-4282
  www.auafoundation.org

- **American Gastroenterological Association**
  4930 Del Ray Ave.
  Bethesda, MD 20814
  301-654-2055
  www.gastro.org

- **American Geriatrics Society**
  350 Fifth Ave., Suite 801
  New York, NY 10118
  212-308-1414
  www.americangeriatrics.org

- **American Heart Association**
  7272 Greenville Ave.
  Dallas, TX 75231
  800-AHA-USA-1 (242-8721), 301-223-2307
  www.americanheart.org

- **American Liver Foundation**
  75 Maiden Lane, Suite 603
  New York, NY 10038
  800-GO-LIVER (465-4837), 212-668-1000
  www.liverfoundation.org

- **American Lung Association**
  61 Broadway, 6th Floor
  New York, NY 10006
  800-LUNGUSA (586-4872), 800-548-8252
  www.lungusa.org

- **American Lyme Disease Foundation**
  P.O. Box 466
  Lyme, CT 06371
  www.aldf.com

- **American Macular Degeneration Foundation**
  PO Box 515
  Northampton, MA 01061-0515
  413-268-7660
  www.macular.org

- **American Pain Foundation**
  201 N. Charles St., Suite 710
  Baltimore, MD 21201-4111
  888-615-PAIN (7246)
  www.painfoundation.org

- **American Physical Therapy Association**
  1111 North Fairfax St.
  Alexandria, VA 22314-1488
  800-999-APTA (2782), 703-684-APTA
  TDD: 703-683-6748
  www.apta.org

- **American Psychological Association**
  750 First St. NE
  Washington, DC 20002-4242
  800-374-2721, 202-336-5500
  www.apa.org

- **American Sleep Apnea Association**
  1424 K St. NW, Suite 302
  Washington, DC 20005
  202-293-3650
  www.sleepapnea.org

- **American Society of Hypertension**
  148 Madison Ave., 5th Floor
  New York, NY 10016
  212-696-9099
  www.ash-us.org

- **American Society of Plastic Surgeons**
  444 E. Algonquin Rd.
  Arlington Heights, IL 60005
  888-4-PLASTIC (475-2784)
  www.plasticsurgery.org

- **American Speech–Language–Hearing Association**
  10801 Rockville Pike
  Rockville, MD 20852
  800-498-2071, 800-638-8255
  www.asha.org

- **American Stroke Association**
  7272 Greenville Ave.
  Dallas, TX 75231
  888-4-STROKE (478-7653)
  www.strokeassociation.org

■ **Anxiety Disorders Association of America**
8730 Georgia Ave., Suite 600
Silver Spring, MD 20910
240-485-1001
www.adaa.org

■ **Arthritis Foundation**
PO Box 7669
Atlanta, GA 30357-0669
800-568-4045
www.arthritis.org

■ **Centers for Disease Control and Prevention**
1600 Clifton Rd.
Atlanta, GA 30333
800-311-3435, 404-639-3311
www.cdc.gov

■ **Colorectal Cancer Network (CCNetwork)**
PO Box 182
Kensington, MD 20895-0182
301-879-1500
www.colorectal-cancer.net

■ **Council for Responsible Nutrition**
1828 L St. NW, Suite 900
Washington, DC, 20036-5114
202-776-7929
www.crnusa.org

■ **The Crohn's & Colitis Foundation of America**
386 Park Ave. S, 17th Floor
New York, NY 10016
800-932-2423
www.ccfa.org

■ **Deafness Research Foundation**
2801 M Street NW
Washington, DC 20007
866-454-3924
TTY: 888-435-6104
www.drf.org

■ **Endocrine Society**
The Hormone Foundation
8401 Connecticut Ave., Suite 900
Chevy Chase, MD 20815-5817
800-HORMONE (467-6663)
www.hormone.org

■ **Herb Research Foundation**
4140 15th St.
Boulder, CO 80304
303-449-2265
www.herbs.org

■ **The Leukemia & Lymphoma Society**
1311 Mamaroneck Ave.
White Plains, NY 10605
800-955-4572, 914-949-5213
www.leukemia-lymphoma.org

■ **Melanoma International Foundation**
250 Mapleflower Rd.
Glenmoore, PA 19343
610-942-3432
www.melanomainternational.org

■ **National Cancer Institute**
Building 31, Room 11A16
9000 Rockville Pike
Bethesda, MD 20892
800-4-CANCER (422-6237)
TTY: 800-332-8615
www.cancer.gov

■ **National Capital Poison Center**
3201 New Mexico Ave., Suite 310
Washington, DC 20016
202-362-3867
Emergency Line: 800-222-1222
www.poison.org

■ **National Headache Foundation**
820 N. Orleans, Suite 217
Chicago, IL 60610
888-NHF-5552 (643-5552)
www.headaches.org

■ **National Institute of Allergy and Infectious Diseases (NIAID)**
6610 Rockledge Dr., MSC 6612
Bethesda, MD 20892-6612
301-496-5717
www.niaid.nih.gov

■ **National Institute of Arthritis and Musculoskeletal and Skin Diseases**
One AMS Circle
Bethesda, MD 20892-3675
877-22-NIAMS (226-4267), 301-495-4484
TTY: 301-565-2966
www.niams.nih.gov

■ **National Institute of Diabetes & Digestive & Kidney Diseases**
Building 31, Room 9A04
31 Center Dr., MSC 2560
Bethesda, MD 20892-2560
301-496-3583
www.niddk.nih.gov

■ **National Institute of Mental Health (NIMH)**
6001 Executive Blvd.
Room 8184
Bethesda, MD 20892-9663
866-615-NIMH (6464), 301-443-4513
TTY: 301-443-8431
www.nimh.nih.gov

■ **National Institute of Neurological Disorders and Stroke**

PO Box 5801
Bethesda, MD 20824
800-352-9424, 301-496-5751
TTY: 301-468-5981
www.ninds.nih.gov

■ **National Institute on Aging**

Building 31, Room 5C27
31 Center Dr., MSC 2292
Bethesda, MD 20892
301-496-1752
www.nia.nih.gov

■ **National Institute on Alcohol Abuse and Alcoholism (NIAAA)**

5635 Fishers Lane, MSC 9304
Bethesda, MD 20892-9304
301-443-3860
www.niaaa.nih.gov

■ **National Kidney Foundation**

30 East 33rd St.
New York, NY 10016
800-622-9010, 212-889-2210
www.kidney.org

■ **National Library of Medicine**

8600 Rockville Pike
Bethesda, MD 20894
888-FIND-NLM (346-3656), 301-594-5983
www.nlm.nih.gov

■ **National Multiple Sclerosis Society**

733 Third Ave.
New York, NY 10017
800-FIGHT-MS (344-4867)
www.nmss.org

■ **National Osteoporosis Foundation**

1232 22nd St. NW
Washington, DC 20037-1292
202-223-2226
www.nof.org

■ **National Prostate Cancer Coalition**

1154 15th St. NW
Washington, DC 20005
888-245-9455, 202-463-9455
www.4npcc.org

■ **The National Psoriasis Foundation**

6600 SW 92nd Ave., Suite 300
Portland, OR 97223-7195
800-723-9166, 503-244-7404
www.psoriasis.org

■ **The National Safety Council**

1121 Spring Lake Dr.
Itasca, IL 60143-3201
630-285-1121
www.nsc.org

■ **National Sleep Foundation**

1522 K St. NW, Suite 500
Washington, DC 20005
202-347-3471
www.sleepfoundation.org

■ **National Spinal Cord Injury Association**

6701 Democracy Blvd., Suite 300-9
Bethesda, MD 20817
800-962-9629
www.spinalcord.org

■ **National Stroke Association**

9707 E. Easter Lane
Englewood, CO 80112
800-STROKES (787-6537), 303-649-9299
www.stroke.org

■ **The National Women's Health Information Center**

8270 Willow Oaks Corporate Dr.
Fairfax, VA 22031
800-994-WOMAN (9662)
www.4woman.gov

■ **Parkinson's Disease Foundation**

1359 Broadway, Suite 1509
New York, NY 10018
800-457-6676
www.pdf.org

■ **The Skin Cancer Foundation**

245 Fifth Ave., Suite 1403
New York, NY 10016
800-SKIN-490 (754-6490)
www.skincancer.org

■ **The Susan G. Komen Breast Cancer Foundation**

5005 LBJ Freeway, Suite 250
Dallas, TX 75244
972-855-1600
www.komen.org

■ **United Network for Organ Sharing**

PO Box 2484
Richmond, VA 23218
804-782-4800
www.unos.org

■ **US Food and Drug Administration**

5600 Fishers Lane
Rockville, MD 20857-0001
888-INFO-FDA (463-6332)
www.fda.gov

Index

for heartburn relief, 208
to prevent sinusitis, 35
and skin care, 22
Weight. *See* Obesity
Whooping cough (pertussis), vaccine
for, 148–149
Wine. *See* Alcohol
Women. *See also* Cervical cancer;
Menopause; Ovarian cancer;
Pregnancy
aspirin, dosages for, 190
aspirin, daily, after menopause, 320
cholesterol-lowering drugs and, 100,
102
colorectal cancer risk and
supplements, 323
crying by, 134
fatigue as symptom of heart disease,
140–141

heart disease in, testing for, 276,
311–312
hypertension and OTC painkillers, 322
hysterectomy, alternatives to, 316–318
midlife crises, traps to avoid, 312–313
mini-strokes, risk of, 190
osteoporosis and supplements, 323
overprescription of drugs in ER for,
104–105
reactions to drugs in, 94–96, 96
symptoms of heart attack in, 175, 312
testosterone levels in, 313–314
undiagnosed heart attacks, 174–175
uterine fibroids, treatment of, 317–318
vitamin E and risk of heart attack or
stroke, 190
Women's Health Initiative (WHI), 190,
318, 320, 323
Worry, health effects of, 133–134. *See*

also Stress
Wound care, 166–167
honey for, 167
oxygen to reduce infection, 165–166
Wrinkles
acupuncture to reduce, 219–220
treatments for, 20–22

Y

Yoga
for back pain, 262–263
instant-energy breathing, 200–201
for pain relief, 214
to relieve headaches from stress, 141
and weight loss, 234

Z

Zinc, dangers of, 199
Zoos, petting, bacteria in, 154–155